AF544986

FRONTIERS IN MULTIPLE SCLEROSIS
VOLUME 2

FRONTIERS IN MULTIPLE SCLEROSIS

VOLUME 2

Edited by

AKSEL SIVA, MD
Professor of Neurology
Istanbul University
Cerrahpaşa School of Medicine
Istanbul, Turkey

JÜRG KESSELRING, MD
Professor of Neurology and Neurorehabilitation
University of Bern
Head of Department of Neurology
Rehabilitation Centre
Klinik Valens
Valens, Switzerland

ALAN J THOMPSON, MD, FRCP, FRCPI
Garfield Weston Professor of Clinical Neurology
and Neurorehabilitation
Institute of Neurology
University College London
London, UK

MARTIN DUNITZ

First published in the UK in 1999 by

Martin Dunitz Ltd
The Livery House
7–9 Pratt Street
London NW1 0AE

A CIP catalogue record for this book is available from the British Library.

ISBN 1-85317-506-4

Distributed in the United States by:
Blackwell Science Inc.
Commerce Place, 350 Main Street
Malden, MA 02148, USA
Tel: 1-800-215-1000

Distributed in Canada by:
Login Brothers Book Company
324 Salteaux Crescent
Winnipeg, Manitoba, R3J 3T2
Canada
Tel: 204-224-4068

Distributed in Brazil by:
Ernesto Reichmann Distribuidora de Livros, Ltda
Rua Coronel Marques 335, Tatuape 03440-000
Sao Paulo,
Brazil

Composition by Scribe Design
Printed and bound in the UK

Contents

List of contributors

Oded Abramsky MD PhD
Department of Neurology
Hadassah-Hebrew University Hospital
Jerusalem
Israel

Ingrid V Allen MRIA DSc MD FRCPath
Research and Development Office
for the Health and Personal
Social Services in Northern Ireland
2–12 Linehall Street
Belfast BT2
United Kingdom

Oluf Andersen MD
Institute of Clinical Neuroscience/Neurology
Sahlgrenska University Hospital
SE 41345 Göteborg
Sweden

Daniel C Anthony PhD
Department of Pharmacology
University of Oxford
Mansfield Road
Oxford OX1 3QT
UK

Juan J Archelos MD
Max Planck Institute of Psychiatry
Kraepelinstrasse 10
80804 Munich
Germany

Lance D Blumhardt PhD
Division of Clinical Neurology
University Hospital
Queen's Medical Centre
Nottingham NG7 2HH
UK

Henrik Brønnum-Hansen MSc
The Danish Institute for Clinical Epidemiology
Svanmøllevej 25
DK 2100 Copenhagen
Denmark

Michel Clanet MD
Federation de Neurologie
CHU Toulouse Purpan
31059 Toulouse Cedex
France

Giancarlo Comi MD
Multiple Sclerosis Centre
San Raffaele Hospital
University of Milan
Milan 20132
Italy

D Alastair S Compston PhD FRCP
University of Cambridge Neurology Unit
Addenbrooke's Hospital
Hills Road
Cambridge CB2
UK

Christian Confavreux MD
Department of Neurology and EDMUS
Coordinating Center
Hôpital de l'Antiquaille
69321 Lyon Cedex 05
France

George W Ellison MD
Department of Neurology
UCLA School of Medicine
Reed Neurological Research Center
710 Westwood Plaza
Los Angeles
CA 90095-1769
USA

Mefkure Eraksoy MD
Department of Neurology
University of Istanbul
Istanbul Faculty of Medicine
Capa, Istanbul
Turkey

Margaret M Esiri PhD
Department of Pharmacology
University of Oxford
Mansfield Road
Oxford OX1 3QT
UK

Massimo Filippi MD
Multiple Sclerosis Centre
San Raffaele Hospital
University of Milan
Milan 20132
Italy

Hans Peter Hartung MD
Department of Neurology
Karl-Franzens Universität
8036 Graz
Auenbruggerplatz 22
Austria

Boris Kallman MD
Clinical Research Group for MS and
Neuroimmunology
Julius Maximilians Universität
Josef Schneider Strasse 11
Würzburg D97080
Germany

Orhun Kantarci MD
Department of Neurology
Istanbul University
Cerrahpasa School of Medicine
Istanbul
Turkey

Rana Karabudak MD
Hacettepe University Hospital
Department of Neurology
Sihhiye 06100 Ankara
Turkey

Dimitrios M Karussis MD PhD
Department of Neurology
Hadassah-Hebrew University Hospital
Jerusalem
Israel

Jürg Kesselring MD PhD
Chefarzt Neurologie
Klinik Valens
CH-7317 Valens
Switzerland

Nils Koch-Henriksen MD MSc
The Danish MS Registry
Rigshospitalet
DK 2200 Copenhagen and
Department of Neurology
Aalborg Hospital North
DK 9100 Aalborg
Denmark

Nitza Lahat PhD
Division of Neuroimmunology and MS Center
Department of Neurology and Immunology
Research Unit
Carmel Medical Center
Faculty of Medicine Technion
7 Michal Street
Haifa 34362
Israel

Barbara D Leake PhD
Department of Neurology
UCLA School of Medicine
Reed Neurological Research Center
710 Westwood Plaza
Los Angeles
CA 90095-1769
USA

Letizia Leocani MD
Multiple Sclerosis Centre
San Raffaele Hospital
University of Milan
Milan 20132
Italy

David KB Li MD
Division of Diagnostic Radiology
Department of Radiology
Vancouver Hospital and Health Sciences Centre
Vancouver
Canada

Fred D Lublin MD
Multiple Sclerosis Center
Allegheny University of the Health Sciences

Vittorio Martinelli MD
Multiple Sclerosis Centre
San Raffaele Hospital
University of Milan
Milan 20132
Italy

Gianvito Martino MD
Multiple Sclerosis Centre
San Raffaele Hospital
University of Milan
Milan 20132
Italy

M Ray Mickey PhD
Department of Neurology
UCLA School of Medicine
Reed Neurological Research Center
710 Westwood Plaza
Los Angeles
CA 90095-1769
USA

Ariel Miller MD PhD
Division of Neuroimmunology and MS Center
Department of Neurology and Immunology
Research Unit
Carmel Medical Center
Faculty of Medicine Technion
7 Michal Street
Haifa 34362
Israel

David Miller MD
Institute of Neurology
Queen Square
London WC1N
UK

Xavier Montalban MD
Unit of Clinical Neuroimmunology
HGU Vall d'Hebron, EUI-5a Planta, 08035
Barcelona,
Spain

Lawrence W Myers MD
Department of Neurology
UCLA School of Medicine
Reed Neurological Research Center
710 Westwood Plaza
Los Angeles
CA 90095-1769
USA

Tomas Olsson MD
Neuroimmunology Unit
Department of Medicine
Center for Molecular Medicine
Karolinska Hospital
S 17176 Stockholm
Sweden

Donald W Paty MD FRCPC
Division of Neurology
Department of Medicine
The University of British Columbia
Vancouver
Canada

V Hugh Perry PhD
Department of Pharmacology
University of Oxford
Mansfield Road
Oxford OX1 3QT
UK

Chris H Polman MD PhD
Department of Neurology
Free University Hospital
PO Box 7057
1007 MB Amsterdam
The Netherlands

Anthony T Reder MD
Hacettepe University Hospital
Department of Neurology
Sihhiye 06100 Ankara
Turkey

Peter Rieckmann MD
Clinical Research Group for MS and Neuroimmunology
Julius Maximilians Universität
Josef Schneider Strasse 11
Würzburg D97080
Germany

Neil P Robertson MD
University of Cambridge Neurology Unit
Addenbrooke's Hospital
Hills Road
Cambridge CB2
UK

Mariemma Rodegher MD
Multiple Sclerosis Centre
San Raffaele Hospital
University of Milan
Milan 20132
Italy

Marco Rovaris MD
Multiple Sclerosis Centre
San Raffaele Hospital
University of Milan
Milan 20132
Italy

Sarah Shapiro PhD
Division of Neuroimmunology and MS Center
Department of Neurology and Immunology Research Unit
Carmel Medical Center
Faculty of Medicine Technion
7 Michael Street
Haifa 34362, Israel

Aksel Siva MD
Department of Neurology
Istanbul University
Cerrahpasa School of Medicine
Istanbul
Turkey

Alan J Thompson MD FRCP FRCPI
The National Hospital
Queen Square
London WC1N
UK

Brian G Weinshenker MD
Mayo Clinic/Mayo Foundation
Rochester
Minnesota 55905
USA

Preface

Science becomes productive when accompanied by creative thinking, and the results found are fruitful if they evoke new ideas and improve understanding. A number of highly acclaimed multiple sclerosis researchers have put together their expertise to bring us volume two of *Frontiers in Multiple Sclerosis*. In most chapters the reader will find not merely results, but also the philosophy behind their work, as well as ideas that lead to new thinking and concepts.

This book is loosely based on a series of plenary lectures and satellite symposia that took place at the *13th Congress of the European Committee on Treatment and Research in Multiple Sclerosis*, held in Istanbul on November 2–5, 1997. However, instead of being a proceedings book it has evolved into a reference book, as most chapters were written or updated in 1998. This book contains very recent data and includes some, as yet, unpublished results. The sequence of chapters, each unique in its content, is arranged with the aim of keeping the interest of the reader 'alive' throughout the book.

It is inevitable that such a book cannot cover all areas of the huge subject matter, but we believe that the reader will find the new understanding and changing concepts that arise in multiple sclerosis at the edge of the next millenium. The rapid advances in molecular genetics and immunology are well reflected in the field of inflammatory-demyelinating diseases of the central nervous system and our understanding of multiple sclerosis within the last 'decade of brain' has gained new dimensions.

We are grateful to all who contributed to this book and wish to express our thanks to the staff of Martin Dunitz Publishers, especially to our managing editor Yasmin Khan-Chowdhury, editorial assistant Jenny Cranwell, commissioning editor Alan Burgess and to our publisher Martin Dunitz, for all their efforts in the production of this book.

Aksel Siva
Jurg Kesselring
Alan J Thompson

October 1998

1

An introduction to the clinical spectrum of inflammatory demyelinating disorders of the central nervous system

Aksel Siva and Orhun Kantarci

INTRODUCTION

'Multiple sclerosis—more than one disease?' was the title of an epidemiology study carried out in Norway in 1985, and the authors had concluded that multiple sclerosis (MS) may have two different forms as the remitting and progressive types, which behave differently when considered epidemiologically and clinically.[1] Although the variation in the clinical presentation and the course of MS has long been well recognized, the clinical, imaging, pathological and immunogenetic studies looking into the different forms of what we call 'MS' and of various other idiopathic inflammatory diseases of the central nervous system (CNS) that fall within the same clinical spectrum are relatively recent.[2–6] The concept of 'What is and what is not MS?' and that MS might cover a group of disorders rather than being a single disease is emerging as a current understanding.[7–9]

Until the early 1980s our understanding of MS was more straightforward as a demyelinating disease with some clinical variations but not as prominent disease forms within a spectrum.[10] The diagnosis of MS then, had been guided by the diagnostic criteria of Schumacher, which relied entirely on clinical features and viewed MS as a clinical disease disseminated in time and space.[11] In 1983, a committee modified the Schumacher's diagnostic criteria of MS by including paraclinical criteria such as neuroimaging and neurophysiology, and further introduced the laboratory concept of supportive cerebrospinal fluid (CSF) studies, namely the increased immunoglobulin G (IgG) level and/or the presence of oligoclonal bands (OCB) in the diagnosis of MS.[12]

Computerized tomography (CT) was soon replaced by magnetic resonance imaging (MRI) as the paraclinical neuroimaging modality in the diagnosis of MS with its introduction into clinical practice. The initial 'observational' MRI studies describing the MRI patterns of disease[13–15] were followed by 'longitudinal' studies with and without gadolinium, which reported that MS was an ongoing disease with neuroimaging showing more common activity than could be detected clinically.[16–18] The differences between the primary and secondary progressive forms of MS as well as the so-called benign form were also noted.[3,19]

The demonstration of brain lesions consistent with demyelination in the unaffected monozygotic twin or in other family members of an MS patient in MRI suggested the existence of an asymptomatic form of the disease.[20–22] Autopsy studies revealing MS lesions in people without any history of a neurological disorder[23] further pointed out to the possibility of having 'morphological' (imaging/histology) disease without corresponding clinical signs or symptoms, classified as asymptomatic and subclinical MS. Likewise, finding of oligoclonal bands in the CSF in some of the clinically healthy twins discordant for MS or in the healthy nontwin siblings of MS patients[24,25] may also be accepted as an evidence to the nonclinical existence of MS.

This morphological, but not clinical, expression of inflammatory demyelination might be placed to one end of the spectrum as 'nonphasic, asymptomatic, mono/polyregional disease' (Table 1.1).

Brain lesions consistent with inflammation–demyelination were also demonstrated in the MRIs of patients presenting with clinically isolated syndromes suggestive of multiple sclerosis such as optic neuritis, a brainstem syndrome or transverse myelitis.[26] These observations have shown that such isolated syndromes are morphologically more widespread than could be detected on clinical grounds. This type of presentation may find place in the spectrum as 'monophasic, monosymptomatic, polyregional disease'. It is well known that only some of these patients will develop further CNS symptoms and fulfil the clinical criteria of classical relapsing–remitting MS; the 'polyphasic, polysymptomatic, polyregional disease'. Others will have either none or single corresponding lesions in MRI, hence remain 'monoregional' and these patients are known to have a lower rate of conversion to relapsing remitting MS.[27,28]

Another disease which is 'monophasic, polysymptomatic, polyregional' is acute disseminated encephalomyelitis (ADEM). The evolution and the course of this disease seems to be self-limited and it is often accepted that it may not be possible to differentiate by neuroimaging (the initial MRI) between 'MS' and ADEM.[29] In our experience, however, the

Table 1.1 The temporospatial behavior of the inflammatory demyelinating diseases of the central nervous system

Dissemination in time	Dissemination in space		
Nonphasic (asymptomatic)	Monoregional (focal)*	Polyregional (multifocal)*	
	Monosymptomatic		Polysymptomatic
Monophasic	Optic neuritis Brainstem syndrome Myelitis	(Optic neuritis) (Brainstem syndrome) (Myelitis)	Acute disseminated encephalitis
Multiphasic	Recurrent optic neuritis Recurrent myelitis	(Recurrent optic neuritis) (Recurrent myelitis)	Relapsing–remitting multiple sclerosis Neuromyelitis optica
Progressive	Progressive optic neuritis Progressive myelitis	(Progressive optic neuritis) (Progressive myelitis)	Fulminant multiple sclerosis Progressive multiple sclerosis

* The clinical presentation of monoregional and polyregional disease is the same, indicated in parentheses, but morphologically its behavior is different.

extent of the inflammatory reaction in these patients, as can be seen morphologically in MRI, gives the impression of being more prominent and widespread compared with that seen in either the initial attack of the classical 'relapsing–remitting MS' or with the other isolated demyelinating syndromes of the CNS. Similarly there is another subgroup of patients who present with large 'tumor-like lesions' that are histologically shown to have demyelinating disease at biopsy.[30,31] Like ADEM, most of these patients do not develop 'MS' when they are followed on clinical grounds.[30] These types of presentations should also be considered as having the 'monophasic, polysymptomatic, mono/polyregional disease' yet with a different (more prominent?) immunological behavior. This concept requires further support from longitudinal clinical and immunopathological studies.

Seven to 15% of patients with MS are known to have a clinically progressive course from onset (primary progressive MS) with some of them having a tendency to involve predominantly one part of the CNS, most often the spinal cord;[32] 'progressive, mono/polysymptomatic, mono/polyregional disease'. On the other hand, patients with a mono- or polyphasic form may later develop progressive disease, i.e. secondary progressive MS. In patients with a mono- or polyphasic disease course, however, an ongoing subclinical activity might be detected by neuroimaging or by probable immunological markers of activity, i.e. 'biologically[33] progressive' disease.

Most patients with the 'classical relapsing–remitting MS' have symptoms consistent with the involvement of different regions of the CNS-axis, while some will have a tendency for the involvement of the same particular regions, as is seen in the Devic's form of presentation. However, some cases the brain is not involved and lesions consistent with demyelination—typical of MS—may be demonstrated only in the spinal cord as reported at autopsy or biopsy.[34–36] This 'site preference' needs explanation. The observation of the more frequent involvement of the optic nerves and the spinal cord in MS patients in Japan, 'oriental MS',[37,38] may also be considered within this concept.

As described, the clinical, biological and morphological behaviour of inflammatory demyelinating disorders of the CNS within the spectrum differ. Whether these various expressions are based on the extent or difference of the aetiopathogenetic mechanisms, remains a question to be answered.

THE HETEROGENEITY IN THE GENETIC ASPECTS OF THE SPECTRUM

An association between MS susceptibility and the class II major histocompatibility complex (MHC) alleles DR15 and DQ6 and their corresponding genotypes DRB1*1501, DRB5*1501-DQA1*0102-DQB1*0602 has been reported for northern European and north American Caucasian MS patients.[39] Recently a nonhuman leukocyte antigen (HLA) genetic susceptibility to MS was suggested by the finding of chromosome 19q13.2 single locus and multilocus haplotype associations with MS in Caucasian and racially different Chinese patient samples that may have indicated an effect from a nearby disease susceptibility locus.[40]

In another recent study conducted in a sample of Japanese MS patients, it was shown that the western type of MS is associated with DRB1*1501 and DRB5*0101, while the Asian type is not.[41] This supports further the role of the immunogenetic background in the development and clinical expression of MS. In an earlier study the haplotype DRw17(3), DQw2 was reported to be found more commonly in relapsing–remitting MS than the primary progressive form and this observation of immunogenetic heterogeneity between these two groups, together with the clinical, epidemiological and imaging differences, were suggested as supportive for their separation as different disease entities.[4] The influence of HLA-DR and -DQ alleles (DRB1*1501) on progression to MS following clinically isolated syndromes in MRI-positive patients was also reported.[42] An association between the haplotypes DR1,DQ5 and DR17,DQ2 and a poor prognosis has been shown in another north

European study.[43] Although these findings need to be confirmed in larger studies, they may still indicate that genetics is influential as a cofactor in the behavioural expression and progression of the inflammatory demyelinating disorders within the spectrum.

THE HETEROGENEITY IN THE IMMUNOLOGY OF THE SPECTRUM

The heterogeneity of the clinical spectrum of disorders covered under the heading 'Multiple Sclerosis' might be due to variability in the immunopathological mechanisms. Considering the aspects of immunology of MS, certain points in the reaction chain can be identified to account for the heterogeneity in the outcome, hence the observed clinical spectrum.

A considerable amount of information about the immunology of inflammatory-demyelinating diseases is based on animal models, so hypothesizing that the animal models may represent the human model to a certain extent, the following discussion will consider the two models together.

The first stage assumption is that the inactive autoaggressive T-lymphocytes specific for autoantigens of the nervous system pre-exist outside the CNS where they are suppressed.[44–46] Why and how these cells pre-exist is unknown. It can be hypothesized that susceptibility to MS, which may in part be genetically determined, lies here.

In developing MS, these cells either escape control or are activated by stimuli unknown to date. A nonspecific approach would be the stimulatory effect of viral or bacterial superantigens, which are capable of activating many different clones of T cells simultaneously owing to superantigen binding site sharing among different clones. The staphylococcal superantigen-induced relapses in experimental autoimmune encephalomyelitis (EAE) exemplifies this situation.[47] However, the best placement of this hypothesis in MS would be in the possible explanation of observed relapses during nonspecific infections. Another and more specific stimulatory effect would be observed within the concept of molecular mimicry as such that several viral and bacterial peptides were identified as activators of myelin basic protein (MBP)-specific T cells.[48] This could provide an explanation for both the initial attack and relapses in MS. Together these suggested initial mechanisms seem to only account for dissemination in time, but the specific type of mimicry may also determine the tissue that will be involved. Furthermore, in a situation with continuous superantigenic stimulation of the autoreactive T-cell lines, one would expect the disease to progress with no time to remit. In patients with sphincter symptoms and ongoing subclinical urinary infections who have a progressive course, such a mechanism could be questioned.

In the next stage following activation of the T cells, adhesion molecule expression is amplified allowing for the cells to roll along and penetrate the endothelium. The endothelial adhesion and penetration, hence the blood–brain barrier (BBB) breakdown, has been suggested to be an ongoing process rather than an episodic one in progressive MS. This concept was supported by the observation of raised concentrations of soluble E-selectin in primary progressive MS, regardless of the amount of inflammation, while not being as such in either relapsing or secondary types.[49] How to relate this finding to the low number of lesions and the smaller amount of gadolinium-diethylene-triamine-pentaacetic acid (Gd-DPTA) uptake observed in primary progressive MS, as defined in MRI studies,[3] is a controversial issue.

The T cells sensitized by foreign pathogens but able to react with both the pathogenic and the CNS autoantigens are expected to migrate towards antigens presented by cells expressing MHC-II including perivascular macrophages, microglia and even astrocytes. The antigen-presenting cells express MHC-II also in situations that are not known to be immune mediated, such as infarcts and Alzheimer's disease.[50] This suggests that this antigen presentation becomes a pathologically important factor in MS only in the presence of specific, presensitized, active autoreactive T cells.

In EAE, both oligodendroglial antigens of MBP, proteolipid protein (PLP), myelin-associated glycoprotein (MAG) and myelin oligodendrocyte glycoprotein (MOG), and the astroglial antigen of S100β are shown to be provocative.[51,52] The specific types of antigens presented have certain localizational values within the lesion and within CNS in a broad sense. Suggested to have an interactive function between the oligodendrocyte and the axon, the periaxonally located glycoprotein MAG is located both in the CNS and the peripheral nervous system (PNS), probably related to demyelinating diseases with involvement of the CNS and PNS simultaneously.[53] Being the major protein constituents of the myelin (55% of the myelin proteins), MBP and PLP antigens located within the thick myelin, functioning in the compaction of the structure are more often encountered in the brainstem and spinal cord.[54] The relatively rare (0.05% of the myelin proteins) but highly immunogenic surface antigen MOG is encountered more often within the periventricular and cerebellar white matter.[54,55] In one study it was also suggested that anti-PLP antibodies are more readily encountered in the CSF of primary progressive cases,[56] while in another study T-cell reactivity to PLP was demonstrated in relapsing–remitting and secondary progressive cases but not in primary progressive cases.[57] Taken together, and as spinal cord involvement is common in primary progressive MS,[32,35,36] the site preference observed in the progressive forms might be attributed to the type of antigen involved. At this level of inflammation, the chain of reactions seems to be a part of the nonspecific common pathway except for the type of antigens presented and T cells presensitized against these antigens, which may be of partial help in the understanding of the concept of dissemination in space.

The early MHC-II expression is later amplified by the proinflammatory cytokines (i.e. interferon gamma (INF-γ, tumor necrosis factor alpha (TNF-α) and lymphotoxin) and a full-blown immune response follows with the involvement of macrophages, microglia and B-cell production of specific antibodies. The extent of the antibody response probably contributes to the amount of demyelination that will occur (e.g. the demyelination observed with the T cells alone was further increased by the coadministration of anti-MOG antibodies).[58] The increase in the number of plasma cells while the number of T cells and macrophages are dropping, as observed in late chronic MS, suggests a more pronounced role of the antibody response in demyelination than the early cellular attacks directed to myelin.[59]

The whole chain of reactions slows down and arrests at a certain stage, limiting the demyelination so that the clinical-imaging features stabilize. What determines this halting is unknown, but it is probably not a single factor. The more ready apoptosis of the autoreactive T cells within the CNS[60] is one of the self-limiting factors; however, since the extent of the demyelination is determined mainly by the later stages of the inflammatory chain only the igniting factor is discarded by this mechanism. On the other hand, as reviewed by Hohlfeld, since a resistance against the autoreactive T cells is gained afterwards in the EAE model, virtually cleaning the CNS from the provocative T cells, this apoptotic mechanism may in part explain the monophasic nature of some of the observed disorders within the spectrum of MS.[61] A relapse would then be explained by either complete resistance with a new attack by a totally different clone of T cells or incomplete resistance formation. The amount of resistance would depend on the extent of the initial inflammation, and a strong antigenic stimulus with a full-blown inflammatory reaction would be expected to provoke a higher resistance formation than a weak stimulus. Whether this would explain the gained resistance in situations such as ADEM or no resistance in progressive MS is questionable.

Besides the apoptotic mechanisms suggested, a systemic increase in the downregulatory cytokines (e.g. transforming growth factor beta (TGF-β)) was observed in MS.[62] This would suggest that the halting might be caused by mechanisms operating outside the CNS. The balance between the ongoing activation and the rate of suppression could help to explain the progressive nature of some of the disorders within the spectrum.

THE HETEROGENEITY IN THE PATHOLOGY OF THE SPECTRUM

In neuropathological terms, MS is defined as an inflammatory demyelinating disease of the CNS that is characterized by chronic perivenous inflammation, multifocal plaque-like demyelination, and reactive glial scar formation. This neuropathological definition, however, not only includes the typical cases of chronic MS, but also atypical cases of acute or monophasic manifestations of this disease,[63] i.e. the inflammatory demyelinating disorders within the spectrum. The demonstration of inflammation, despite differences in severity and extent in primary as well as secondary progressive forms of the disease, was suggested as evidence for similarity in the pathological process of these clinically distinct forms.[5] In a recent study, however, it was reported that the different patterns of demyelination and oligodendrocyte destruction observed in various forms and stages of MS emphasize the pathologic heterogeneity, and it was suggested that the pathogenetic mechanisms leading to demyelination may be fundamentally distinct in different groups of MS.[6] These authors further hypothesized that combinations of different susceptibility genes may dictate the individual's immunopathogenetic response to the inciting injury and account for specific subtypes of the disease which share a common pathological end point of myelin destruction by a variety of different immunological mechanisms.

The relative preservation of oligodendrocytes and the oligodendrocyte proliferation early in the disease may compensate for the demyelination.[64] In the later stages, as in most typical cases, oligodendrocytes are reduced in number. The change in the microenvironment around the oligodendrocyte by continuous inflammation and demyelination byproducts are proposed to be responsible for this decrease in number, hence the impairment of remyelination.[65] The extent of this change might be related to the amount of inflammation and the number and duration of repetitive insults, hence suggesting a probable correlation of the prognostic factors defined in the natural history studies with the impaired remyelination. Thus, different forms of MS might be partly related to different patterns of remyelination capabilities.

The balance between demyelination and remyelination is not the only pathological process thought to be responsible for the evaluation or chronicity of MS lesions. Axonal pathologic changes in MS have been known since Charcot and were believed to be secondary to demyelination until recently. It was suggested that the loss of myelin in the chronic stages that leads to progressive axonal loss might be responsible for the accumulating disability observed in MS patients.[66] Wallerian degeneration of axonal projections as a result of transection was also reported as another possible mechanism of axonal degeneration observed in normal-appearing white matter outside of demyelinating lesions.[67,68] Ferguson et al. recently found evidence of axonal injury throughout acute lesions as well as along the margins of active chronic lesions and suggested that this was an episodic event rather than progressive.[69] Trapp et al. confirmed these findings by showing that transected axons are common in the active lesions of MS and that this damage may be associated with inflammation.[70] From this emerging axonal point of view, just as it was questioned for remyelination, it would be appropriate to discuss how this different axonal involvement pattern would help explain some of the variation observed within the clinical spectrum.

FUTURE ASPECTS

Today MS seems not to be delineating a 'clinical' disease anymore, but rather covering a spectrum of primary inflammatory demyelinating disorders—with or without accompanying primary axonal loss—that may be diagnosed morphologically and/or biologically. Recognizing this behavioral variation and whether the pathogenetic mechanisms involved are similar or not currently needs to be confirmed. This may influence the design of both the epidemiologic and immunogenetic studies as well as future therapeutic trials. Another clinical implication will be the selection of patients for the currently approved long-term treatments, such as the interferon-beta (INF-β) and glatiramer acetate, as well as for other emerging therapies. As these treatments have relatively substantial side-effects and costs, it will be very important to verify the different disease forms within the spectrum that may respond best and thus the patients who will benefit most.

REFERENCES

1. Larsen JP, Kvaale G, Riise T et al. Multiple sclerosis—more than one disease? *Acta Neurol Scand* 1985; **72**: 145–150.
2. Olerup O, Hillert J, Frederikson S et al. Primarily chronic progressive and relapsing/remitting multiple sclerosis: two immunogenetically distinct disease entities. *Proc Natl Acad Sci USA* 1989; **86**: 7113–7117.
3. Thompson AJ, Kermode AG, Wicks D et al. Major differences in the dynamics of primary and secondary progressive multiple sclerosis. *Ann Neurol* 1991; **29**: 53–62.
4. Hillert J, Grönning M, Nyland H et al. An immunogenetic heterogeneity in multiple sclerosis. *J Neurol Neurosurg Psychiatry* 1992; **55**: 887–890.
5. Revesz T, Kidd D, Thompson AJ et al. A comparison of the pathology of primary and secondary progressive multiple sclerosis. *Brain* 1994; **117**: 759–765.
6. Lucchinetti CF, Brück W, Rodriguez M, Lassmann H. Distinct patterns of multiple sclerosis pathology indicates heterogeneity in pathogenesis. *Brain Pathol* 1996; **6**: 259–274.
7. Weinshenker BG. Natural history of multiple sclerosis. *Ann Neurol* 1994; **36**: S6–S11.
8. Weinshenker BG. The natural history of multiple sclerosis. *Neurol Clin* 1995; **13**: 119–146.
9. McDonald WI, Thompson AJ. How many kinds of multiple sclerosis are there? In: Thompson AJ, Polman C, Hohlfeld R, eds. *Multiple Sclerosis: Clinical Challenges and Controversies*. London: Martin Dunitz, 1997; 35–42.
10. Reder AT, Antel JP. Clinical spectrum of multiple sclerosis. *Neurol Clin* 1983; **1**: 573–599.
11. Schumacher GA, Beebe GW, Kibler RF et al. Problems of experimental trials of therapy in multiple sclerosis. *Ann NY Acad Sci* 1965; **122**: 552–568.
12. Poser CM, Paty DW, Scheinberg L. New diagnostic criteria for multiple sclerosis: guidelines for research protocols. *Ann Neurol* 1983; **13**: 227–231.
13. Jacobs L, Kinkel WR, Polachini I, Kinkel RP. Correlations of nuclear magnetic resonance imaging, computerized tomography, and clinical profiles in multiple sclerosis. *Neurology* 1986; **36**: 27–34.
14. Paty DW, Oger JJ, Kastrukoff LF et al. MRI in the diagnosis of MS: a prospective study with comparison of clinical evaluation, evoked potentials, oligoclonal banding, and CT. *Neurology* 1988; **38**: 180–185.
15. Uhlenbrock D, Seidel D, Gehlen W et al. MR imaging in multiple sclerosis comparison with clinical, CSF, and visual evoked potential findings. *AJNR* 1988; **9**: 59–67.
16. Miller DH, Rudge P, Johnson G et al. Serial gadolinium enhanced magnetic resonance imaging in multiple sclerosis. *Brain* 1988; **111**: 927–939.
17. Issac C, Li DKB, Genton M et al. Multiple sclerosis: a serial study using MRI in relapsing patients. *Neurology* 1988; **38**: 1511–1515.
18. Harris JO, Frank JA, Patronas NJ et al. Serial gadolinium enhanced magnetic resonance imaging scans in patients with early relapsing–remitting multiple sclerosis: implications for clinical trials. *Ann Neurol* 1991; **29**: 1058–1065.
19. Thompson AJ, Kermode AG, MacManus DG et al. Patterns of disease activity in multiple sclerosis: clinical and magnetic resonance imaging study. *BMJ* 1990; **300**: 631–634.
20. Uitdehaag BMJ, Polman CH, Valk J et al. Magnetic resonance imaging studies in multiple sclerosis twins. *J Neurol Neurosurg Psychiatry* 1989; **52**: 1417–1419.
21. Sadovnick AD, Armstrong H, Rice GPA et al. A population-based study of multiple sclerosis in twins: update. *Ann Neurol* 1993; **33**: 281–285.
22. Mumford CJ, Wood NW, Kellar WH et al. The British Isles survey of multiple sclerosis in twins. *Neurology* 1994; **44**: 11–15.
23. Gilbert JJ, Sadler M. Unsuspected multiple sclerosis. *Arch Neurol* 1983; **40**: 533–536.
24. Xu X, McFarlin DE. Oligoclonal bands in the cerebrospinal fluid: twins with MS. *Neurology* 1984; **34**: 769–774.

25. Duquette P, Charest L. Cerebrospinal fluid findings in healthy siblings of multiple sclerosis patients. *Neurology* 1986; **36**: 727–729.
26. Ormerod IEC, Miller DH, Mcdonald WI et al. The role of NMR imaging in the assessment of multiple sclerosis and isolated neurological lesions. A quantitative study. *Brain* 1987; **110**: 1576–1616.
27. Miller DH, Ormerod IE, McDonald WI et al. The early risk of multiple sclerosis after optic neuritis. *J Neurol Neurosurg Psychiatry* 1988; **51**: 1569–1571.
28. Morrissey SP, Miller DH, Kendall BE et al. The significance of brain magnetic resonance imaging abnormalities at presentation with clinically isolated syndromes suggestive of multiple sclerosis. A 5-year follow-up study. *Brain* 1993; **116**: 135–146.
29. Kesselring J, Miller DH, Robb SA et al. Acute disseminated encephalomyelitis MRI findings and the distinction from multiple sclerosis. *Brain* 1990; **113**: 291–302.
30. Kepes JJ. Large focal tumor-like demyelinating lesions of the brain: intermediate entity between multiple sclerosis and acute disseminated encephalomyelitis? A study of 31 patients. *Ann Neurol* 1993; **33**: 18–27.
31. Youl BD, Kermode AG, Thompson AJ et al. Destructive lesions in demyelinating disease. *J Neurol Neurosurg Psychiatry* 1991; **54**: 288–292.
32. Thompson AJ, Polman C, Miller DH et al. Primary progressive multiple sclerosis. *Brain* 1997; **120**: 1085–1096.
33. Paty DW. Biologic versus clinical MS (correspondence). *Neurology* 1989; **39**: 151.
34. Ikuta F, Zimmerman HM. Distribution of plaques in seventy autopsy cases of multiple sclerosis in the United States. *Neurology* 1976; **26**: 26–28.
35. Weinshenker BG, Gilbert JJ, Ebers GC. Some clinical and pathologic observations on chronic myelopathy: a variant of multiple sclerosis. *J Neurol Neurosurg Psychiatry* 1990; **53**: 146–149.
36. Thorpe JW, Kidd D, Moseley IF et al. Spinal MRI in patients with suspected multiple sclerosis and negative brain MRI. *Brain* 1996; **119**: 709–714.
37. Okinaka S, Tsubaki Y, Kuroiwa Y et al. Multiple sclerosis and allied diseases in Japan. Clinical characteristics. *Neurology* 1958; **8**: 756–763.
38. Shibasaki H, Kuroda Y, Kuroiwa Y. Clinical studies of multiple sclerosis in Japan: classical multiple sclerosis and Devic's disease. *J Neurol Sci* 1974; **23**: 215–222.
39. Sawcer S, Robertson N, Compston A. Genetic epidemiology of multiple sclerosis. In: Thompson AJ, Polman C, Hohlfeld R, eds. *Multiple Sclerosis: Clinical Challenges and Controversies*. London: Martin Dunitz, 1997; 13–34.
40. Barcellos L, Thomson G, Carington M et al. Chromosome 19 single-locus and multilocus haplotype associations with multiple sclerosis. Evidence of a new susceptibility locus in Caucasian and Chinese patients. *JAMA* 1997; **278**: 1256–1261.
41. Kira J-I, Kanai T, Nishimura Y et al. Western versus Asian types of multiple sclerosis immunologenetically and clinically distinct disorders. *Ann Neurol* 1996; **40**: 569–574.
42. Kelly MA, Cavan DA, Penny MA et al. The influence of HLA-DR and -DQ alleles on progression to multiple sclerosis following a clinically isolated syndrome. *Human Immunol* 1993; **37**: 185–191.
43. Runmarker B, Martinsson T, Wahlstörm J et al. HLA and prognosis in multiple sclerosis. *J Neurol* 1994; **241**: 385–390.
44. Schluesener HJ, Wekerle H. Autoaggressive T lymphocyte lines recognizing the encephalitogenic region of myelin basic protein: in vitro selection from unprimed rat T lymphocyte populations. *J Immunol* 1985; **135**: 3128–3133.
45. Burns J, Rosenzweig A, Zweimann B et al. Isolation of myelin basic protein-reactive T-cell lines from normal human blood. *Cell Immunol* 1983; **81**: 435–440.
46. Genain CP, Lee-Paritz D, Nguyen M-H et al. In healthy primates, circulating autoreactive T cells mediate autoimmune disease. *J Clin Invest* 1994; **94**: 1339–1345. (Comment in: *J Clin Invest* 1994; **94**: 921–922.)
47. Brocke S, Gaur A, Piercy C et al. Induction of relapsing paralysis in experimental autoimmune encephalomyelitis by bacterial superantigen. *Nature* 1993; **365**: 642–644.
48. Wuscherpfennig KW, Strominger JL. Molecular mimicry in T cell-mediated autoimmunity: viral peptides activate human T cell clones specific for myelin basic protein. *Cell* 1995; **80**: 695–705.
49. Giovannoni G, Thorpe JW, Kidd D et al. Soluble E-selectin in multiple sclerosis: raised concentrations in patients with primary progressive disease. *J Neurol Neurosurg Psychiatry* 1996; **60**: 20–26.

50. McGeer RL, Itagaki S, Tago H et al. Reactive microglia in patients with senile dementia of the Alzheimer type are positive for the histocompatibility glycoprotein HLA-DR. *Neurosci Let* 1987; **79**: 195–200.
51. Wekerle H, Kojima K, Lannes-Vieira J et al. Animal models. *Ann Neurol* 1994; **36 Suppl**: S47–S53.
52. Kojima K, Berger T, Lassmann H et al. Experimental autoimmune panencephalitis and uveoretinitis transferred to the Lewis rat by T lymphocytes specific for the S100β molecule, a calcium binding protein of astroglia. *J Exp Med* 1994; **180**: 817–829.
53. Sergott RC, Brown MJ, Lisak RP et al. Antibody to myelin associated glycoprotein produces central nervous system demyelination. *Neurology* 1988; **38**: 422.
54. Lassmann H, Vass K. Are current immunological concepts of multiple sclerosis reflected by the immunopathology of its lesions? *Springer Semin Immunopathol* 1995; **17**: 77–87.
55. Linington C, Lassmann H. Antibody responses in chronic allergic encephalomyelitis: correlation of serum demyelinating activity with antibody titre to the myelin/oligodendrocyte protein (MOG). *J Neuroimmunol* 1987; **17**: 61.
56. Warren KG, Catz I. Relative frequency of autoantibodies to myelin basic protein and proteolipid protein in optic neuritis and multiple sclerosis cerebrospinal fluid. *J Neurol Sci* 1994; **121**: 468–473.
57. Greer JM, Csurhes PA, Cameron KD et al. Increased immunereactivity to two overlapping peptides of myelin proteolipid protein in multiple sclerosis. *Brain* 1997; **120**: 1447–1460.
58. Linington C, Bradl M, Lassmann H et al. Augmentation of demyelination in rat acute allergic encephalomyelitis by circulating mouse monoclonal antibodies directed against a myelin/oligodendrocyte glycoprotein. *Am J Pathol* 1988; **130**: 443–454.
59. Lassmann H, Suchanek G, Ozawa K. Histopathology and the blood–cerebrospinal fluid barrier in multiple sclerosis. *Ann Neurol* 1994; **36 Suppl**: S42–S46.
60. Bauer J, Wekerle H, Lassmann H. Apoptosis in brain-specific autoimmune disease. *Curr Opin Immunol* 1995; **7**: 839–843.
61. Hohlfeld R. Biotechnical agents for the immunotherapy of multiple sclerosis. Principles, problems and perspectives. *Brain* 1997; **120**: 865–916.
62. Rieckmann P, Albrecht M, Kitze B et al. Cytokine mRNA levels in mononuclear blood cells from patients with multiple sclerosis. *Neurology* 1994; **44**: 1523–1526.
63. Lassmann H. Pathology and experimental models. In Kesselring J, ed. *Multiple Sclerosis*. Cambridge: Cambridge University Press, 1997: 7–29.
64. Prineas JW, Barnard RO, Revesz T et al. Multiple sclerosis: pathology of recurrent lesions. *Brain* 1993; **116**: 681.
65. McLaurin JA, Yong VW. Oligodendrocytes and myelin. *Neurol Clin* 1995; **13**: 23–49.
66. McDonald WI, Miller DH, Barnes D. The pathological evaluation of multiple sclerosis. *Neuropathol Appl Neurobiol* 1992; **18**: 319–334.
67. Davie CA, Barker GJ, Webb S et al. Persistent functional deficit in multiple sclerosis and autosomal cerebellar ataxia is associated with axon loss. *Brain* 1995; **118**: 1583–1592.
68. Narayanan S, Fu L, Pioro E et al. Imaging of axonal damage multiple sclerosis: spatial imaging of magnetic imaging lesions. *Ann Neurol* 1997; **41**: 385–391.
69. Ferguson B, Matyszak MK, Esiri MM et al. Axonal damage in acute multiple sclerosis. *Brain* 1997; **120**: 393–399.
70. Trapp BD, Peterson J, Ransohoff RM et al. Axonal transection in the lesions of multiple sclerosis. *N Engl J Med* 1998; **338**: 278–285.

2

Asymptomatic multiple sclerosis: what does it mean?

Ingrid V Allen

Asymptomatic multiple sclerosis (MS) can be defined in a variety of ways, but essentially there are three major categories for consideration:

- clinically silent disease that is diagnosed by chance, usually through neuroimaging or at autopsy;
- discrete lesions that are undetected in the course of the disease, either clinically or through neuroimaging, but which are apparent at autopsy;
- diffuse abnormalities in the normal-appearing white matter in MS, detected neuropathologically or by neuroimaging and which are of unknown significance.

In the first category the disease itself is clinically silent and affected individuals present usually at autopsy or through neuroimaging, with classical MS plaques in the central nervous system which have apparently been symptom free. Recognition of this form of MS, though rare, is well substantiated by several investigators, with 51 such cases reported in the literature.[1–16] The reported studies are of necessity retrospective and, on a population basis, represent a highly selected sample in which autopsy was carried out for conditions unrelated to MS. In one of the largest series reported by Engell,[13] from the Danish MS register, 18 cases of MS were first identified, but five were rejected because MS may have been obscured by neurological symptoms of other conditions. In the remaining 13 cases, neuropathological examination was undertaken for neoplastic or vascular disease, and in these MS was considered to be clinically silent. Two key points emerge from the Danish study, firstly in relationship to the overall incidence of clinically silent MS, and secondly regarding the pathophysiological basis of the syndrome. In this study the mean frequency in three series of 16 000 neuropathological examinations was 0.08%. The authors, extrapolating from this figure, calculate that in an MS susceptible population, some 25% of MS cases are asymptomatic. This figure, however, may be too high, firstly because minor neurological symptoms may be ignored or misinterpreted, and secondly because of the age distribution of MS cases at autopsy, which differs significantly from the overall age distribution at death. The study, however, raises the interesting possibility that there may be a significant number of undiagnosed cases of MS (as opposed to wrongly diagnosed cases) in communities in which MS has a high incidence.

It is still not entirely clear why some cases of MS are clinically silent, although several hypotheses have been advanced. These theories include consideration of the anatomy of the lesions, the degree of oligodendrocyte and axonal pathology, and the extent of myelin repair. The key factor seems to be the anatomical location of the lesions, with the predominant distribution of plaques in the reported cases sited in the periventricular region. This location seems more important than the number or size of plaques. The absence of clinical signs in periventricular lesions is well substantiated and is supported by other studies, e.g. silent periventricular lesions have been demonstrated in isolated optic neuritis.[17] In a detailed neuropathological study of 11 autopsy cases of clinically silent MS, several issues of relevance to this syndrome have been addressed.[18] Lesions were scattered throughout the central nervous system, but 39% of all lesions were periventricular as emphasized in earlier studies. In addition, fewer infratentorial lesions were found, as compared with classic cases, and this factor also may be relevant to the absence of clinical signs. Variation in axonal and oligodendrocyte pathology within individual lesions may also affect the development of clinical signs, although the difference in these features within individual lesions in asymptomatic and classic cases is less clear.

In classic MS, particularly in the advanced stages of the disease, it is difficult to assign specific clinical symptoms and signs to specific discrete lesions. Nevertheless, studies of clinical MS using neuroimaging indicate that the number of lesions is often greater than the clinical symptomatology would suggest, and it has long been recognized that many more neuropathological lesions are identified at autopsy than have been suspected clinically or by neuroimaging. Therefore the relative sensitivity of the various investigations has to be considered in this context. Clearly neurological investigation depends on testing anatomical and physiological systems and may not be the most sensitive mechanism for identifying lesions which cross, or only partially affect, individual systems. Magnetic resonance imaging (MRI) is clearly a much more sensitive diagnostic tool, yet even this technique has been shown to underdiagnose pathological lesions. In a pathological and MRI study of cortical lesions in MS (D Kidd et al, unpub. data), in one case the two techniques were correlated. MRI identified 134 lesions of which 58 were subcortical and two were purely cortical; subsequent neuropathological examination of the brain slices revealed 328 lesions of which 108 were cortical and involving the subjacent white matter. This study confirms earlier work that involvement of the grey matter is common in MS; such lesions are under-reported by MRI.

Perhaps the most poorly understood asymptomatic MS lesions are diffuse abnormalities, affecting the normal-appearing white and grey matter, and defined using histological, histochemical, biochemical and neuroimaging techniques. These diffuse abnormalities, often not associated with overt demyelination, may have significance for neural function and disease progression. For example, a histological study of normal-appearing white matter (NAWM) samples showed that over 70% had some histological abnormality.[19] The most common abnormality was astrocytic gliosis, though unsuspected demyelination, vascular hyalinization and perivascular cellular infiltration were also noted. Further abnormalities in non-demyelinated white matter in MS have been defined in several molecular studies, but few of these studies have focused primarily on the NAWM and it is therefore difficult to deduce if the reported abnormalities are focal or diffuse. Reports of lysosomal enzyme activation in NAWM indicate a diffuse but selective increase.[20–22] Studies related to antigen presentation, adhesion molecule upregulation, and cytokine activation, however, suggest a more restricted reaction, with abnormalities in NAWM adjacent to plaques.[23–25].

Complementary studies with MRI and magnetic resonance spectroscopy support the pathological conclusion of diffuse abnormality in the NAWM. Early studies suggested significant differences in MS in NAWM for T_1 and T_2 relaxation times[26] and further studies suggest increased water self-diffusion in NAWM.[27] continued NAWM abnormality during and after adrenocorticotropic hormone treatment in MS,[28] and microscopic disease in NAWM.[29]

Biochemical abnormality has been confirmed by nuclear magnetic resonance proton spectroscopy,[30] and these findings are suggestive of diffuse disease with axonal damage.[31,32]

Two recent MRI studies suggest diffuse abnormality in NAWM and, on serial scanning, these abnormalities are correlated to new lesion formation.[33,34] In summary, diffuse but poorly defined abnormalities in the NAWM are recognized. These abnormalities may have significance for new lesion formation and disease progression but require further study.

REFERENCES

1. McAlpine D, Compston ND, Lumsden CE. *Multiple sclerosis.* Edinburgh: Churchill Livingstone, 1955.
2. Georgi W. Multiple Sklerose. *Schweiz Med Wschr* 1961; **91**: 606–607.
3. Russell DS. Trauma and multiple sclerosis. *Lancet* 1964; **1**: 978.
4. Vost A, Wolochow DA, Howell DA. Incidence of infarcts of the brain in heart disease. *J Pathol Bact* 1964; **88**: 463–470.
5. Mackay RP, Hirano A. Forms of benign multiple sclerosis, report of two 'clinically silent' cases discovered at autopsy. *Arch Neurol* 1967; **17**: 588–600.
6. Morariu M, Klutzow WF. Subclinical multiple sclerosis. *J Neurol* 1976; **213**: 71–76.
7. Weber W, Ulrich J. Multiple sclerosis, diffuse lymphoplasmocytic encephalitis and Alzheimer's disease in a patient with progressive dementia. *Eur Neurol* 1976; **14**: 266–274.
8. Castaigne P, Lhermitte F, Escourolle R et al. Les scléroses en plaques asymptomatiques. *Rev Neurol* 1981; **137**: 729–739.
9. Gilbert JJ, Sadler M. Unsuspected multiple sclerosis. *Arch Neurol* 1983; **40**: 533–536.
10. Phadke JG, Best PV. Atypical and clinically silent multiple sclerosis: a report of 12 cases discovered unexpectedly at necroscopy. *J Neurol Neurosurg Psychiatry* 1983; **46**: 414–420.
11. Rao TV et al. Multiple sclerosis with an associated diffuse oligodendroglioma. *National Institute of Mental Health and Neuroscience Journal* 1986; **4**: 105–110.
12. Auer RN, Gallagher JC, Butt JC. Solitary asymptomatic plaque of demyelination in the medulla oblongata. *Clin Neuropathol* 1988; **7**: 225–227.
13. Engell T. A clinical patho-anatomical study of clinically silent multiple sclerosis. *Acta Neurol Scand* 1989; **79**: 428–430.
14. Shankar SK et al. Balo's concentric sclerosis: a variant of multiple sclerosis associated with oligodendroglioma. *Neurosurgery* 1989; **25**: 982–986.
15. Barkhof F, Scheltens P, Kamphorst W. Pre- and post-mortem MR imaging of unsuspected multiple sclerosis in a patient with Alzheimer's disease. *J Neurol Sci* 1993; **117**: 175–178.
16. Heinsen H, Lockemann U, Püschel K. Unsuspected (clinically silent) multiple sclerosis. Quantitative investigations in one autoptic case. *Int J Leg Med* 1995; **107**: 263–266.
17. Jacobs I, Kinkel PR, Kinkel WR. Silent brain lesions in patients with isolated optic neuritis. *Arch Neurol* 1986; **43**: 452–455.
18. Mews I, Bergmann M, Bunkowski S et al. Oligodendrocyte and axon pathology in clinically silent multiple sclerosis lesions. *Multiple Sclerosis* 1998; **4**: 85–90.
19. Allen IV, McKeown SR. A histological histochemical and biochemical study of the macroscopically normal white matter in multiple sclerosis. *J Neurolol Sci* 1979; **41**: 81–91.
20. McKeown SR, Allen IV. The cellular origin of lysosomal enzymes in the plaque in multiple sclerosis: a combined histological and biochemical study. *Neuropath Appl Neurobiol* 1978; **4**: 471–482.
21. McKeown SR, Allen IV. The fragility of cerebral lysosomes in multiple sclerosis. *Neuropath Appl Neurobiol* 1979; **5**: 405–415.
22. Huterer SJ, Tourtellotte WW, Wherett JR. Alterations in the activity of phospholipases A (2) in postmortem white-matter from patient with multiple sclerosis. *Neurochem Res* 1995; **20**: 1335–1343.
23. Li H, Newcombe J, Groome NP et al. Characterisation and distribution of phagocytic macrophages in multiple sclerosis plaques. *Neuropath Appl Neurobiol* 1993; **19**: 214–223.
24. Li H, Cuzner ML, Newcombe J. Microglia-derived macrophages in early multiple sclerosis plaques. *Neuropath Appl Neurobiol* 1996; **22** 207–215.
25. Battistini L, Fischer FR, Raine CS et al. CD1b is expressed in multiple sclerosis lesions. *J Neuroimmunol* 1996; **67**: 145–151.

26. Miller DH, Johnson G, Tofts PS et al. Precise relaxation time measurements of normal-appearing white matter in inflammatory central nervous system disease. *Magn Reson Med* 1989; **11**: 331–336.
27. Christiansen P, Gideon P, Thomsen C et al. Increased water self-diffusion in chronic plaques and in apparently normal white matter in patients with multiple sclerosis. *Acta Neurologica Scandinavica* 1993; **87(3)**: 195–199.
28. Armspach JP, Gounot D, Namer IJ et al. Quantitative cerebral magnetic resonance imaging during ACTH treatment of multiple sclerosis. *Magn Reson Imaging* 1993; **11**: 1147–1153.
29. Loevner LA, Grossman RI, Cohen JA et al. Microscopic disease in normal-appearing white matter on conventional MR images in patients with multiple sclerosis: assessment with magnetization–transfer measurements. *Radiology* 1995; **196**: 511–515.
30. Tourbah A, Stievenart JL, Ibazizen MT et al. In-vivo localized NMR proton spectroscopy of normal appearing white-matter in patients with multiple-sclerosis. *J Neuroradiol*. 1996; **3(2)**: 49–55.
31. Rooney WD, Goodkin DE, Schuff N et al. H MRSI of normal appearing white matter in multiple sclerosis. *Multiple Sclerosis* 1997; **3**: 231–237.
32. Schiepers C, Van Hecke P, Vandenberghe R et al. Positron emission tomography, magnetic resonance imaging and proton NMR spectroscopy of white matter in multiple sclerosis. *Multiple Sclerosis* 1997; **3**: 8–17.
33. Goodkin DE, Rooney W, Sloan R et al. PD, T1, Gadolinium (Gd^+) intensities, T2 and MTRs are chronically diffusely abnormal in MS brain and on monthly MRI scans are related to the appearance of new Gd^+ lesions in normal-appearing white matter (NAWM). *Neurology* 1998; **50 (suppl 2)**: 36.
34. Comi G, Rocca MA, Rovaris M et al. Magnetization transfer changes in the normal-appearing white matter precede the appearance of enhancing lesions in patients with multiple sclerosis. *Neurology* 1998; **50 (suppl 2)**: 36.

3

Monophasic isolated inflammatory demyelinating syndromes

Chris H Polman

CLINICAL PRESENTATION

The classical initial manifestation of inflammatory demyelinating disease is a so-called 'clinically isolated syndrome' presenting as subacute dysfunction of the optic nerve, brain or spinal cord, which in most cases spontaneously shows complete or incomplete recovery (first relapse of relapsing–remitting multiple sclerosis (MS)). Only a small number of patients (10%) develop slowly progressive disability without relapses and remissions (primary progressive disease). Of those initially presenting with a relapse the most common clinical manifestations are sensory (40%), visual (25%), motor (20%), brainstem and cerebellar (15%) and bladder (10%) symptoms.

In most cases objective confirmation of neurological dysfunction can easily be obtained by a neurologist (paresis, ataxia, internuclear ophthalmoplegia, abnormal reflexes), but sometimes, particularly in cases with special presentations (e.g. Lhermitte's sign, vertigo, bladder dysfunction), this can be more difficult.

DIAGNOSTIC WORK-UP

At the initial presentation, when by definition the criterion of dissociation in time has not been fulfilled, there is quite a large differential diagnosis, including other inflammatory diseases (like vasculitis, Sjögren's syndrome), infectious diseases (like neuroborreliosis, neurosyphilis), sarcoidosis, cerebrovascular disease and, depending on the clinical site of presentation, also compressive disease and vitamin B_{12} deficiency.

In general it is recommended to perform brain magnetic resonance imaging (MRI), blood analysis (ESR, serology of *Borrelia* and syphilis, antinuclear antibody (ANA), anticardiolipin antibody, vitamin B_{12}) and cerebrospinal fluid (CSF) analysis (cell count, total protein, IgG-index, oligoclonal banding) in all patients and spinal MRI and complete ophthalmological evaluation for those presenting with spinal and optic symptomatology respectively.

Brain MR is highly sensitive in detecting both MS lesions and other conditions that may present with the same clinical picture as that encountered in MS. The typical pattern of discrete, multifocal white matter areas of increased signal on T2-weighted scans, however, has a low specificity. Sometimes lesions, when large and isolated, may be confused with a tumor, but some infectious diseases (e.g. HTLV-1, Lyme's disease), neurosarcoidosis and cerebral vasculitides especially can be very difficult to distinguish from MS. Preliminary evidence suggests that the pattern of enhancement with gadolinium (lesions, meninges) or the imaging characteristics of the spinal cord (presence and aspect of lesions, swelling or atrophy) may help in differentiation.

Conventional criteria for diagnosing MS require clinical demonstration of dissociation both in time and in space; MR may provide additional information by showing radiological dissemination in space (multiple lesions) and time (both enhancing and nonenhancing lesions) at first presentation. Under these conditions MR clearly documents some of the limitations of clinical assessment: many lesions can be present in the absence of typical symptoms (medical history) or signs (even when the lesions are located in the optic nerve or spinal cord).

At the initial presentation it can be extremely difficult to distinguish between MS and another inflammatory demyelinating disease, acute disseminated encephalomyelitis (ADEM).[1] Typically ADEM patients present with widespread neurological abnormalities, including multifocal signs in the brain, spinal cord and optic nerves that may include drowsiness or seizures. The condition is usually precipitated by a viral infection. In the acute phase, MRI of the brain and spinal cord shows high signal T2 lesions, although the underlying pathology may be oedema with minimal demyelination. This may explain the resolution of these lesions on serial scanning, while in MS usually new lesions develop. In addition the two diseases may be discriminated since CSF oligoclonal bands are found only infrequently in ADEM.

There has been a lot of debate whether—in the absence of a very effective treatment—patients with an initial presentation suggestive of inflammatory demyelinating disease should be diagnosed vigorously and whether during initial care patients should be told that they have a high probability of developing MS.[2] One study prospectively assessed the effect of diagnostic information on patients' sense of well-being. It was found that, although there is quite some interindividual variation dependent on the results of the diagnostic work-up, overall it seemed to benefit patients.[3]

PROGNOSIS

According to Runmarker and Andersen, who followed an incidence cohort of 308 MS patients during at least 25 years of disease, the type of disease course was the most important clinical parameter to predict the long-term prognosis, with primary progressive patients experiencing a more severe course.[4] In patients with an acute onset, low onset age, high degree of remission at first exacerbation, symptoms from afferent nerve fibres and onset symptoms from only one region (as compared with polyregional symptoms) of the CNS were factors significantly associated with a more favourable long-term prognosis. Comparable data were obtained in a Canadian natural history study on factors that predict outcome.[5,6] Brain MRI has been shown to greatly enhance the ability to predict which patients with a clinically isolated syndrome are likely to develop MS. The presence of 'clinically silent' brain lesions on MRI at the time of presentation increases the risk of conversion to MS, largely irrespective of this clinically isolated syndrome manifesting as an optic neuritis, a brainstem syndrome or a spinal cord syndrome.[7,8] Many studies have shown that the risk of MS, at least within the first 5 years, is low (< 10%) with normal brain MRI and much higher (50–70%) in those with brain lesions. Morrissey et al.[8] demonstrated that the PPV (positive predictive value) of an abnormal MR-scan (minimum four T2-lesions) in patients presenting with isolated syndromes suggestive for MS for development of clinically definite MS within 5 years is 65%, while the NPV (negative predictive value) of a normal brain MR scan is 97%. As the number and load of lesions increase, the risk of progression becomes greater;[7] in one study a moderate correlation was found between quantitated T2 lesion load at presentation and disability after 5 years.[9]

To improve specificity and sensitivity various criteria have been adapted. Paty's criteria (minimum of four lesions, or three of which one is periventricular), being prospectively evaluated in patients with clinically isolated syndromes, showed high sensitivity but relatively low specificity. Fazekas criteria (three lesions or more), with at least two characteristics (infratentorial, periventricular or at least 6 mm), being retrospectively evaluated in patients with established MS, showed both high sensitivity and specificity. A study by Tas et al. demonstrated that the combination of gadolinium-enhancing lesions and nonenhancing lesions on the same scan increases the likelihood for early progression from a clinically isolated syndrome to clinically definite MS.[10] In a recent multicentre study under the auspices of MAGNIMS (a CEC programme entitled 'Development of optimal magnetic resonance techniques to monitor treatments for preventing disability in MS') a number of MR imaging criteria were compared with regard to their value of predicting conversion to MS. A model which included gadolinium-enhancement, juxtacortical, infratentorial and periventricular lesion location had a very high PPV (92%) for conversion to MS.[11]

In contrast to almost all other studies, one recent study suggests that abnormal CSF IgG levels correlate more strongly than abnormal MRI with the subsequent development of clinically definite MS.[12]

TREATMENT

The Optic Neuritis Treatment Trial prospectively studied the effect of three treatment regimens (intravenous methylprednisolone 1000 mg for 3 subsequent days followed by oral prednisone; oral prednisone; placebo) on 389 patients with acute monosymptomatic optic neuritis who did not meet diagnostic criteria for definite MS at that time, both with regard to outcome of the presenting episode as to frequency of future episodes.[7] It was found that, compared with the placebo regimen, the intravenous regimen showed more rapid recovery but no long-term benefit, most of the difference in rate of recovery being observed in the first 2 weeks. Unexpectedly, the study found as a secondary outcome parameter that the intravenous group had a lower rate of development of MS within the first 2 years than did the placebo or prednisone group, most of this treatment effect being observed in the patients with abnormal MRI at study entry (reduction in development of definite MS from 36% after 2 years in the placebo group to 16% in the intravenous group). This treatment effect no longer persisted after the third year of follow-up.

Treatment of clinically isolated syndromes suggestive for MS can be particularly attractive because it is assumed that early (immune) intervention has the highest likelihood of arresting the disease. At this moment there are two studies investigating whether interferon beta, when started immediately after the first episode, can have a favourable impact on the future course of the disease. Irrespective of the outcome of these studies it is very important, given the large variability in MS prognosis, to select for treatment those patients that are likely to show progression and to save patients with low risk from unnecessary treatment side-effects.

REFERENCES

1. Grand Rounds Hammersmith Hospitals. Distinguishing acute disseminated encephalomyelitis from multiple sclerosis. *BMJ* 1996; **313**: 802–804.
2. Editorial. What to tell patients with their first attack of multiple sclerosis. *Eur Neurol* 1996; **36**: 183–190.
3. Mushlin AI, Mooney C, Grow V et al. The value of diagnostic information to patients with suspected multiple sclerosis. *Arch Neurol* 1994; **51**: 67–72.
4. Runmarker B, Andersen O. Prognostic factors in a multiple sclerosis incidence cohort with twenty-five years follow-up. *Brain* 1993; **116**: 117–134.
5. Weinshenker BG, Bass B, Rice GPA et al. The natural history of multiple sclerosis: a geographically based study: predictive value of the early clinical course. *Brain* 1989; **112**: 1419–1428.
6. Weinshenker BG, Rice GPA, Noseworthy JH et al. The natural history of multiple sclerosis: a

geographically based study: multivariate analysis of predictive factors and models of outcome. *Brain* 1991; **114**: 1045–1056.
7. Beck RW, Cleary PA, Anderson MM et al. A randomisation controlled trial of corticosteroids in the treatment of acute optic neuritis. *New Engl J Med* 1992; **326**: 581–588.
8. Morrissey SP, Miller D, Kendall BE et al. The significance of brain magnetic resonance imaging abnormalities at presentation with clinically isolated syndromes suggestive of multiple sclerosis. *Brain* 1993; **116**: 135–146.
9. Filippi M, Horsfield MA, Morrissey SP et al. Quantitative brain MRI lesion load predicts the course of clinically isolated syndromes suggestive of multiple sclerosis. *Neurology* 1994; **44**: 635–641.
10. Tas MW, Barkhof F, van Walderveen MAAA et al. The effect of gadolinium on the sensitivity and specificity of MR imaging in the initial diagnosis of multiple sclerosis. *AJNR* 1995; **16**: 259–264.
11. Barkhof F, Filippi M, Miller DH et al. Comparison of MR imaging criteria at first presentation to predict conversion to clinically definite multiple sclerosis. *Brain* 1997; **120**: 2059–2069.
12. Jacobs LD, Kaba SE, Miller CM et al. Correlation of clinical, magnetic resonance imaging, and cerebrospinal fluid findings in optic neuritis. *Ann Neurol* 1997; **41**: 392–398.

4

How early can we estimate transition into the progressive course from relapsing–remitting multiple sclerosis?

Giancarlo Comi, Vittorio Martinelli, Massimo Filippi, Letizia Leocani, Mariemma Rodegher, Marco Rovaris and Gianvito Martino

INTRODUCTION

Multiple sclerosis (MS) is a disease characterized by a largely unpredictable course in the single patient. Some patients experience a rapid and continuous deterioration of neurological functions from disease onset, but others have more or less frequent relapses followed by a complete—or almost complete—recovery for many years, and start to deteriorate only after 10–20 years or never accumulate significant disability. In about 85% of the patients the disease starts with a relapsing–remitting (RR) course; 50% of these patients convert to a secondary progressive (SP) course within 10 years, 70% within 20 years, and 90–95% during their life.[1–4] The conversion to a progressive course is associated with an irreversible impairment/disability and with a more rapid deterioration of neurological functions.[4] There are converging evidences from pathological, immunological, neurophysiological and magnetic resonance imaging (MRI) studies indicating that the pathogenetic mechanisms underlying the RR and the SP phases of MS can be different, thus indicating the importance to have early markers of the shift from the RR to the SP course in order to tailor the treatment, which could be quite different in the two phases of the disease.

In this review we will focus on the pathological, immunological, neurophysiological and MRI abnormalities observed in the two phases of the disease and on the potential markers of the conversion from RR to SP course. There are essentially two types of markers: (a) markers of pathological changes occurring in the central nervous system (CNS), such as MRI and neurophysiological parameters, or products of the pathologic processes like the levels of myelin basic protein (MBP) or MBP-like material in the body fluids; (b) markers of immunological changes occurring in the peripheral blood and/or in the cerebrospinal fluid (CSF). The possibility that either one or the other type of marker can be useful for an early detection of the shift from RR to SP course depends on the pathogenetic mechanisms underlying this transition, which are mostly still unknown.

CLINICAL MARKERS

One of the major obstacles in reviewing the studies performed in this field is the high variability in the definition of the clinical forms and of the clinical stages of MS. Only recently a consensus has been reached on the classification of MS courses, as the result of an international survey involving 125 members of the international MS clinical research community.[5] In this consensus, progression is defined as 'a gradual, nearly continuous, worsening baseline with minor fluctuations but no distinct relapses'; phases of plateau of variable duration and also phases of minor improvement can be accepted as part of the progressive phase. It is interesting to note that the term 'worsening' was not better defined, thus implying that either the deterioration of pre-existing signs or the appearance of new signs (when they are persistent and not related to a relapse) determine the classification of a course as progressive. The pros of the criteria proposed by Lublin and Reingold[5] are their simplicity, because the classification of the courses is based on the variable combination over time of only two parameters: relapses and progression. The cons are that the term 'progressive' can be misleading because it describes only the modality of neurological deterioration: patients classified as 'nonprogressive' may have a progression of the disease due to an incomplete recovery from relapses. Nevertheless, in this review we will refer to this classification.

In RR MS patients no single demographic or clinical characteristic is strongly predictive of an imminent evolution to a SP course. Usually the secondary progression phase starts when disability ranges from an expanded disability status scale (EDSS)[6] of 3 to 4,[7] but some RR patients may enter the progressive phase when their EDSS is beyond 6.[8] The higher risk of entering a progressive phase of the disease for patients with EDSS from 3 to 5 is indirectly pointed out by the higher risk of confirmed deterioration for this group of patients.[9] The yearly risk of developing progressive MS is not constant over time, but it reaches a peak dependent on the age at onset of the disease, then declines.[4,8] Other clinical characteristics which have some predictive value for a future progressive course include male gender, a later age at onset, corticospinal and cerebellar involvement, increased number of relapses in the first 5 years and a shorter interval between the first and the second relapse.[7]

It is difficult to estimate prospectively the exact time a patient enters the progressive phase for many reasons:

(a) the disability scales are imprecise and not sensitive enough to small changes of the neurological status
(b) the persistence of the deterioration must be confirmed by two consecutive neurological evaluations, at least 6 months apart
(c) it must be excluded that the neurological changes are due to undetected relapses (which is extremely difficult in patients who have already accumulated a certain level of disability)
(d) phases of plateau are frequently observed in the progressive course and require a long observation period to classify patients in the SP group.

PATHOLOGICAL FINDINGS

Multiple sclerosis is characterized by destruction of myelin sheaths during the active disease process, which leads to the formation of large demyelinated plaques. During the early relapsing–remitting stage of disease evolution, extensive remyelination is usually observed, which explains the full recovery characterizing most of the bouts in this phase of the disease.[10–15] Remyelination depends upon the availability of oligodendrocytes or their progenitor cells within the lesions.[16,17] In the late chronic stage of the disease, repair of myelin is sparse and, if present at all, restricted to a small rim at the plaque edges. It is as yet unclear which cells in the CNS accomplish remyelination. They could in part be recruited from oligodendrocytes that have survived the acute phase of demyelination.[17] However, recent experimental data suggest that mature, terminally differentiated oligodendrocytes are incapable of synthesizing new myelin.[18] In contrast, in most experimental situations, remyelinating cells are derived from the pool of undifferentiated glial precursor cells, which are present even in the adult CNS tissue and can also be found in low numbers in demyelinated plaques. Thus, it is suggested that the failure of myelin repair in late chronic MS lesions could be due to a depletion of this progenitor cell pool, which is likely to occur in areas of repeated demyelinating episodes.[12,13,19,20] The recurrence of inflammation in the same area stresses the oligodendrocytes and their death may be due to the action of gamma/delta lymphocytes[21] or to aspecific processes: an antigen-aspecific bystander mechanism due to the liberation of cytokines, proteolytic or lipolytic enzymes or other toxic macrophage products or complement components.[22] Some observations support this interpretation:

(a) Prineas et al.[12] found that, in about 20% of shadow plaques, fresh lesions are located within or overlap the remyelinated tissue; in these areas oligodendrocytes are reduced in number, if compared with areas without signs of inflammation in the same shadow plaque
(b) in the encephalomyelitis induced by the Theiler's virus about 1/3 of remyelinated plaques show recurrent demyelinative activity[23]
(c) MRI studies have shown that 20–40% of active lesions are recurrent or enlarging lesions[24,25]
(d) we observed[26] that magnetization transfer ratio, a marker of destructive pathology, is lower in recurrent lesions than in new lesions, thus suggesting that the superimposition of temporally discrete lesions may result in a permanent pathological damage.

On the other hand, some oligodendrocyte progenitor cells can be found even in old demyelinated scars of MS patients. A diversity between the immune targets of the pathogenetic processes underlying the early relapsing and the late chronic phases of the disease could in part explain the above-mentioned pathological differences. The two major target candidates are oligodendrocytes and myelin components. Conceivably, both are involved in the disease, which would explain clinical heterogeneity of MS by virtue of target heterogeneity. However, in the chronic form of MS, oligodendrocytes seem to represent the primary target of the pathological process, and are almost completely lost in demyelinating areas, so that no spontaneous remyelination takes place. In contrast, in the acute relapsing–remitting form of the disease, the persistence of oligos in demyelinating areas in which remyelination takes place, suggests that the primary targets in this form are myelin components such as myelin basic protein (MBP), proteolipid protein (PLP), myelin oligodendrocyte-associated protein (MOG) or others. This latter disease form, which accounts for more than 80% of MS patients, might therefore benefit from therapies aimed at stimulating oligodendrocytes to remyelinate.[27,28] Besides the intrinsic, immediate effects of demyelination on nervous conduction, it can be also speculated that repetitive bouts of acute inflammation/demyelination in response to various pathogenetic mechanisms may also exert their harmful effects by making distal extensions of the glial cells vulnerable, and by causing the presentation of novel antigens to the immune system. Moreover, in response to a local inflammatory reaction, a switch may occur in the differentiation of common glial cell progenitors, leading to preferential differentiation into type II astrocytes. Astrocyte hyperplasia and scarring is a prominent feature of MS lesions, a potentially relevant factor since astrocytes have been reported to interfere with axon outgrowth in the adult CNS. Oligodendrocyte depletion and astrocyte proliferation may therefore compromise the clinical picture, ultimately leading to the complete and permanent inhibition of axonal conduction, that is the key feature of the chronic phase of MS. Thus, one important factor in the clinical evolution of the disease lies in the ability of oligodendrocytes to proliferate, differentiate and produce remyelination.

The pathological patterns observed in MS, although heterogeneous, are not mutually exclusive; different immunological mechanisms may result in a common final pathological end point. In fact, it has been found, in post-mortem studies, that the same pattern of immunopathological abnormalities is present in most of the MS plaques of a given patient, suggesting that changes of the immune system at the peripheral level might be more important than local changes within the CNS in determining the shift from RR to SP type of course.

IMMUNOLOGICAL MARKERS

The immunopathological hallmark of MS is the presence within the CNS of inflammatory infiltrates containing few autoreactive T cells and a multitude of pathogenic nonspecific lymphocytes.[29,30] It is currently believed that CNS antigen-specific T cells (directed against myelin components and/or oligodendrocytes) provide the organ specificity of the pathogenetic process and regulate the recirculation within the CNS of nonspecific lymphocytes, which in turn act as effector cells by releasing myelinotoxic substances (complement components, nitric oxide, immunoglobulins, cytokines, etc.). However, the mediators as well as the intracellular mechanisms sustaining central antigen-specific versus peripheral nonantigen-specific expansion of inducer and effector T cells in MS, which might represent useful monitoring markers for the disease progression, are still only partially clarified. From an immunological point of view, possible candidate markers of peripheral nonantigen specific T-cell activation are then the cytokines (mainly those with a proinflammatory profile) while possible markers of CNS-confined immune-mediated specific events are products of myelin degradation.

It is well documented that mouse and human $CD4^+$ (and $CD8^+$) T cells comprise three cell subsets which differ in their cytokine secretion profile. T helper 1 (Th1) cells secrete interleukin (IL)-2, interferon-γ (IFN-γ), and tumor necrosis factor-α (TNF-α) whereas T helper 2 (Th2) produce IL-4, IL-5, and IL-10. Their precursor cells, named Th0 cells, can produce IL-2, IFN-γ and IL-4 simultaneously,[31,32] and their switch towards a Th1 or Th2 phenotype is mainly orchestrated by IL-12 and IL-4, respectively. While Th2 cytokines play a predominant role in allergic reactions and parasitic infections, Th1 cytokines are considered to be involved in the induction of experimental autoimmune diseases (i.e. experimental allergic encephalomyelitis, insulin-dependent diabetes mellitus, collagen-induced arthritis)[33,34] as well as human organ-specific autoimmune diseases (i.e. Hashimoto's thyroiditis, Graves' disease, rheumatoid arthritis, and MS).[34] To support the central role of Th1 (proinflammatory)-cytokines in orchestrating nonantigen-specific T-cell activation in peripheral lymphocytes from MS patients are the finding that nonantigen-specific priming can be induced in T cells from MS patients by the combined action of IFN-γ, TNF-α, IL-2, and IL-6[35] and the in vivo evidence that cytokines are crucial in the development of MS (clinical course of MS worsens when patients are treated with IFN-γ;[36,37] TNF-α and IFN-γ are present in demyelinating plaques;[38,39] TNF-α, and IFN-γ circulating levels increase during active phases of MS).[40]

Cytokines might then represent not only possible surrogate markers for monitoring MS but also a marker for monitoring the transition between early relapsing MS to chronic disease. The RR phase of the disease is, in fact, characterized by intense inflammation in which Th1-cytokines play a decisive role, while the SP form shows scarce inflammation mainly confined to the CNS. However, studies on Th1 cytokines in MS lead to conflicting results. Sharief and Hentges[41] reported that increased levels of TNF-α in CSF from MS patients predict and parallel the progressive course. These results have not been confirmed subsequently.[42] Nicoletti et al.[43] reported increased levels of IL-12 in the blood of SP MS patients. Balashov et al.[44] confirmed the elevation of IL-12 in SP MS and, interestingly, found normal levels in RR MS. They attributed the increased levels of IL-12 to an upregulation of CD40 ligand on $CD4^+$ cells which stimulated non-T cells to secrete IL-12. This selective increase of IL-12 in SP MS patients has to be confirmed by further studies, considering that the activity of other IL-12-associated Th1 cytokines (e.g. IFN-γ) has been found to be related to the disease course in some studies but unrelated in others.[40]

Brain-derived myelin-like material might represent the CNS-confined specific events occurring during demyelination in MS and therefore might be a potential marker for the disease course in MS. One of the major limitations in considering brain-derived material as a marker of MS course is that this material is mostly present within the areas of demyelination or alternatively in the cerebrospinal fluid compartment which is however scarcely accessible. Again, studies aimed to find this material outside the CNS have produced conflicting results. However, Whitaker et al.[45] reported increased urinary levels of MBP-like material (MBPLM) in a large group of MS patients along which SP patients showed the highest values. These results were partially confirmed in a subsequent study in which Whitaker and collaborators[46] reported that the increase of MBPLM preceded the clinical transition of MS patients from a RR to a SP course. However, it has been observed that interindividual variability of urinary MBPLM levels was high and that a partial overlapping between progressive and nonprogressive cases occurred thus limiting the prognostic value of this parameter.

In conclusion, various immunological markers have been evaluated, but at present there are no definitive studies supporting a substantial difference in the immunological profile between RR and SP MS patients. Although some of the markers proposed might represent reasonable candidates for differentiating the immunological profile of RR and SP MS, none of them has at present a clear predictive value for the imminent evolution from one type of MS course to the other.

MAGNETIC RESONANCE MARKERS

The correlations between MS lesion loads on conventional, T2-weighted brain MRI and clinical findings are still controversial,[47] although it has been reported[48] that brain MRI lesion load at the onset of the disease (i.e. in clinically isolated syndromes suggestive of MS) is predictive of both conversion to clinically definite MS and subsequent development of clinical disability. When comparing patients with SP MS and patients with 'benign' disease course (i.e. patients with long disease duration and mild or no clinical disability), brain MRI lesion volumes were significantly lower for the latter patients[49] but this difference was not present between SP MS and RR MS patients.[50] On the other hand, when considering disease activity in terms of enhancing lesions on gadolinium-enhanced MRI scans, although the frequency of enhancement differed significantly among the different clinical forms of MS and was a good predictor of both short-term and long-term clinical activity,[51] in patients with both SP MS and RR MS the average number of enhancing lesions detectable on monthly scans was similar (i.e. 20 lesions) and it was significantly higher than in patients with benign MS (i.e. 9 lesions).[52] However, in a recent study,[53] it was found that patients with SP MS and severe disability had a lower number of enhancing lesions per month than patients with mild RR MS, while the yearly change of lesion burden on T2-weighted brain MRI was similar in the two groups. These data suggest that the rate of enhancement decreases in the more advanced phases of MS. This may indicate that the failure of the reparative mechanisms within chronic lesions is important in determining clinical disability. This is in keeping with studies with newer, nonconventional MRI techniques providing measures with a higher pathological specificity than T2-weighted scans. The burden of hypointense lesions on unenhanced T1-weighted scans,[50,54] that represent areas of severe demyelination and/or axonal loss, is higher in patients with severe disability, and its increase is significantly correlated with clinical worsening in MS patients. Several studies showed strong correlations between clinical disability and degree of spinal cord,[55,56] cerebellar[57] and brain[58] atrophy, which implicates axonal loss. This relationship has also been confirmed in longitudinal studies;[58,59] in details, Filippi et al.[59] found that the cervical spinal cord cross-sectional area did not change on follow-up scans in patients with benign MS, while it was significantly reduced in patients with SP MS. Using the histogram analysis of magnetization transfer (MT)-weighted images, a technique which provides information about the normal-appearing white matter (NAWM), we also found (unpublished data) that both macroscopic and microscopic brain damage are more severe in patients with SP MS, and MT measures correlate with clinical disability better than conventional MRI parameters. From all these data it is clear that nonconventional MR markers of brain tissue disruption may help us in differentiating MS clinical courses and in monitoring disease evolution; however, the lack of prospective studies in RR MS patients at the onset of their transition into a progressive phase of the disease does not yet provide us with a MR measure that could be used as a reliable predictor of this transition.

NEUROPHYSIOLOGICAL MARKERS

The frequency and severity of multimodal evoked potentials abnormalities is lower in patients with a first episode suggestive of MS, increases in patients with RR MS and is extremely high in patients with SP MS.[49,60–62] Filippi et al.[49] compared a group of patients with benign MS with a group of patients with SP MS; the two groups were matched for age and duration of disease, but had a clear difference in the level of disability (mean EDSS of 1.9 and 6.1, respectively). For all evoked potential modalities the frequency of abnormalities was significantly higher in SP MS compared to benign MS; moreover the response in at least one EP modality was absent in 92% of SP MS versus 8% of benign MS. In patients with SP MS there is a good correlation between global disability and degree of evoked potential abnormalities.[63] Longitudinal studies have demonstrated a significant correlation between clinical and evoked potential changes.[64–68] These observations indicate that conduction abnormalities along afferent and efferent pathways, revealed by evoked potentials, are constantly present in disabled patients, but they can also be observed in patients with no or minimal disability, owing to the high sensitivity of these neurophysiological techniques in detecting subclinical damage.[60] These findings result in a low discrimination value between RR and SP MS. The use of conventional scores to quantify the neurophysiological changes could increase the ability of evoked potentials to reveal MS patients at high risk for entering the SP course. Further studies are needed to clarify this possibility; at present evoked potentials are not useful from this point of view.

CONCLUSIONS

About 85% of MS patients start with a relapsing–remitting course and about 90% of them enter into the progressive phase of the disease during their life. The SP course is almost always associated with a relevant disability. There are clear implications for the patient who enters a progressive phase of the disease: the prognosis worsens and there is an impact on his or her working activity, personal life and general expectations. The mechanisms underlying the transition from RR to SP course are still obscure, but there is growing evidence that the two phases of the disease might be characterized by different pathological and immunological findings which partially overlap during the transition phase. Thus, treatments which are active during the RR course may be ineffective during the SP course and vice versa. Moreover, there are changes in the risk–benefit ratio for treatments: the increased risk of severe disability and death can make feasible a treatment that is not indicated in the RR phase because of the high risk of severe adverse events. Early markers of the transition from RR to SP type are therefore important. Unfortunately, no single immunological, neuroradiological or neurophysiological marker turned out to be satisfactory. This is mainly because we do not really know what is the trigger event leading to the progression phase of the disease and because the transition into the progressive phase of the disease is—in the majority of cases—a retrospective finding, which usually does not allow an evaluation of the usefulness of the putative markers. The follow-up of patients in the placebo group of some recent large clinical trials could give useful information about clinical, immunological and MRI changes related to the conversion from RR to SP courses. An interesting indication could also arise from some new MR techniques, characterized by a better pathological specificity than traditional MRI measures, but a key role will be probably played by further immunological and pathological studies.

REFERENCES

1. Müller R. Studies on disseminated sclerosis. With special reference to symptomatology, course and prognosis. *Acta Med Scand* 1949; **133 Suppl**: 222.
2. Kurtzke JK, Beebe GW, Nagler B et al. Studies on the natural history of multiple sclerosis. VIII. Early prognostic features of the later course of the illness. *J Chronic Dis* 1977; **30**: 819–830.
3. Confavreux C, Aimard G, Devic M. Course and prognosis of multiple sclerosis assessed by the computerized data processing of 349 patients. *Brain* 1980; **103**: 281–300.
4. Weinshenker BG, Bass B, Rice GPA et al. The natural history of multiple sclerosis: a geographically based study. 2. Predictive value of the early clinical course. *Brain* 1989; **112**: 1419–1428.
5. Lublin FD, Reingold SC. The National Multiple Sclerosis Society (USA; Advisory Committee on Clinical Trials of New Agents in Multiple Sclerosis). Defining the clinical course of multiple sclerosis: results of an international survey. *Neurology* 1996; **46**: 907–911.
6. Kurtzke JF. Rating neurologic impairment in multiple sclerosis: an expanded disability status scale (EDSS). *Neurology* 1983; **33**: 1444–1452.
7. Weinshenker BG. Natural history of multiple sclerosis. *Ann Neurol* 1994; **36**: S6–S11.
8. Runmarker B, Andersen O. Prognostic factors in a multiple sclerosis incidence cohort with twenty-five years of follow-up. *Brain* 1993; **116**: 117–134.
9. Weinshenker BG, Issa M, Baskerville J. Long-term and short-term outcome of multiple sclerosis. *Arch Neurol* 1996; **53**: 353–358.
10. Lassmann H. Comparative neuropathology of chronic experimental allergic encephalomyelitis and multiple sclerosis. *Schriftenr Neurol* 1983; **25**: 1–135.
11. Prineas JW. The neuropathology of multiple sclerosis. In: Koetsier JA, ed. *Handbook of Clinical Neurology*. Amsterdam: Elsevier Science 1985; 213–258.
12. Prineas JW, Barnard RO, Revesz T et al. Multiple sclerosis. Pathology of recurrent lesions. *Brain* 1993; **116**: 681–693.
13. Prineas JW, Barnard RO, Kwon EE et al. Multiple sclerosis: remyelination of nascent lesions. *Ann Neurol* 1993; **33**: 137–151.
14. Raine CS, Wu E. Multiple sclerosis: remyelination in acute lesions. *J Neuropath Exp Neurol* 1993; **52**: 199–204.
15. Rodriguez M. Central nervous system demyelination and remyelination in multiple sclerosis and viral models of disease. *J Neuroimmunol* 1992; **40**: 255–263.
16. Brück W, Schmied M, Suchanek G et al. Oligodendrocytes in the early course of multiple sclerosis. *Ann Neurol* 1994; **35**: 65–73.
17. Ozawa K, Suchanek G, Breitschopf H et al. Patterns of oligodendroglia pathology in multiple sclerosis. *Brain* 1994; **117**: 1311–1322.
18. Targett MP, Sussman J, Scolding N et al. Failure to achieve remyelination of demyelinative rat axons following transplantation of glial cells obtained from the adult human brain. *Neuropath Appl Neurobiol* 1996; **22**: 199–206.
19. Ludwin SK. Central nervous system demyelination and remyelination in the mouse: an ultrastructural study of cuprizone toxicity. *Lab Invest* 1978; **39**: 597–612.
20. Linington C, Engelhardt B, Kapocs G et al. Induction of persistently demyelinated lesions in the rat following the repeated adoptive transfer of encephalitogenic T-cells and demyelinating antibodies. *J Neuroimmunol* 1992; **40**: 219–224.
21. Winsnieski HM, Bloom BR. Primary demyelination as a nonspecific consequence of a cell mediate immune reaction. *J Exp Med* 1975; **141**: 346–359.
22. Sato S, Quarles RH, Brady RO. Susceptibility of the myelin-associated glycoprotein and basic protein is a neutral protease in highly purified myelin from human and rat brain. *J Neurochem* 1982; **89**: 97–105.
23. Dal Canto MC, Lipton HL. Recurrent demyelination in chronic central nervous system infection produced by Theiler's murine encephalomyelitis virus. *J Neurol Sci* 1979; **42**: 391–405.
24. Koopmann RA, Li DKB, Grochowski E et al. Benign versus chronic progressive multiple sclerosis: magnetic resonance imaging features. *Ann Neurol* 1989; **25**: 74–81.

25. Thompson AJ, Kermode AG, Loicks D. Major differences in the dynamics of primary and secondary progressive multiple sclerosis. *Ann Neurol* 1991; **29**: 53–62.
26. Campi A, Filippi M, Comi G et al. Magnetisation transfer ratios of contrast-enhancing and nonenhancing lesions in multiple sclerosis. *Neuroradiology* 1996; **38**: 115–119.
27. Lucchinetti CF, Bruck W, Rodriguez M et al. Distinct pattern of multiple sclerosis pathology indicates heterogeneity on pathogenesis. *Brain Pathol* 1996; **6**: 259–274.
28. Miller DJ, Asakura K, Rodriguez M. Central nervous system remyelination: clinical application of basic neuroscience principles. *Brain Pathol* 1996; **6**: 331–344.
29. Martin R, McFarland HF, McFarlin DE. Immunological aspects of demyelinating disease. *Annu Rev Immunol* 1992; **10**: 153–187.
30. Steinman L. A few autoreactive cells in an autoimmune infiltrate control a vast population of nonspecific cells: a tale of smart bombs and the infantry. *Proc Natl Acad Sci USA* 1996; **93**: 2253–2256.
31. Mosmann TR, Cherwinski H, Bond MW et al. Two types of murine helper T cell clone. I. Definition according to profiles of lymphokine activities and secreted proteins. *J Immunol* 1986; **136**: 2348–2357.
32. Erard F, Wild M-T, Garcia-Sanz JA et al. Switch of CD8 T cells to noncytolytic CD8-CD4– cells that make TH2 cytokines and helper B cells. *Science* 1993; **260**: 1802–1805.
33. Baron JL, Madri JA, Ruddle NH et al. Surface expression of alpha 4 integrin by CD4 T cells is required for their entry into brain parenchyma. *J Exp Med* 1993; **177**: 57–68.
34. Nakajima H, Takamori H, Hiyama Y et al. The effect of treatment with interferon-gamma on type II collagen-induced arthritis. *Clin Exp Immunol* 1990; **81**: 441–445.
35. Martino G, Grohovaz F, Brambilla E et al. Cytokine regulation of antigen-independent T cell activation by two separate calcium signaling pathways in multiple sclerosis. *Ann Neurol* 1998 (in press).
36. Panitch HS, Hirsch RL, Haley AS et al. Exacerbation of multiple sclerosis in patients treated with gamma interferon. *Lancet* 1987; **i**: 893–895.
37. Panitch HS, Hirsch RL, Schindler A et al. Treatment of multiple sclerosis with gamma interferon: exacerbations associated with activation of the immune system. *Neurology* 1987; **37**: 1097–1102.
38. Selmaj KW, Raine CS, Cannella B et al. Identification of lymphotoxin and tumor necrosis factor in multiple sclerosis lesions. *J Clin Inv* 1991; **87**: 949–954.
39. Martino G, Grimaldi LME. The pathogenetic role for interferon-γ in multiple sclerosis. In: Reder A, ed. *Interferon Therapy of Multiple Sclerosis*. New York: Marcel Dekker, 1996; 193–214.
40. Beck J, Rondot P, Catinot L et al. Increased production of interferon gamma and tumor necrosis factor precedes clinical manifestation in multiple sclerosis: do cytokines trigger off exacerbations? *Acta Neurol Scand* 1988; **78**: 318–323.
41. Sharief MK, Hentges R. Association between tumor necrosis factor-alpha and disease progression in patients with multiple sclerosis. *New Engl J Med* 1991; **325**: 467–472. [Comment in: *New Engl J Med* 1992; **326**: 272–273.]
42. Noseworthy JH, Rodriguez M, Nia-Siang J et al. TNF-alpha in multiple sclerosis. *Neurology* 1993; **43**: A355.
43. Nicoletti F, Patti F, DiMarco R et al. Circulating serum levels of IL-1ra in patients with relapsing remitting multiple sclerosis are normal during remission phases but significantly increased either during exacerbations or in response to IFN-beta treatment. *Cytokine* 1996; **8**: 395–400.
44. Balashov KE, Smith DR, Khoury SJ et al. Increased interleukin 12 production in progressive multiple sclerosis: induction by activated CD4+ T cells via CD40 ligand. *Proc Natl Acad Sci USA* 1997; **94**: 599–603.
45. Whitaker JN, Williams PH, Layton BA et al. Correlation of clinical features and findings on cranial magnetic resonance imaging with urinary myelin basic protein-like material in patients with multiple sclerosis. *Ann Neurol* 1994; **35**: 577–585.
46. Whitaker JN, Kachelhofer RD, Bradley EL et al. Urinary myelin basic protein-like material as a correlate of the progression of multiple sclerosis. *Ann Neurol* 1995; **38**: 625–632.
47. Filippi M, Miller DH. MRI in the differential diagnosis and monitoring the treatment of multiple sclerosis. *Curr Opin Neurol* 1996; **9**: 176–186.
48. Filippi M, Horsfield MA, Morrissey et al. Quantitative brain MRI lesion load predicts the course of clinically isolated syndromes suggestive of multiple sclerosis. *Neurology* 1994; **44**: 635–641.

49. Filippi M, Campi A, Mammi S et al. Brain magnetic resonance imaging and multimodal evoked potentials in benign and secondary progressive multiple sclerosis. *J Neurol Neurosurg Psychiatry* 1995; **58**: 31–37.
50. Van Walderveen MAA, Barkhof F, Hommes OR et al. Correlating MRI and clinical disease activity in multiple sclerosis: relevance of hypointense lesions on short TR/short TE (T_1-weighted) spin-echo images. *Neurology* 1995; **45**: 1684–1690.
51. Smith ME, Stone LA, Albert PS et al. Clinical worsening in multiple sclerosis is associated with increased frequency and area of gadopentetate dimeglumine-enhancing magnetic resonance imaging lesions. *Ann Neurol* 1993; **33**: 480–489.
52. Miller DH. Magnetic resonance in monitoring the treatment of multiple sclerosis. *Ann Neurol* 1994; **36**: S91–S94.
53. Filippi M, Rossi P, Campi A et al. Serial contrast-enhanced MR in patients with multiple sclerosis and varying levels of disability. *AJNR* 1997; **18**: 1549–1556.
54. Truyen L, van Waesberghe JHTM, van Walderveen MAA et al. Accumulation of hypointense lesions ("black holes") on T1 spin-echo MRI correlates with disease progression in multiple sclerosis. *Neurology* 1997; **47**: 1469–1476.
55. Filippi M, Campi A, Colombo B et al. A spinal cord MRI study of benign and secondary progressive multiple sclerosis. *J Neurol* 1996; **243**: 502–506.
56. Losseff NA, Webb SL, O'Riordan JI et al. Spinal cord atrophy and disability in multiple sclerosis. A new reproducible and sensitive MRI method with potential to monitor disease progression. *Brain* 1996; **119**: 701–708.
57. Davie CA, Barker GJ, Webb S et al. Persistent functional deficit in multiple sclerosis and autosomal dominant cerebellar ataxia is associated with axonal loss. *Brain* 1995; **118**: 1583–1592.
58. Losseff NA, Wang L, Lai HM et al. Progressive cerebral atrophy in multiple sclerosis. A serial MRI study. *Brain* 1996; **119**: 2009–2019.
59. Filippi M, Colombo B, Rovaris M et al. A longitudinal magnetic resonance imaging study of the cervical cord in multiple sclerosis. *J Neuroimaging* 1997; **7**: 78–80.
60. Comi G, Martinelli V, Medaglini S et al. Correlation between multimodal evoked potentials and magnetic resonance imaging in multiple sclerosis. *J Neurol* 1989; **236**: 4–8.
61. Filippini G, Comi G, Cosi V et al. Sensitivities and predictive values of paraclinical tests for diagnosing multiple sclerosis. *J Neurol* 1994; **24**: 132–137.
62. Lee KH, Hashimoto SA, Hooge JP et al. Magnetic resonance imaging of the head in the diagnosis of multiple sclerosis: a prospective two years follow up with comparison of clinical evaluation, evoked potentials, oligoclonal banding, and CT. *Neurology* 1991; **41**: 657–660.
63. Martinelli V, Comi G. Il valore prognostico dei potenziali evocati nella sclerosi multipla. In: Comi G, ed. *I Potenziali Evocati Nella Sclerosi Multipla*. Italy: Springer-Verlag, 1995; 105–116.
64. De Weerd AW, Jonkman EJ. Changes in visual and short latency somatosensory evoked potentials in patients with multiple sclerosis. In: Courjon J, Mauguiére F, Revol N, eds. *Clinical Applications of Evoked Potentials in Neurology*. New York: Raven Press, 1982; 527–534.
65. Walsh JC, Garrick R, Cameron J et al. Evoked potentials changes in clinically definite multiple sclerosis: a two year follow up study. *J Neurol Neurosurg Psychiat* 1982; **454**: 494–500.
66. Ghezzi A, Zaffaroni M, Caputo D et al. Evaluation of evoked potentials and lymphocyte subsets as possible markers of multiple sclerosis: one year follow-up of 30 patients. *J Neurol Neurosurg Psychiatry* 1986; **49**: 913–919.
67. Nuwer MR, Packwood JW, Myers LW et al. Evoked potentials predict the clinical changes in a multiple sclerosis drug study. *Neurology* 1987; **37**: 1754–1761.
68. Andersen T, Siden A. Multimodality evoked potentials and neurological phenomenology in patients with multiple sclerosis and potentially related conditions. *Electromyogr Clin Neurophysiol* 1991; **31**: 109–117.

5

Differences between primary and secondary progressive multiple sclerosis

Alan J Thompson

INTRODUCTION

At first glance there are obvious differences between primary and secondary progressive multiple sclerosis (MS). The rarer primary progressive group is characterized by slow deterioration over time without any relapses or remissions while the secondary progressive group begins with relapses and remissions followed by slow irreversible deterioration that may or may not be associated with relapses. However, the real issue is how fundamental these apparent differences are.[1–3] In other words, are primary and secondary progressive MS different diseases or simply different aspects of a clinicopathological spectrum and, secondly, are the underlying mechanisms of deterioration different in the two groups? The latter is perhaps the more important question as it requires a thorough understanding of the pathological processes responsible for irreversible deterioration.

It is perhaps useful at the onset to attempt to define some of the key terms which are often used interchangeably causing unnecessary confusion. MS may result in neurological change (impairment) which may in turn affect function or the ability to carry out tasks (i.e. cause disability). Irreversible deterioration, which may mean irreversible changes in impairment alone or impairment and disability depending on how severe it is, can result from two mechanisms: incomplete recovery from relapse (incomplete remission) or slow progression (Fig. 5.1).

It has been suggested that while relapses are invariably associated with inflammatory demyelination, progression may result from axonal loss, though of course these two processes are very closely related. In this chapter the term progression will be restricted to irreversible deterioration which is independent of relapse activity.

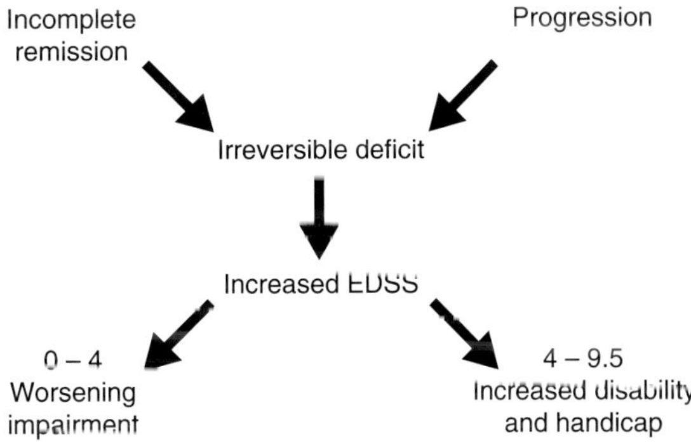

Figure 5.1 Relationship between mechanisms of irreversible recovery, change in EDSS and impairment, disability and handicap.

CONFOUNDING FACTORS

When comparing primary and secondary progressive MS there are a number of confounding factors which need to be taken into account:

(a) the variety of poorly defined terms which have been used in the past for patients with progressive MS make comparisons difficult
(b) difficulty with defining and diagnosing primary progressive MS
(c) difficulty with identifying the onset of the progressive phase in secondary progressive MS
(d) difficulty matching patients with primary and secondary progressive MS for age, disease duration and disability.

The most frequently used term in the past has been 'chronic progressive multiple sclerosis' but this has meant different things in different studies. The terms 'relapsing progressive' and 'progressive relapsing' have also been used.[4,5] In an attempt to clarify the situation Lublin and Reingold[6] carried out a consensus study which arrived at four definitions: relapsing–remitting MS; secondary progressive MS; primary progressive MS; and progressive relapsing MS, which relates to those patients whose disease has progressed from onset but who have clear acute relapses without full recovery. These consensus definitions are of some help but are not universally used and are thought by some to be an oversimplification. There is no doubt that within the secondary progressive group there are patients who, after a period of relapses and remissions, develop slowly progressive deterioration without any further relapses while others continue to have relapses, and there is also a group whose progression appears to begin from an incomplete recovery from relapse. On the other hand, in the primary progressive category there are patients who have a single relapse many years (often 10–20) before the onset of the progressive phase and others who have a single relapse or remission during their progression. This group has been labelled transitional progressive MS.[7–9] Finally there is a small group of patients whose frequent relapses give the appearance of rapidly progressive disease and who may be erroneously described as having primary progressive MS. In a recent study of interobserver variation in classifying MS the area of greatest difficulty related to distinguishing between primary and secondary progressive MS.[10]

Diagnosing primary progressive MS also poses problems, both in relation to distinguishing it from other progressive neurological syndromes and in excluding patients who have had any relapse activity in the past.[11] This may help explain the differences between the percentages of primary progressive patient seen in various studies, which range from 7% to 18%. This frequency may also be affected by the way in which data is collected. In the Weinshenker study an initial percentage of 18% was quoted when the data was analysed retrospectively, while in the prospective study it fell to 7.7%.[12] This difficulty is well illustrated in the recruitment to a recent study of interferon (IFN) beta-1a in primary progressive MS.[13] Of the 117 patients referred with a definite diagnosis of primary progressive MS only 38 were entered into the study. Of the remaining 79, 50% did not have primary progressive MS and 10% did not have MS at all. One of the major difficulties relates to the Poser criteria, which require evidence of involvement of two or more areas of the central nervous system at separate times. This is difficult to demonstrate in primary progressive MS.[3]

The third factor relates to the difficulty in identifying when a patient has moved from the relapsing–remitting phase of the disease into the secondary progressive phase (a difficulty which has been highlighted by the recent prescribing conditions for IFN-β). Again there are marked differences between studies as to when this is likely to happen,[12,14,15] perhaps confounded because—according to one study—up to 40% of patients may move from one disease category to another during their lifetime.[16]

Finally, as will be discussed later, patients with primary progressive MS usually have a later age of onset and deteriorate quite rapidly, while those with secondary progressive disease present earlier but have a variable period of relapses and remissions before they develop slow progression. Thus, while it may be possible to match the two groups for age and disability, the secondary progressive group will tend to have a longer disease duration from initial presentation making direct comparisons difficult.

CLINICAL DIFFERENCES BETWEEN PRIMARY AND SECONDARY PROGRESSIVE MS

Primary progressive MS has been reviewed recently in two papers[1,3] (Table 5.1). Of the differences shown, of interest is the loss of the female predominance in the primary progressive group, which is found in most studies including the recent MAGNIMS study, which includes 158 patients with primary progressive MS, 51% of which are male.[8] Some of the other differences are less clear cut. Although it is well established that the age of onset of primary progressive MS is later than that of relapsing–remitting MS, it is very similar to the onset of the secondary progressive phase, which has prompted Minderhoud et al. to suggest that the diseases are the same apart from the relapsing–remitting period in the secondary progressive group.[17] Almost all patients with primary progressive MS present with a progressive cord syndrome, usually a paraparesis but occasionally a hemiparesis, while in the secondary progressive patient onset is more likely to be related to optic neuritis or sensory disturbance. However, the progression in this group tends to relate to progressive deterioration in mobility, most of which relates to spinal cord disease. In a similar vein, it is reported that primary progressive disease has a worse prognosis for developing disability than patients with relapsing–remitting MS. However, this is again accounted for since the secondary progressive patients have an initial relapsing–remitting period of some 5–15 years and, if one compares primary and secondary progressive MS, the rate of deterioration as measured by reaching an expanded disability status scale (EDSS) of 6 and 9 is identical.[14]

Another potential clinical distinction which has been made between primary and secondary progressive MS is the relative lack of cognitive dysfunction in patients with the former. In 1995 Comi and colleagues compared 17 patients with secondary progressive MS and 14 with primary progressive disease.[18] The groups were of similar age and disability but the secondary progressive group had a longer disease duration. They found that while nine of the secondary progressive patients were cognitively impaired (above two standard deviations in three of more of the 12 tests carried out) only one of the primary progressive patients was impaired. This does not mean to say that patients with primary progressive MS do not have cognitive impairment, and a recent study

Table 5.1 Progressive MS

	Primary	Secondary
Sex distribution	Equal	Female preponderance
Age at onset (yrs)	35–40	35–40*
Clinical pattern	Predominately paraparesis	Presentation variable subsequently paraparesis common

*Of progressive phase

by Camp et al.[19] has looked at 62 patients with either primary progressive MS (43 patients) or progressive transitional MS (19 patients) using the short repeatable battery[20] with a verbal spatial reasoning test (VESPAR)[21] and the Montgomery and Asberg depression rating scale (MADRS)[22] in both the patient group and controls matched for age, sex and estimated pre-morbid IQ.[19] They demonstrated widespread cognitive dysfunction in the patient group which was significant on tests of verbal memory, attention, verbal fluency and spatial reasoning.[19]

GENETICS AND IMMUNOLOGY

Differences between primary and secondary progressive MS in relation to immunological abnormalities and genetic profile have been reviewed elsewhere.[3] There is little conclusive evidence in either area. The initial suggestion that DQP1 was more commonly seen in primary progressive MS[23] has not been confirmed.[24] Intrafamilial comparisons of the clinical course have been reported recently in sibling pairs with MS.[25] The authors obtained an overall significant κ value of 0.150 [$P = > 0.02$] for both primary progressive disease and relapsing–remitting disease indicating significant intrafamilial concordance for disease course. However, by inference there were a significant number of families (38 of 166) in which one sibling had relapsing–remitting MS while the other had primary progressive disease.

Immunological abnormalities are even less clear. Although some markers of progression have been identified none have been confirmed and few have compared primary and secondary progressive MS. One report, which needs to be confirmed, suggests that increased serum levels of soluble E-selectin and endothelial adhesion molecule are seen only in patients with primary progressive MS.[26]

PATHOLOGY

A comparison of a small number of cases of primary and secondary progressive MS was reported in 1994 which focused exclusively on the pattern and extent of inflammation.[27] This was a retrospective study of four cases of primary and five cases of secondary progressive MS. A total of 578 lesions was analysed and inflammation, as judged by perivascular cuffing and increased cellularity of the parenchyma, was seen in both groups but was significantly more marked in patients with secondary progressive disease. More recently, exciting and somewhat provocative work has been published based on extensive biopsy and some autopsy material gathered in a collaboration between Vienna and the Mayo Clinic.[28] The authors have studied a total of 72 biopsies from MS patients and have attempted to carry out both a structural and a histochemical classification, particularly relating to the fate of the oligodendrocyte and axon. They have suggested it might be possible to distinguish clinical groups on the basis of this and, furthermore, they have suggested that in primary progressive MS oligodendrocyte destruction may occur both within the plaque and also in a narrow rim of normal-appearing white matter (NAWM) around it; at the latter site there was no demyelination. However, the number of observations on which this is based is very small and the three cases were somewhat atypical in that they had a rapidly progressing course, the patients dying within 2 years of onset (Lucchinetti and Bruck, personal communication). None the less there is considerable potential to study possible pathological differences between primary and secondary progressive MS within this unique tissue collection.

MAGNETIC RESONANCE IMAGING (MRI)

Much of the current discussion on primary and secondary progressive MS has stemmed from MRI studies carried out almost 10 years ago.[29,30] These showed consistent differences between the two groups in that patients with primary progressive MS have fewer lesions on brain MRI, and those lesions which were present tended to be small. Perhaps more importantly these lesions rarely, if ever, enhanced with

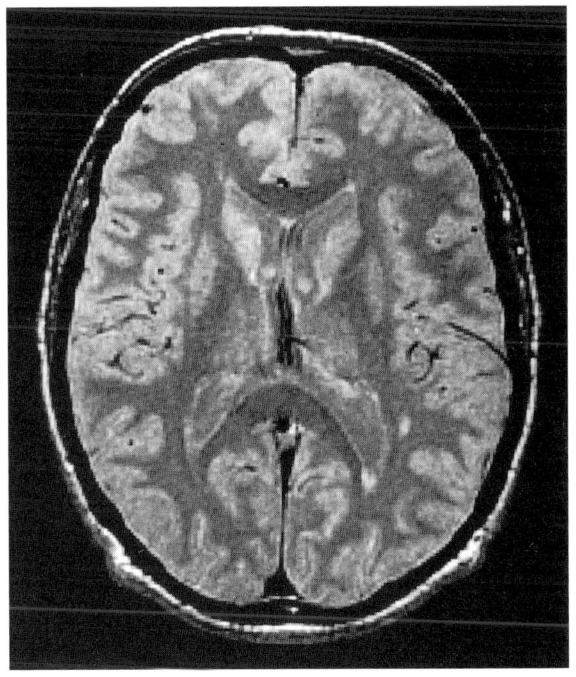

(a)

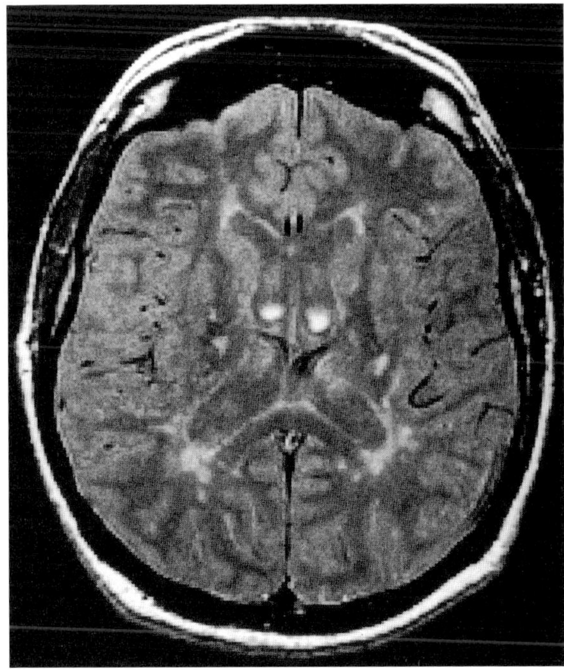

(b)

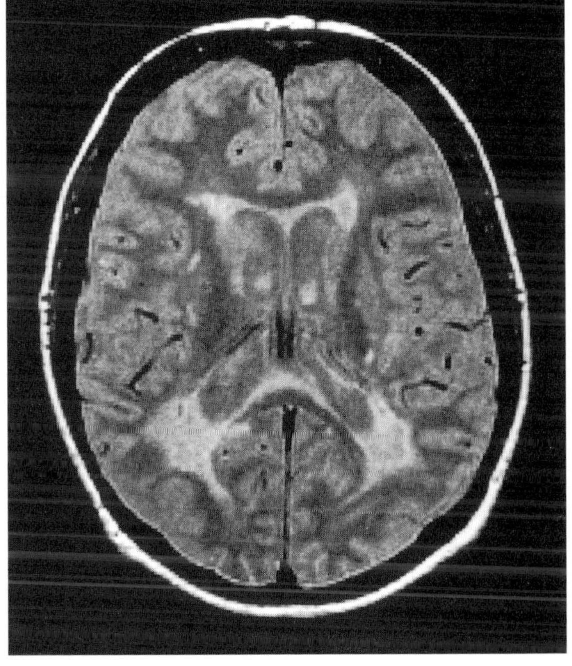

(c)

Figure 5.2 T2-weighted MRI scans of patients with primary progressive MS (a and b) and secondary progressive MS (c). (a) presented with a spastic paraparesis while (b) presented with cerebellar syndrome. The scans demonstrate a small lesion load in (a), increasing in (b), but much greater in (c).

gadolinium, lending further evidence to the suggestion that this is a less inflammatory form of MS. Recent studies have shown that if triple-dose gadolinium is given then a somewhat higher proportion of lesions enhance and slightly more new lesions are detected on cross-sectional and serial evaluation in primary progressive MS,[31,32] though this is not a universal finding.[33] The recent MAGNIMS study[8] has also found that within the primary progressive group there is a difference between those with a progressive cord syndrome when compared to those with progressive ataxia, visual loss, etc. in that the latter group tend to have more lesions on MRI of the brain (Fig. 5.2).

One of the striking features of the primary progressive group, therefore, is the discrepancy between the paucity of MR abnormality of the brain and their disability. This discrepancy has not been explained with improved imaging of the cord; no difference in the number and extent of lesions in the cord between the primary and secondary progressive group was seen either on cross-sectional[34] or serial evaluation.[35] A more promising approach has been the evaluation of spinal cord atrophy,[34] particularly at the C2 level,[36] which is highly reproducible,[37] and has demonstrated a strong correlation with disability, most marked in the primary progressive group. Furthermore, a recent study has demonstrated that the primary progressive patients show a greater change over time in cord atrophy than is seen in the secondary progressive patients.[38] These findings suggest that axonal loss makes a greater contribution to the development of disability in the primary progressive group.

Another important area that warrants further investigation of the underlying mechanisms of disease progression is the so-called NAWM, previously shown to be far from normal.[39] This has been investigated with MR spectroscopy, and it has been demonstrated that the N-acetyl aspartate (NAA) concentration (a marker of axonal function) in NAWM in primary progressive MS is lower than that seen in the benign group, though a direct comparison between primary and secondary progressive MS has not yet been carried out.[40] Other MR techniques which may be useful in looking for pathological differences between these groups include magnetization transfer ratio, transverse magnetization decay curve analysis and T1 analysis.

CONCLUSIONS

Reviewing our current state of knowledge of primary and secondary progressive MS, it is reasonable to conclude that although there are several differences between the two groups they tend to be either inconclusive or relative rather than absolute and to suggest that we are looking at a spectrum of disease activity rather than at clinically independent disease entities.

What about the mechanisms underlying deterioration in the two groups? Looking at this from a purely clinical perspective it is obvious that patients with secondary progressive MS may deteriorate either as a result of incomplete remission (for those who are continuing to have superimposed relapses) and progression, while in the primary progressive group it is progression alone. The pathological mechanisms underlying this deterioration, particularly possible differences between the two groups, remains unclear. It may be useful to address each of the three main areas of disease activity—inflammation, demyelination and axonal loss—when considering this question.

Inflammation is clearly important in secondary progressive MS and would appear to precede, at least on MRI, other aspects of disease activity. The role of inflammation is less clear in primary progressive MS; it appears to be less relevant and rather than preceding demyelination it may occur as a consequence of it. This is the logical conclusion from the biopsy data, but it needs to be clearly demonstrated, possibly through further MRI studies.

The second issue is whether or not demyelination may occur in the absence of inflammation—a phenomenon, which if it occurs, is more likely to be seen in the primary progressive group. The role of axonal loss is obviously crucial as it inevitably leads to irreversible deficit once a critical level had been reached. Could this occur in the absence of inflammation or even demyelination in primary progressive disease while in the secondary progressive it is seen only in areas of severe inflammatory demyelination? These questions need to be answered in future studies. The rapid advances in more pathologically specific MR techniques and the increased availability of pathological tissue will probably resolve these important issues, which are fundamental to our understanding of MS and its treatment, within the next decade.

REFERENCES

1. McDonnell GV, Hawkins SA. Primary progressive multiple sclerosis: a distinct syndrome? *Multiple Sclerosis* 1996; **2**: 141.
2. McDonald WI, Thompson AJ. How many kinds of multiple sclerosis are there? In: Thompson AJ, Polman CH, Hohlfeld R, eds. *Multiple Sclerosis: Clinical Challenges and Controversies*. London: Martin Dunitz, 1997; 35–42.
3. Thompson AJ, Polman CH, Miller DH et al. Primary progressive multiple sclerosis. *Brain* 1997; **120**: 1085–1096.
4. McAlpine D. Course and prognosis. In: McAlpine D, Lumsden CE, Acheson ED, eds. *Multiple Sclerosis. A reappraisal*. Edinburgh and London: E & S Livingstone, 1965; 179–196.
5. McAlpine D. Course and prognosis. In: McAlpine D, Compston ND, Lumsden CE, eds. *Multiple Sclerosis*. Edinburgh and London: E & S Livingstone: 1955; 135–155.
6. Lublin FD, Reingold SC. Defining the clinical course of multiple sclerosis: Results of an international survey. *Neurology* 1996; **46**: 907–111.
7. Filippi M, Campi A, Martinelli V et al. Transitional progressive multiple sclerosis: MRI and MTI findings. *Acta Neurol Scand* 1995; **92**: 178–182.
8. Stevenson VL, Thompson AJ, Miller DH et al. Primary progressive and transitional multiple sclerosis: a cross-sectional clinical and MRI study. *J Neurol* 1997; **244**: S77 [abstract].
9. Gayou A, Brochet B, Dousset V. Transitional progressive multiple sclerosis: a clinical and imaging study. *J Neurol Neurosurg Psychiatry* 1997; **63**: 396–398.
10. Ford HL, Johnson MH, Rigby AS. Variation between observers in classifying multiple sclerosis. *J Neurol Neurosurg Psychiatry* 1996; **62**: 418.
11. McDonnell GV, Hawkins SA. Practical problems in the classification of primary progressive multiple sclerosis (PPMS). *J Neurol* 1997; **244**: S63 [abstract].
12. Weinshenker BG, Bass B, Rice GP et al. The natural history of multiple sclerosis: a geographically based study. 2. Predictive value of the early clinical course. *Brain* 1989; **112**: 1419–1428.
13. Leary SM, Miller DH, Thompson AJ. Design of a study of interferon beta-1a in primary progressive multiple sclerosis. *J Neurol* 1997; **244**: S63 [abstract]
14. Runmarker B, Andersen O. Prognostic factors in a multiple sclerosis incidence cohort with twenty-five years of follow-up. *Brain* 1993; **116**: 117–134.
15. Confavreux C, Aimard G, Devic M. Course and prognosis of multiple sclerosis assessed by the computerized data processing of 349 patients. *Brain* 1980; **103**: 281–300.
16. Goodkin DE, Hertsgaard D, Rudick RA. Exacerbation rates and adherence to disease type in a prospectively followed-up population with multiple sclerosis. Implications for clinical trials. *Arch Neurol* 1989; **46**: 1107–1112.
17. Minderhoud JM, van der Hoeven JH, Prange AJ. Course and prognosis of chronic progressive multiple sclerosis. Results of an epidemiological study. *Acta Neurol Scand* 1988; **78**: 10–15.
18. Comi, G, Filippi M, Martinelli V et al. Brain MRI correlates of cognitive impairment in primary and secondary progressive multiple sclerosis. *J Neuro Sci* 1995; **132**: 222–227.
19. Camp SJ, Langdon DW, Stevenson VL et al. Cognitive function in primary progressive MS: a controlled study with MR correlates. *Multiple Sclerosis* 1997; **3**: 302 [abstract].
20. Rao SM. *Neurobehavioural Aspects of Multiple Sclerosis*. New York: Oxford University Press, 1990.
21. Langdon DW, Warrington EK. *VESPAR: A Verbal and Spatial Reasoning Test*. Hove: Lawrence Erlbaum, 1995.
22. Montgomery SA, Asberg M. A new depression scale designed to be sensitive to change. *Br J Psychiatry* 1979; **134**: 382–389.
23. Olerup O, Hillert J, Fredrikson S et al. Primarily chronic progressive and relapsing/remitting multiple sclerosis: two immunogenetically distinct disease entities. *Proct Natl Acad Sci USA* 1989; **86**: 7113–7117.
24. Hillert J, Gronning M, Nyland H et al. An immunogenetic heterogeneity in multiple sclerosis. *J Neurol Neurosurg Psychiatry* 1992; **55**: 887–890.
25. Robertson NP, Clayton D, Fraser M et al. Clinical concordance in sibling pairs with multiple sclerosis. *Neurology* 1996; **47**: 347–352.
26. Giovannoni G, Thorpe JW, Kidd D et al. Soluble E-selectin in multiple sclerosis: raised concentrations in patients with primary progressive disease. *J Neurol Neurosurg Psychiatry* 1996; **60**: 20–26.
27. Revesz T, Kidd D, Thompson AJ et al. A comparison of the pathology of primary and secondary progressive multiple sclerosis. *Brain* 1994; **117**: 759–765.

28. Lucchinetti CF, Bruck W, Rodriguez M et al. Distinct patterns of multiple sclerosis pathology indicates heterogeneity of pathogenesis. *Brain Pathol* 1996; **6**: 259–274.
29. Thompson AJ, Kermode AG, MacManus DG et al. Pathogenesis of progressive multiple sclerosis. *Lancet* 1989; **i**: 1322–1323.
30. Thompson AJ, Kermode AG, Wicks D et al. Major differences in the dynamics of primary and secondary progressive multiple sclerosis. *Ann Neurol* 1991; **29**: 53–62.
31. Filippi M, Yousry T, Campi A et al. Comparison of triple dose versus standard dose gadolinium-DTPA for detection of MRI enhancing lesions in patients with MS. *Neurology* 1996; **46**: 379–384.
32. Filippi M, Rovaris M, Gasperini C et al. A preliminary study comparing the sensitivity of serial monthly enhanced MRI after standard and triple dose gadolinium-DTPA for monitoring disease activity in primary progressive MS. *J Neurol* 1998 (in press).
33. Silver NC, Good CD, Barker GJ et al. Sensitivity of contrast enhanced MRI in multiple sclerosis: effects of gadolinium dose, magnetisation transfer contrast and delayed imaging. *Brain* 1997; **120**: 1149–1161.
34. Kidd D, Thorpe JW, Thompson AJ et al. Spinal cord MRI using multi-array coils and fast spin echo. II. Findings in multiple sclerosis. *Neurology* 1993; **43**: 2632–2637.
35. Kidd D, Thorpe JW, Kendall BE et al. MRI dynamics of brain and spinal cord in progressive multiple sclerosis. *J Neurol Neurosurg Psychiatry* 1996; **60**: 15–19.
36. Losseff NA, Webb SL, O'Riordan JI et al. Spinal cord atrophy and disability in multiple sclerosis. A new reproducible and sensitive MRI method with potential to monitor disease progression. *Brain* 1996; **119**: 701–708.
37. Leary SM, Parker GJM, Stevenson VL et al. Quality assurance for serial studies of spinal cord atrophy. *Multiple Sclerosis* 1997; **3**: 279 [abstract].
38. Stevenson VL, Leary SM, Losseff NA et al. Serial measurement of spinal cord atrophy in multiple sclerosis: a potential tool for monitoring disease progression. *Neurology* 1998 (in press).
39. Allen IV, McKeown SR. A histological, histochemical and biochemical study of the macroscopically normal white matter in multiple sclerosis. *J Neuro Sci* 1979; **41**: 81–91.
40. Davie CA, Barker GJ, Thompson AJ et al. ^{1}H Magnetic resonance spectroscopy of chronic cerebral white matter lesions and normal appearing white matter in multiple sclerosis. *J Neurol Neurosurg Psychiatry* 1997; **63**: 736–742.

6

Multiple sclerosis: one disease or many?

Brian G Weinshenker and David Miller

INTRODUCTION

Disease is defined in *Dorland's Medical Dictionary* as 'a definite morbid process having a characteristic train of symptoms; ... its etiology, pathology, and prognosis may be known or unknown'. The homogeneity of multiple sclerosis (MS) as a disease entity has been a long debated issue. AB Baker MD, former Chairman of the Department of Neurology at the University of Minnesota and founder of the American Academy of Neurology, wrote in 1968 that 'in all probability, what is generally known as multiple sclerosis is not a single disease but a group of diseases with certain clinical similarities ... From the standpoint of clinical research, the present state of affairs is not satisfactory. In order to conduct clinical research in MS, it is imperative that very rigid criteria for diagnosing this disease be developed'.[1] This statement foreshadowed the development of a series of research diagnostic criteria for MS, the most recent of which, the Poser criteria,[2] constitute the basis for the diagnosis of MS in clinical practice. These criteria are heavily based on the principle that MS tends to affect multiple regions in the central nervous system and tends to have a relapsing–remitting course. The general principle of 'dissemination in time and space' is the underpinning of all of the formal diagnostic criteria for MS that have been proposed. However, several problems exist with current diagnostic criteria for MS. While these criteria do increase the specificity of the diagnosis of MS, many other entities, including multiple cerebral infarcts and vasculitis, satisfy these diagnostic criteria. While these criteria are accompanied by the caveat that no other diagnosis should better explain the syndrome, this is often a difficult caveat to translate into practice. A false positive rate of 5–10% is present in the hands of even experienced neurologists. These criteria do not account for the relative specificity of some clinical syndromes, such as optic neuritis, sensory useless hand, paroxysmal tonic spasms, and the lack of specificity of other syndromes such as hemiparesis and ataxia. These diagnostic criteria are not readily applied to the clinical situations of acute fulminant demyelination syndromes or primary progressive MS. By the current acceptance of the Poser criteria as the basis for the diagnosis of MS, our understanding of the spectrum of idiopathic inflammatory demyelinating disease (IIDD) of the central nervous system is limited by excluding monophasic demyelinating syndromes and acute nonremitting fulminant demyelinating syndromes. These criteria have led to clinical investigations to 'prevent conversion to MS', this conversion being based on the scientifically arbitrary concept that MS begins with the second clinical event. Although the second episode may be important for diagnosis, its precise timing is of relatively trivial clinical importance. Finally, by creating various categories based on degrees of clinical certainty (e.g. clinically definite, laboratory-supported definite, etc.) these criteria confuse primary physicians and patients, who find it difficult to understand these terms.

Doctor Baker made one other critical point in his review: 'only at autopsy can MS be diagnosed with a great degree of confidence'.[1] Thus, the final arbiter of the diagnosis is the demonstration at autopsy of inflammation and demyelination without specific cause, such as an underlying viral infection (e.g. progressive multifocal leukoencephalopathy). Accordingly, one might reasonably propose the redefinition of MS as an IIDD of the central nervous system. Clearly, almost all cases will not have pathological material available at the time of diagnosis. The diagnosis of an IIDD is based on the likelihood that the setting, nature and pace of the symptoms, radiological findings, other paraclinical and cerebrospinal fluid (CSF) findings, as well as response to treatment is consistent with MS, not exclusively on the principle of 'dissemination in time and space'. For patients where the diagnosis is in doubt, particularly those whose disability is severe or progressive, serious consideration should be given to brain biopsy.

Any proposed definition should be regarded as tentative and subject to revision as more definitive criteria become available based on immunological, genetic or other pathophysiological studies. There are many examples of diseases where diagnostic criteria have been modified based on the types of criteria, either to collapse several disorders into one 'lump' or to expand the numbers of diseases originally classified as a single disorder ('split'). Discoveries in the area of molecular genetics perhaps provide the best example. Duchenne's and Becker's muscular dystrophies have been collapsed based on genetic data into 'dystrophinopathies', the extent of disease simply reflecting the degree of disruption of gene function according to the specific mutation in the same gene.[3] Conversely, the dominantly inherited idiopathic ataxias have been reclassified largely based on the discovery of distinct genes causing the diseases.[4] Genetics has not been the only driving force in reclassification of diseases. Another autoimmune neurological disease, polymyositis, which overlaps in terms of muscle involvement with dermatomyositis, has now been convincingly differentiated based on the evidence of complement activation and, therefore, a humoral pathophysiological mechanism in dermatomyositis. Polymyositis, on the other hand, is believed to be T-cell mediated.[5]

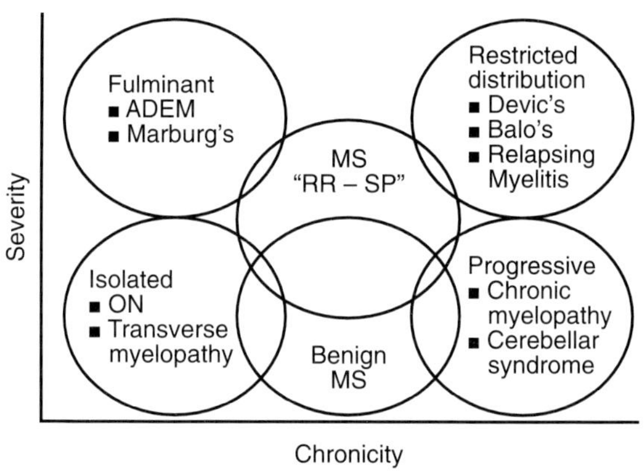

Figure 6.1 The spectrum of the idiopathic inflammatory demyelinating diseases of the CNS according to chronicity and severity.

The spectrum of the idiopathic inflammatory demyelinating diseases is illustrated in the Venn diagram in Fig. 6.1. The differences are based on the chronicity and severity, the latter depending on one or more of the extent, location and histopathological severity of the process.

Prototypic MS is generally regarded as embracing both relapsing–remitting and secondary progressive MS as the latter develops in more than 50% of those with relapsing–remitting disease. Benign MS appears to overlap and is differentiated mainly based on its favourable course, relatively few attacks and MRI lesions and tendency not to enter a secondary progressive phase.[6,7] Primary progressive MS is more problematic. A history of prior relapses may be difficult to obtain, particularly if they occurred a decade or more before the onset of progressive illness. The differences between primary progressive MS and prototypic MS are largely quantitative rather than qualitative. Patients with primary progressive MS usually have typical lesions on MRI scan of the brain, but they are fewer than in patients with relapsing–remitting or secondary progressive MS. Patients with primary progressive MS tend to have a greater spinal cord burden of disability and relatively less cerebral burden, although there is overlap. Some patients with primary progressive MS clinically have many cerebral lesions, comparable to those with secondary progressive MS. It is unclear whether the absence of relapses is the best way to distinguish between those with primary progressive MS and those with prototypic MS. (Primary progressive MS is discussed in Chapter 5 in this volume.)

Patients with monosymptomatic inflammatory demyelinating disease (e.g. 'isolated' optic neuritis or transverse myelitis) commonly develop attacks which subsequently lead to the diagnosis of MS. It is uncertain whether patients with an apparent monophasic course are on the most benign end of a continuum of patients with prototypic MS, or whether those who never develop a relapse suffer from a monophasic autoimmune disease and have a very limited form of acute disseminated encephalomyelitis. The distinction from those with a relapsing form of IIDD may be analogous to the distinction between Guillain–Barré syndrome (AIDP, or acute inflammatory demyelinating polyneuropathy) and chronic inflammatory demyelinating polyneuropathy (CIDP).

In this chapter we will discuss several special entities not discussed in other chapters of this book, namely Marburg's variant of MS, Balo's concentric sclerosis, focal inflammatory demyelinating mass lesions, Devic's disease or neuromyelitis optica, acute disseminated encephalomyelitis, and spinal-predominant MS. Special attention will be paid to the following characteristics which serve to separate these entities from MS: clinical features, CSF findings, MRI findings and pathology. It is unknown whether the differences represent extremes of a continuous distribution or distinct entities. For example, the severity of pathological injury and the presence of severe axonal injury in Devic's disease and Marburg's variant may simply reflect the severity of the inflammatory process or perhaps the level of expression of various inflammatory mediators such as cytokines. In some instances (e.g. Devic's disease), the restricted distribution of lesions may reflect the distribution of a putative autoantigen or potentially selective tropism of a putative causative virus.

To decide whether we should 'split' or 'lump' in the MS field will depend upon more definitive pathophysiological information. In the meantime, a more contemporary designation for the disease that we currently call MS and its variants might be 'an idiopathic inflammatory demyelinating disease of the central nervous system (IIDD)'. This designation would parallel the use of more descriptive terminology for other diseases. For example, rather than Guillain–Barré syndrome, we now tend to use the more descriptive term acute inflammatory demyelinating polyneuropathy or AIDP. Furthermore, a less restrictive concept of MS as an IIDD would allow for less constrained ascertainment of cases by individuals who currently restrict their practice to patients with Poser criteria-defined MS.

MARBURG VARIANT OF MULTIPLE SCLEROSIS

This entity was first described by Otto Marburg in 1906.[8] There are many subsequent reports of similar cases.[9–11] This variant is a rapidly progressive, nonremitting illness with extensive, often multifocal, lesions typically involving the cerebral hemispheres but also involving brainstem and optic nerves. Marburg's original patient was a 30-year-old woman who developed a confusional state, headaches, vomiting, gait unsteadiness and, subsequently, a left hemiparesis. After an illness of 26 days, she died. Pathology confirmed supratentorial white matter demyelination.[8] Others have observed brainstem involvement.

Although there is undoubtedly reporting bias, this variant appears to be often—perhaps usually—fatal. However, there was a recent report of a patient with the Marburg variant of MS who, after responding to corticosteroids, had a typical relapsing–remitting course of MS.[12] Lesions on MRI scans tend to be extensive and confluent. Homogeneous enhancement is common and ring enhancement may occasionally be seen. The CSF findings are variable and often reveal a low-grade mononuclear pleocytosis, similar to that encountered in MS. Oligoclonal bands are typically absent.

The pathology is generally widespread demyelination often with massive macrophage infiltration. Furthermore, there is evidence of acute axonal injury and/or necrosis with occasional microcavitation. Immunological derangements in these relatively rare cases have not been well documented. The degree of demyelination and the extent of axonal injury and necrosis seem to differentiate the Marburg variant from acute disseminated encephalomyelitis. However, it is often difficult to distinguish between these entities on clinical grounds (see below). Furthermore, as the pathology has generally been studied in fatal cases, the full spectrum of this entity has probably not been appreciated.

The pathogenesis of the syndrome has not been studied comprehensively. Recently, there was a report from Canada of one patient with the Marburg variant of MS who had a substantial abnormality in the composition of myelin basic protein.[13] There was a marked excess of a less cationic deiminated form of myelin basic protein, presumably a result of a post-translational modification of myelin basic protein in which arginine residues are converted to citrulline residues. The authors speculate that this abnormality may interfere with the normal compaction of white matter. Similar findings, quantitatively less severe, have been described in patients with prototypic MS.[14] The authors speculate that the more severe abnormalities encountered in this patient may account for the greater severity of his illness.

A few patients have been reported to respond to corticosteroids. As noted above, one patient, after responding satisfactorily to steroids, went on to have the typical relapsing–remitting course seen in prototypic multiple sclerosis.[12] Rodriguez et al. reported occasional patients with Marburg variant of MS who did not respond to corticosteroids but who seem to respond to plasma exchange.[15] There is an ongoing trial of the effectiveness of plasma exchange in acute fulminant inflammatory demyelinating syndromes at the Mayo Clinic.

BALO'S CONCENTRIC SCLEROSIS

Balo's concentric sclerosis is defined by its characteristic pathology which consists of concentric lamellae of demyelinated and partially myelinated axons. This entity was first described by Balo in 1928.[16] Balo described a 23-year-old Hungarian patient who presented with an acute illness consisting of right hemiparesis, aphasia and papilloedema, and died within 8 months. Several subsequent reports of a similar entity have been described, commonly in patients of Asian ethnic background.[17,18] Several patients recently diagnosed with this entity, based on a rather characteristic MRI appearance, have subsequently proven to have the typical pathological changes of Balo's concentric sclerosis at autopsy, suggesting that it might be possible to identify this entity during life.[17–19] The typical MRI changes consist of concentric rings or a whorled appearance on T2-weighted images and on gadolinium-enhanced T1-weighted images.

Balo's concentric sclerosis, similar to Marburg's variant of MS, tends to be a rapidly progressive monophasic illness that some have suggested is a variant of acute disseminated encephalomyelitis. It has been commonly reported to cause death within weeks to months, but occasional cases have been described to have prolonged survival.[19] Almost all cases have involved supratentorial white matter, usually exclusively. The clinical presentation is usually headache, aphasia, cognitive or behavioural dysfunction, and/or seizures. Spinal fluid studies often reveal a mononuclear inflammatory reaction and oligoclonal bands are often present.

Pathologically, the disease process spares the optic nerves, brainstem, cerebellum and spinal cord. The characteristic pathological findings are alternating rings of myelin preservation and myelin loss.

The pathogenesis of Balo's concentric sclerosis is not well understood. The only differentiating feature from MS is the lamellar pattern of pathology. Some have suggested that this may indicate a demyelinating process, perhaps a virus, which is periodically inhibited by antibodies. Potentially some other humoral demyelinating factor diffusing from a central focus which is periodically inhibited by an opposing anti-inflammatory or antidemyelinating factor could produce a similar pattern. Moore et al. have suggested that this entity represents remyelination in plaque borders after successive episodes of demyelination.[20] Yao et al. suggest that this entity represents different stages of ongoing myelin breakdown.[21]

MS PRESENTING AS A MASS LESION

Many patients who present with a suspected tumor and were diagnosed based on brain biopsy as having an IIDD are described in the clinical or MRI literature. There are over 50 such case reports or small case series.[22–24] The presentation is generally headache, aphasia, disturbance in consciousness, or seizures. Neuroimaging reveals unifocal or multifocal enhancing lesions, occasionally with associated mass effect and brain edema. Brain biopsy is generally necessary to confirm the diagnosis. Masdeu et al. described 'the open ring sign'.[25] In lesions which abut grey matter, the rim of enhancement tends to be most prominent at the leading edge of demyelination in the white matter and least prominent where the lesions abut the cortical mantle or deep grey matter structures. Masdeu and colleagues were able to show that this sign generally differentiated acute demyelinating lesions from brain tumors. MR spectroscopy may offer some promise for differentiating brain tumor from demyelination in the future.

Pathology usually distinguishes tumor from acute demyelination. The presence of extensive macrophage infiltration is unusual in tumours and should strongly suggest demyelinating disease. However, occasional biopsy samples may lead to diagnostic confusion given the hypercellular nature of these lesions and associated alterations in astrocyte morphology. Frequently, reactive astrocytosis is misinterpreted as evidence for glioma, which may lead inappropriately to radiotherapy. Occasionally, lymphoma is a diagnostic consideration based on pathology, considering the collection of lymphocytes; staining for light chain isotype can determine if there is a monoclonal origin for the lymphocytic infiltrate, that would suggest lymphoma. The demonstration of extensive myelin loss and relative axonal preservation is very helpful in the pathological assessment when an adequate sample is provided.

ACUTE DISSEMINATED ENCEPHALOMYELITIS

Acute disseminated encephalomyelitis (ADEM) is, in its classical form, a monophasic inflammatory/demyelinating disease of the central nervous system which is thought to be immunologically mediated. It is encountered more frequently in children than in adults, a point of distinction from classical MS.

In most cases the neurological syndrome develops a few days or weeks after an infectious event. It is thought that the cellular and/or human immune response to viral or bacterial antigens cross-reacts with myelin antigens leading to immune-mediated demyelination. The inciting infection may be due to an identifiable specific agent such as rubeola, varicella, Epstein–Barr virus, or mycoplasma pneumonia. Alternatively, it may follow a nonspecific upper respiratory tract or gastrointestinal infection, or occasionally vaccination. In the past, it was a more common event following smallpox vaccination or anti-rabies vaccination using killed rabies virus produced in rabbit brain tissue.

Clinical features include fever, encephalopathy with obtundation, coma and seizures, ataxia, optic neuritis and transverse myelitis. Whereas optic neuritis is usually unilateral in MS, it is more characteristically bilateral in postinfectious ADEM. In the acute phase there may be optic disc swelling. Spinal cord involvement not infrequently results in a more or less complete deficit, with flaccid, areflexic paraplegia and a clear sensory level. Upper cervical cord or medullary involvement can lead to quadriplegia, dysphagia, aspiration and respiratory failure, and assisted ventilation may be required.

Pathologically, widespread perivascular foci of inflammation and demyelination are the characteristic hallmarks. Both the brain and spinal cord may be involved. Multiple small and widespread lesions may be found, or larger more confluent areas of demyelination can occur, with a tendency to symmetry in the cerebral hemispheres.[26] Both white matter and grey matter may be affected, though white matter involvement predominates. Mass effect from both brain and spinal cord lesions may be encountered.[27] MRI reveals multifocal white matter cerebral lesions, which may be asymmetrical and indistinguishable from the appearances seen in the classical multiple sclerosis.[28] During the acute phase, and providing that there is no concurrent corticosteroid administration, most lesions exhibit gadolinium enhancement.[29] This suggests a monophasic process with most lesions being acute, and contrasts with the more usual situation in MS where only a minority of lesions exhibit enhancement at any time. Other patients with ADEM can exhibit a striking symmetry of abnormalities, which can involve the cerebral and/or cerebellar white matter.[28] Patients with acute transverse myelitis typically show MRI evidence of swelling and T2 signal hyperintensity extending over multiple segments during the acute phase. Follow-up MRI in ADEM often shows striking resolution of abnormalities over months to years. Only a few patients have been followed long term, but this experience suggests that new MRI lesions are infrequent, consistent with a monophasic process.

The CSF during the acute illness typically shows a moderate to marked mononuclear pleocytosis, with an elevation in the CSF protein but normal glucose. Oligoclonal bands may be present, but not necessarily so; in one series they were reported in three of seven patients.[28] In one patient, the bands were reported to disappear on follow-up,[28] a feature which is not expected in MS.

Treatment of ADEM usually consists of a short course of high dose corticosteroids, often intravenous methylprednisolone with or without an oral corticosteroid taper. Clinical improvement has been reported in patients with a particularly acute, fulminant clinical presentation treated with plasma exchange,[30] and in a patient with recurrent acute disseminated encephalomyelitis intravenous immunoglobulin was helpful.[31]

The difficulty in making a firm distinction between monophasic ADEM and multiphasic MS is apparent when one considers the following clinical scenarios:

(a) while ADEM is usually postinfectious, MS relapses also follow infections fairly often
(b) adult patients with a clinically isolated syndrome characteristic of MS (e.g. unilateral optic neuritis or partial myelitis) may occasionally exhibit predominantly enhancing brain lesions during acute presentation, yet may go on to develop MS at follow-up
(c) although encephalopathic features or cerebral lesions with mass effect are well recognized in ADEM, these features are also occasionally seen in otherwise typical MS
(d) patients who present with a clinical picture characteristic of ADEM, may occasionally

proceed to have one or several relapses during ensuing months or years.[32]

In summary, although a combination of clinical and investigative features, especially in children, can point towards a higher probability of a monophasic inflammatory demyelinating disease (ADEM), a firm distinction from multiphasic disease (MS) is often not possible. Prolonged follow-up can help to distinguish between monophasic and multiphasic disease, although even this does not provide an absolute distinction. In a few patients the second relapse of MS occurs after an interval of 30 years or more.

DEVIC'S NEUROMYELITIS OPTICA

The definition of what is included under the synonym Devic's neuromyelitis optica is far from clear. Sometimes it has been regarded as a specific disease entity and at other times as a syndrome with multiple causes. The term Devic's neuromyelitis optica has been applied not only to a narrow group of patients with monophasic bilateral optic neuritis and complete transverse myelitis occurring in a post-infectious situation, in whom the probable diagnosis is ADEM, but also to a heterogeneous group of acute, relapsing syndromes with only clinical involvement confined to the optic nerves and spinal cord in common; the latter rather 'loose' definition would inevitably include a significant number of patients with MS who have had relapses exclusive to the spinal cord and optic nerves.

It seems preferable that Devic's neuromyelitis optica should be regarded as a syndrome rather than a disease. Multiple specific causes can produce acute or subacute, monophasic or multiphasic, episodes of clinical disturbance isolated to the optic nerves and spinal cord. These include collagen vascular disorders such as systemic lupus erythematosus (SLE) and the antiphospholipid antibody syndrome, acute disseminated encephalomyelitis, multiple sclerosis, neurosarcoidosis, and following pulmonary tuberculosis. Nevertheless, a significant number of cases do not have an underlying, predisposing disease.

Pathological reports have included a range of abnormalities. In some patients, disseminated demyelinating lesions beyond the spinal cord and optic nerves have been reported.[33] Other studies such as that reported by Mandler et al.,[34] have emphasized the lack of involvement of the brain. A striking sparing of the brain (apart from the medulla) was also apparent in the clinicopathological report of identical twin sisters described by McAlpine in *Brain* in 1938.[35] Both had presented in their 20s with remarkably similar relapsing episodes of optic neuritis and myelitis, which led to severe disability and death after 18 and 26 months. Some pathological reports have emphasized the presence of extensive necrosis and cavitation in the spinal cord in some patients.[34,35] More typical areas of inflammation and demyelination are also seen in the cord and optic nerves.

O'Riordan et al. defined Devic's syndrome as the occurrence of either a monophasic or multiphasic disorder with acute episodes of optic neuritis and *complete* transverse myelitis without other central nervous system manifestations.[36] A key element of this definition is that there should be an episode of more or less *complete* transverse myelitis, as it is rare to see an acute complete transverse myelitis in MS. Applying these criteria, 12 cases were identified exhibiting several features distinctive from classical relapsing–remitting MS:

(a) brain MRI was frequently normal
(b) spinal MRI showed swelling of signal change over many segments during the acute myelitis episode, whereas in MS cord lesions are usually only a segment or less in length
(c) the CSF contained oligoclonal bands in only 2 of 12 patients
(d) recovery of vision and motor function was often poor
(e) there was a relatively high proportion of cases among non-Caucasoid ethnic groups.

It is not possible to say at present whether such cases of Devic's syndrome represent a truly different disease, or whether along with MS it is part of a spectrum of inflammatory demyelinating diseases of the central nervous system, which manifests in different ways because of subtle differences in immunogenic or immunopathological mechanisms.

SPINAL MULTIPLE SCLEROSIS

Pathological involvement largely or completely confined to the spinal cord is well recognized in MS.[37] Ikuta and Zimmerman recorded no cerebral plaques in 2 of 70 cases in a postmortem series, and in 9 cases (13%), they reported a pattern of extensive plaques confined largely to the spinal cord and optic nerves.[38] In patients with clinically definite MS, up to 5% have normal brain MRI. Thorpe and colleagues reviewed 20 patients in whom there was a strong clinical suspicion of MS, but who had either normal brain MRI or minor nonspecific abnormalities.[39] The main findings in this study were:

(1) Eleven of the 20 patients had a primary progressive course, usually a progressive spastic paraplegia. A high proportion of patients with this presentation is not too surprising, since a low cerebral lesion load is often encountered in primary progressive MS,[40] particularly the progressive myelopathic variety.
(2) Seven patients had a relapsing–remitting course, with a disease duration which was usually short (< 5 years), although in two patients it was much longer. All patients with a relapsing–remitting course had minimal disability. This suggests that patients with definite relapsing–remitting MS and normal brain imaging may have a relatively good prognosis.
(3) Only one of the 20 patients had a secondary progressive course. It seems that in this subgroup it is particularly unusual to have normal brain imaging.
(4) Visual evoked potentials were abnormal in 10 of 18 patients studied, and CSF oligoclonal bands in 13 of 15 who underwent lumbar puncture. This emphasizes the value of these investigations in diagnostic work up, especially when brain MRI is unhelpful.
(5) All 20 patients exhibited one or more focal cord lesions compatible with demyelination. Spinal MRI lesions in MS are characteristically small, usually < 1 cm long, and only involve part of the cross-section of the spinal cord.[41] Such lesions do not occur with ageing per se,[42] so their presence can be of particular diagnostic value in older patients as well as in those with normal brain imaging.

Other spinal MRI abnormalities found in MS patients (with or without brain MRI abnormalities) have included diffuse signal change in proton density weighted images,[43] and cord atrophy.[44] Both of these features have been associated especially with a progressive course and higher levels of disability.

SUMMARY

This chapter reviews some of the range of clinical syndromes which can manifest in patients with inflammatory demyelinating diseases of the central nervous system. It is still debatable whether these represent a series of different diseases or a single disease with a wide spectrum of manifestations related to different pathogenic mechanisms. With the recent advent of disease-modifying therapies in MS, further elucidation of the aetiology and pathogenic mechanisms of IIDD is imperative.

REFERENCES

1. Baker AB. Problems in the classification of multiple sclerosis. In: Alter M, Kurtzke JF, eds. *The Epidemiology of Multiple Sclerosis*. Springfield, IL: Charles C. Thomas, 1968; 14–25.
2. Poser CM, Paty DW, Scheinberg L, McDonald WI et al. New diagnostic criteria for multiple sclerosis: guidelines for research protocols. *Ann Neurol* 1983; **13**: 227–231.
3. Straub V, Campbell KP. Muscular dystrophies and the dystrophin–glycoprotein complex. *Curr Opin Neurol* 1997; **10**: 168–175.

4. Nance MA. Clinical aspects of CAG repeat diseases. *Brain Pathol* 1997; **7**: 881–900.
5. Dalakas MC, Sivakumar K. The immunopathologic and inflammatory differences between dermatomyositis, polymyositis, and sporadic inclusion body myositis. *Curr Opin Neurol* 1996; **9**: 235–239.
6. Thompson AJ, Hutchinson M, Brazil J et al. A clinical and laboratory study of benign multiple sclerosis. *Q J Med* 1986; **58**: 69–80.
7. Filippi M, Campi A, Martinelli V et al. Brain and spinal cord MR in benign multiple sclerosis: a follow-up study. *J Neurol Sci* 1996; **143**: 143–149.
8. Marburg O. Die sogenannte "akute Multiple Sklerose". *J Psychiatric Neurol* 1906; **27**: 211–312.
9. Johnson MD, Lavin P, Whetsell WO Jr. Fulminant monophasic multiple sclerosis, Marburg's type. *J Neurol Neurosurg Psychiatry* 1990; **53**: 918–921.
10. Mendez MF, Pogacar S. Malignant monophasic multiple sclerosis or "Marburg's disease". *Neurology* 1988; **38**: 1153–1155.
11. Banerjee A, Chopra J, Kumar B. Acute multiple sclerosis: report of a case with neuropathological and neurochemical studies. *Neurol India* 1977; **25**: 233–237.
12. Giubilei F, Sarrantonio A, Tisei P et al. Four-year follow-up of a case of acute multiple sclerosis of the Marburg type. *Italian J Neurol Sci* 1997; **18**: 163–166.
13. Wood DD, Bilbao JM, O'Connors P et al. Acute multiple sclerosis (Marburg type) is associated with developmentally immature myelin basic protein. *Ann Neurol* 1996; **40**: 18–24.
14. Moscarello MA, Wood DD, Ackerley C et al. Myelin in multiple sclerosis is developmentally immature. *J Clin Invest* 1994; **94**: 146–154.
15. Rodriguez M, Karnes WE, Bartleson JD et al. Plasmapheresis in acute episodes of fulminant CNS inflammatory demyelination. *Neurology* 1993; **43**: 1100–1104.
16. Balo J. Encephalitis periaxalis concentrica. *Arch Neurol* 1928; **19**: 242–263.
17. Chen C, Ro LS, Chang CN et al. Serial MRI studies in pathologically verified Balo's concentric sclerosis. *J Comput Assist Tomogr* 1996; **20**: 732–735.
18. Nandini M, Gourie-Devi M, Shankar S et al. Balo's concentric sclerosis diagnosed intravitum on brain biopsy. *Clin Neurol Neurosurg* 1993; **95**: 303–309.
19. Bolay H, Karabudak R, Tacal T et al. Balo's concentric sclerosis: report of two patients. *J Neuroimag* 1996; **6**: 98–103.
20. Moore GR, Neumann PE, Suzuki K et al. Balo's concentric sclerosis: new observations on lesion development. *Ann Neurol* 1985; **17**: 604–611.
21. Yao D, Webster HD, Hudson L et al. Concentric sclerosis (Balo): Morphometric and in situ hybridization study of lesions in six patients. *Ann Neurol* 1994; **35**: 18–30.
22. Rieth K, Di Chiro G, Cromwell L. Primary demyelinating disease stimulating glioma of the corpus callosum. Report of three cases. *Neurosurgery* 1981; **55**: 620–624.
23. Hunter S, Ballinger W, Rubin J. Multiple sclerosis mimicking primary brain tumor. *Arch Pathol Lab Med* 1987; **111**: 464–468.
24. Kepes J. Large focal tumor-like demyelinating lesions of the brain: intermediate entity between multiple sclerosis and acute disseminated encephalomyelitis: a study of 31 patients. *Ann Neurol* 1993; **33**: 18–27.
25. Masdeu JC, Moreira J, Trasi S et al. The open ring. A new imaging sign in demyelinating disease. *J Neuroimag* 1996; **6**: 104–107.
26. Allen IV. Demyelinating diseases. In: Adams JH, Corsellis JAN, Duchen LW, eds. *Greenfield's Neuropathology*, 4th edn. London: Edward Arnold, 1984; 338–384.
27. Youl BD, Kermode AG, Thompson ASJ et al. Destructive lesions in demyelinating disease. *J Neurol Neurosurg Psychiatry* 1991; **54**: 288–292.
28. Kesselring J, Miller DH, Robb SA et al. Acute disseminated encephalomyelitis. MRI findings and the distinction from multiple sclerosis. *Brain* 1990; **113**: 291–302.
29. Mader I, Stock KW, Ettlin T et al. Acute disseminated encephalomyelitis: MR and CT features. *Am J Neuroradiol* 1996; **17**: 104–109.
30. Kanter DS, Horensky D, Sperling RA et al. Plasmapheresis in fulminant acute disseminated encephalomyelitis. *Neurology* 1995; **45**: 824–827.
31. Hahn JS, Siegler DJ, Enzmann D. Intravenous gammaglobulin therapy in recurrent acute disseminated encephalomyelitis. *Neurology* 1996; **46**: 1173–1174.
32. Miller HG, Evans MJ. Prognosis in acute disseminated encephalomyelitis: with a note on neuromyelitis optica. *Q J Med* 1953; **22**: 347–479.
33. Stansbury FC. Neuromyelitis optica (Devic's disease). Presentation of five cases with pathological study and review of the literature. *Arch Ophthalmol* 1949; **42**: 292–335, 465–501.

34. Mandler RN, David LE, Jeffery DR et al. Devic's neuromyelitis optica: a clinicopathological study of 8 patients. *Ann Neurol* 1993; **34**: 162–168.
35. McAlpine D. Familial neuromyelitis optica: its occurrence in identical twins. *Brain* 1938; **61**: 430–448.
36. O'Riordan JI, Gallagher HL, Thompson AJ et al. Clinical, CSF, and MRI findings in Devic's neuromyelitis optica. *J Neurol Neurosurg Psychiatry* 1996; **60**: 382–387.
37. Allen IV, Glover G, Anderson R. Abnormalities in the macroscopically normal white matter in cases of mild or spinal multiple sclerosis (MS). *Acta Neuropathol (Berl)* 1981; **suppl VII**: 176–178.
38. Ikuta F, Zimmerman HM. Distribution of plaques in seventy autopsy cases of multiple sclerosis in the United States. *Neurology* 1976; **26 (suppl)**: 26–28.
39. Thorpe JW, Kidd D, Moseley IF et al. Spinal MRI in patients with suspected multiple sclerosis and negative brain MRI. *Brain* 1996; **119**: 709–714.
40. Thompson AJ, Kermode AG, MacManus DG et al. Patterns of disease activity in multiple sclerosis: a clinical and magnetic resonance imaging study. *BMJ* 1990; **300**: 631–634.
41. Oppenheimer DR. The cervical cord in multiple sclerosis. *Neuropath Appl Neurobiol* 1978; **4**: 293–296.
42. Thorpe JW, Kidd D, Kendall BE et al. Spinal MRI using multi-array coils and fast spin echo. I. Technical aspects and findings in healthy controls. *Neurology* 1993; **43**: 2625–2631.
43. Lycklama a Nijeholt GJ, Barkhof F, Scheltens P et al. MR of the spinal cord in multiple sclerosis: relation to clinical subtype and disability. *Am J Neuroradiol* 1997; **18**: 1041–1044.
44. Losseff NA, Wang L, O'Riordan JI et al. Spinal cord atrophy and disability in multiple sclerosis: a new reproducible and sensitive MRI method with potential to monitor disease progression. *Brain* 1996; **119**: 701–708.

7

Diagnosis of multiple sclerosis 1998: do we need new diagnostic criteria?

Donald W Paty and David KB Li

The established clinical criteria for the diagnosis of multiple sclerosis (MS) depend upon the clinical demonstration of lesions disseminated in both time and space in separate portions of the white matter of the central nervous system (CNS). Patients are also expected to have clinically appropriate MS-like symptoms. The Schumacher criteria clearly defined clinically definite MS (CDMS).[1] The description is an elegant one. However, the Schumacher criteria did not allow for the inclusion of paraclinical studies such as evoked potentials, CT scan, or MRI scan data to be used in the diagnosis. The fundamentals of the Schumacher criteria are as follows:

(1) There should be clinical evidence for lesions that reflect primarily white matter dysfunction disseminated in both time and space. These symptoms should be in a patient in the expected age range (10–50 years).
(2) There must be objective abnormalities on neurological examination preferably, but not exclusively, shown at the time of making the diagnosis.
(3) The dissemination of lesions in time must fit into one of the following patterns:
    (a) at least two clear-cut episodes of functionally significant symptoms each lasting over 24 h and separated by at least 1 month; remission is not necessary;
    (b) slow progressive development of the same disseminated pattern evolving over at least 6 months.
(4) The diagnosis should be made by a competent clinician (preferably a neurologist) and there must be no better explanation for the diagnosis.

A subsequent proposal was made by Poser[2] and his committee to accept paraclinical evidence for dissemination in space. Therefore, for research protocols, solid evoked-potential evidence, CT scan evidence, and more recently magnetic resonance imaging (MRI) evidence for dissemination in space could be accepted for inclusion of patients in research protocols. The concept for the proof of dissemination in time however remained a clinical one.

The Poser[2] criteria, in addition, accepted evidence of oligoclonal banding or increased synthesis of immunoglobulin G (IgG) within the CNS as additional evidence that would allow a classification of laboratory-supported definite multiple sclerosis (LSDMS), again for the inclusion of patients in research protocols.

Subsequent studies of the relationship between LSDMS and the prognosis for CDMS have now shown that the diagnosis of LSDMS almost always leads to a subsequent diagnosis of CDMS.[3]

Autopsy studies by Engell,[4] and Izquierdo et al.[5] have shown that CDMS has a specificity of about 95%. The studies by Lee et al.[3] and others, have shown that the conversion from LSDMS to CDMS increases over time.

The current usage is, therefore, that typical MS-like symptoms supported by the concept of dissemination in space using MRI findings and the presence of immunoglobulin abnormalities in the cerebrospinal fluid predict the eventual diagnosis of CDMS quite accurately.

Clinical signs that increase the likelihood of the diagnosis of MS are previous nonspecific neurological symptoms before an episode of optic neuritis,[6] partial acute transverse myelopathy, or intranuclear ophthalmaplegia. Lhermitte's symptom also increases the likelihood of the diagnosis of MS. The Uhthoff's phenomenon, the useless hand syndrome, and bilateral intranuclear ophthalmaplegia all increase the likelihood of MS being the appropriate diagnosis.

Paroxysmal motor or sensory symptoms can support the diagnosis of MS, but they are too nonspecific to be used as evidence for dissemination in either time or space in the clinical diagnosis. The caveat expressed in the Schumacher criteria are still appropriate, i.e. an experienced neurologist should be convinced that another diagnosis other than MS is not likely.

MRI CRITERIA STRONGLY SUGGESTIVE OF MULTIPLE SCLEROSIS

MRI abnormalities can clearly support the diagnosis of MS. However, one MS abnormality on MRI is probably not enough. The proposal of four lesions, ⩾ 3 mm, in the white matter characteristic of MS or three such lesions, one periventricular, can be considered to be strongly suggestive of MS in the right clinical setting.[6,7] Also, other studies[8] have shown that with increasing numbers of lesions the likelihood of the diagnosis of CDMS in the future also increases.

In addition, there have been several brain locations for individual lesions that have been identified as increasing the specificity for the diagnosis of MS. Lesions that arise from the corpus callosum[9] and infratentorial lesions[10] are such specificity locations. Offenbacher et al.[11] indicated that lesions > 6 mm in diameter were also more specific for MS than smaller lesions. Horowitz et al.[12] also indicated that an oval shape was more specific for MS, particularly oval lesions seen in the parasagittal view that seem to be arising from the corpus callosum or on the superior margin of the lateral ventricle. Others have suggested that open-ring enhancement is also characteristic of MS lesions.[13]

Currently popular usage suggests that, to propose an MRI to be *strongly suggestive* of MS there should be three lesions, at least one periventricular, or four or more lesions. If a lesion of a specific type suggestive of MS or a specific location suggestive of MS is found, in addition to the three or four lesions indicated above, the specificity for MS probably increases.

Kappos et al.[14] have made a proposal that if both enhancing and unenhancing lesions are found in the same scan, the criterion for dissemination in time may be satisfied by this apparent discrepancy in the age of the lesions. Since most enhancements last less than 4 weeks, Kappos' observation was made on the basis that multiple pre-existing (old) lesions are seen in most patients who convert to CDMS within 5 years. If some, but not all, of the lesions enhance, the suggestion is that the lesions are of different ages, therefore supporting the concept of dissemination in time as well as space.

A PROPOSAL FOR A NEW DIAGNOSTIC CATEGORY

We are therefore proposing that a new diagnostic category of MRI-supported definite multiple sclerosis (MSDMS) be added to the categories of CDMS and LSDMS for research protocols.

The new category should apply to patients that have a clinically appropriate symptom with the one event lasting > 24 h.[1] Clinical events highly suggestive of MS are unilateral optic neuritis, sensory loss or positive sensory symptoms, bilateral intranuclear ophthalmaplegia, the useless hand syndrome, or weakness in

Table 7.1 Lesion appearance or locations that increase the MRI specificity for MS

Location of lesion	(a) Corpus callosum	Simon et al.[9]
	(b) Infratentorial	Fazekas et al.[10]
Size	> 6 mm diameter	Fazekas et al.[10]
Shape	Ovoid	Horowitz et al.[12]
Enhancement	Some but not all lesions	Kappos et al.[14]
	Open-ring	Masdeu et al.[13]

Table 7.2 Diagnosis of MS: current criteria (summary)*

	Clinical		Paraclinical (including MRI)		
Criteria (Category)	Time	Space	Time	Space	OB
Schumacher (CDMS)	+	+	0	0	0
Poser (CDMS)	+	0	0	+	0
Poser (LSDMS)‡	+	0	0	+	+
Proposed (MSDMS)‡	+	0	0	+†	0

\+ Required.

0 Not required.

* Caveats: (a) Under age 45; (b) no better explanation.

† Paraclinical evidence must be: (a) MRI only; (b) one or more white matter lesions, or three lesions one being periventricular; (c) one lesion to have a specificity criterion from Table 7.1.

‡ Single episode patient.

Table 7.3 Requirements for meeting the criteria for MRI-supported definite MS (MSDMS) in patients under 45 years of age

Size of lesions	≥ 3 mm diameter
Number of lesions	4 or more, 3 with 1 periventricular
At least 1 specificity feature	(1) 1 or more lesions but not all with enhancement
	(2) Size: > 6 mm diameter
	(3) Shape: oval or flame
	(4) Location: Corpus callosum, infratentorial

one or more extremities associated with pyramidal findings.

If a patient has four lesions, or three lesions with one periventricular, and also has at least one MS-specific location of lesion, quality of lesion, and/or one or two enhancing lesions (less than half of the lesions should be enhancing), the diagnosis of MSDMS could be made.

The caveats are that the patients must be under the age of 45 and a competent physician (preferably a neurologist) must certify that another diagnosis is not likely. Also, the parasagittal view of the brain using proton density and spin-echo T2 sequences visualizing lesions that seem to arise as flames off the corpus callosum should be a part of every MS diagnostic protocol. These newly proposed criteria must now be studied prospectively so their usefulness can be proven.

SUMMARY

We propose a new category for the diagnosis of MS in research protocols: MR-supported definite multiple sclerosis (MRI-supported definite MS (MSDMS)). Such patients should be or have the following features:

(1) be under 45 years of age
(2) have one MS-like clinical episode with appropriate clinical findings, no remission is necessary
(3) an abnormal MRI scan as follows:
  (a) four 3-mm white matter lesions, or three with one periventricular
  (b) at least one specificity finding such as: > 6 mm diameter, oval shape (flame-like), located in or above the corpus callosum or infratentorially, one or more—but not all—enhancing, or one with an open-ring enhancement.

REFERENCES

1. Schumacher GA, Beebe G, Kibler RF et al. Problems of experimental trials of therapy in multiple sclerosis: report by the panel on the evaluation of experimental trials of therapy in multiple sclerosis. *Ann NY Acad Sci* 1965; **122**: 552–568.
2. Poser CM, Paty DW, Scheinberg LC et al. New diagnostic criteria for multiple sclerosis. Guidelines for research protocol. *Ann Neurol* 1983; **13**: 227–231.
3. Lee KH, Hashimoto SA, Hooge JP et al. Magnetic resonance imaging of the head in the diagnosis of MS: a prospective 2-year follow-up with comparison of clinical evaluation, evoked potentials, oligoclonal banding, and CT. *Neurology* 1991; **41**: 657–660.
4. Engell T. A clinico-pathoanatomical study multiple sclerosis diagnosis. *Acta Neurol Scan* 1988; **78**: 39–44.
5. Izquierdo G, Hauw JJ, Lyon-Caen O et al. Value of multiple sclerosis criteria: 70 autopsy-confirmed cases. *Arch Neurol* 1985; **42**: 848–850.
6. Beck RW, Arrington J, Murtagh FR et al. The Optic Neuritis Group. Brain MRI in acute optic neuritis experience of the Optic Neuritis Group. *Arch Neurol* 1993; **50**: 841–846.
7. Paty DW, Oger JJF, Kastrukoff LF et al. Magnetic resonance imaging (MRI) in the diagnosis of multiple sclerosis: a prospective study with comparison of clinical evaluation, evoked potentials, oligoclonal banding and computerized tomography. *Neurology* 1988; **38**: 180–185.
8. Barkoff F, Filippi M, Tas MW et al. Towards specific MR imaging criteria for early MS. *J Neurol* 1994; **241 (suppl 1)**: S150.
9. Simon JH, Holtas SL, Schiffer RB et al. Corpus callosum and subcallosal periventricular lesions in multiple sclerosis: detection with MRI. *Radiology* 1986; **160**: 363–367.
10. Fazekas F, Offenbacher H, Fuchs S et al. Criteria for an increased specificity of MRI interpretation in elderly subjects with suspected MS. *Neurology* 1988; **38**: 1822–1825.
11. Offenbacher H, Fazekas F, Schmidt R et al. Assessment of MRI criteria for a diagnosis of MS. *Neurology* 1993; **43**: 905–909.
12. Horowitz AL, Kaplan RD, Grewe G et al. The ovoid lesion: a new MR observation in patients with multiple sclerosis. *AJNR* 1989; **10**: 303–305.
13. Masdeu JC, Wolfson L, Lantos G et al. Brain white-matter changes in the elderly prone to falling. *Neuroimaging* 1996; **6**: 104–107.
14. Kappos L, Gold R, Heun R et al. MS: Definite at first presentation? The role of Gd-enhanced MRI. *Neurology* 1991; **41**: 168.

8

Prognosis in multiple sclerosis: genetic factors

Neil P Robertson and D Alastair S Compston

INTRODUCTION

The last 10 years has seen an enormous investment in attempting to clarify the relative quantitative contribution of genes to the aetiology of multiple sclerosis (MS), with significant contemporary advances in knowledge being made as a result of the recent family studies, linkage analysis and screens of the human genome. Perhaps the ultimate prognostic goal in clarifying the role of susceptibility genes in this disease will simply be to identify those who will develop clinical manifestations of MS, and any genetic model will have to be compatible with the pattern of disease recurrence observed in relatives. However, in a disease which has such variable expression, it may also be important to establish whether increased knowledge of molecular genetic mechanisms will allow us to predict the course of the disease. We can consider these two aspects of risk as quantitative and qualitative contributions.

QUANTITATIVE RISK

Twins

Twin studies have commonly been used for determining genetic contribution to disease aetiology and despite many potential methodological problems, they probably give an adequate estimate of expected genetic effect. Twin studies, however, are not without their difficulties. In diseases of low frequency such as MS it is necessary to recruit from large population bases or to look for alternative methods of selective recruitment, which may result in ascertainment bias. In addition, inappropriate assignment of zygosity, the recognition of subclinical forms of the disease, variable age at onset and liability for omission of mild or subclinical forms of the disease have all been recognized as potential sources of inaccuracy.

In an attempt to ascertain large numbers investigators have commonly employed twin registers,[1–3] advertisement,[4–7] and clinic populations.[8,9] Most demonstrate an increased concordance rate in monozygous twins of between 21% and 50% compared with 0–17% in dizygous twins (Table 8.1). The largest studies are remarkably consistent with monozygous concordance of around 25%; magnetic resonance demonstrates abnormalities consistent with MS in a further 14% of unaffected monozygotic co-twins.[7,8] Only one study offers longitudinal data that saw the concordance rise from 26% to 30.8% in monozygous twins and from 2% to 5% in the dizygous pairs over 7.5 years,[9] and it seems likely that a longer period of observation of these cohorts will see concordance rates rise further. Note that these observed risks (OR) are

Table 8.1 Twin studies

Authors	Year	Monozygous concordance		Dizygous concordance	
		No.	%	No.	%
Bobowick et al.[1]	1978	2/5	40.0	0/4	0
Williams et al.[4]	1980	6/12	50.0	2/12	17
Heltberg and Holm[2]	1982	4/19	21.1	1/28	4
Kinnunen et al.[3]	1987	2/7	28.6	0/6	0
Uitdehaag et al.[5]	1989	0/4	0.0	0/3	0
Ebers et al[8]	1986	8/26	30.8	2/43	5
Sadovnick et al[9]	1993	5/19	26.3	0/23	0
Mumford et al.[7]	1994	11/44	25.0	2/61	3
French research group[6]	1994	1/17	5.9	1/37	3
Totals		39/153	25.5	8/217	4

not directly comparable to the age-adjusted recurrence risks (AAR) for relatives widely quoted; a similar analysis would provide a concordance figure of around 50% if applied.

The only major, contemporary study to disagree with this trend was from the French Research Group on Multiple Sclerosis,[6] which recruited 116 pairs from a television appeal and reported concordance independent of zygosity in 54 twinships. It is not clear why this study is at odds with the others, but it is of note that the results were based on only 54 of the 116 twinships identified so that over half of the cohort could not be fully evaluated. Also the 95% confidence limits (0–17.1%) are not significantly different to those of the larger Canadian study (13.0–42.5%).[8]

The persistent excess of monozygotic concordance, with the exception of the French Research Group study, provides very powerful support for a genetic contribution to disease aetiology, although genetic factors appear to be neither sufficient nor necessary for disease expression. However, it seems clear from twin studies that genes contribute no more than 50% to the absolute risk, although modifier genes may come into play following manifestation of clinical symptoms and/or signs.

General recurrence risks

The excess frequency at which MS recurs in the relatives of affected individuals has been one of the cardinal features of this complex disease recognized since the early part of the 20th century. However, early investigators failed to record their observations in a manner that allowed easy comparison between studies, and it has only been during the 1990s that systematic studies of large populations have been performed. These contemporary studies, as well as further analyses of important subgroups, have provided considerable insight into the nature of the genetic effect in MS and an effective tool for estimating the practical clinical resources necessary to perform molecular genetic studies.

Table 8.2 Meta-analysis of major contemporary studies[10–12] on crude and age-adjusted recurrence risks for relatives of probands with multiple sclerosis

Relative	Combined results			
	*n**	Total population	Crude risk (%)	AAR (%)†
Probands	2163			
Parent	74	3558	2.08	2.11
Sibling	130	5069	2.56	3.23
Child	19	3318	0.57	2.07
Nephew/niece	25	7820	0.32	1.16
Aunt/uncle	85	8702	0.98	1.01
First cousin	99	16096	0.62	0.87
Total	432	44563	0.97	

**n*, Number of affected relatives.
†AAR, age-adjusted recurrence risk.

One of the major difficulties in interpreting recurrence statistics in familial disease is the variable age at onset of MS, so younger generations may not yet have lived to an age at which they are at risk of expressing the disease. Three large studies have overcome this by the application of statistical models that modify the risk according to the established age at onset profile of the affected population to provide AARs. These are derived from the ORs and attempt to deal with each generation in an even-handed way. The first of these was by Sadovnick and colleagues in 1988 who analysed the pedigrees of 815 consecutive patients who attended the MS clinics in Vancouver, Canada;[10] this was followed by a population based study in Cambridgeshire, England[11] using data from 674 probands; and a further consecutive clinic population of 674 patients from Flanders, Belgium.[12] All these studies are reasonably consistent in risks for first degree relatives with maximum risks for siblings (AAR 2.1–3.9%; OR 1.8–2.86%), followed by children (AAR 1.73–2.54%; OR 0.55–0.60%) and parents (AAR 1.61–2.84%; OR 1.59–2.81%). In addition the increased recurrence even in distant relatives such as aunts and uncles (AAR 0.66–1.89%; OR 0.64–1.85%) and first cousins (AAR 0.37–2.16%; OR 0.37–1.30%) unlikely to have shared a common environment strongly supports a genetic effect. A meta-analysis of these studies which includes data from 2163 probands is shown in Table 8.2. There was no preferential recurrence for maternal or paternal inheritance in any of these studies. The greater differences in recurrence risks existing in more distant relatives between studies probably relate to the quality of information concerning disease status available and the extent to which the pedigrees were investigated. The Flanders study in particular was notable for employing government population records and this is reflected in the mean pedigree sizes which were 14, 17 and 39 for the Vancouver, Cambridgeshire and Flanders study, respectively. It should be understood that risks such as these may not be meaningful for populations not dominated by peoples of north European ancestry as familial

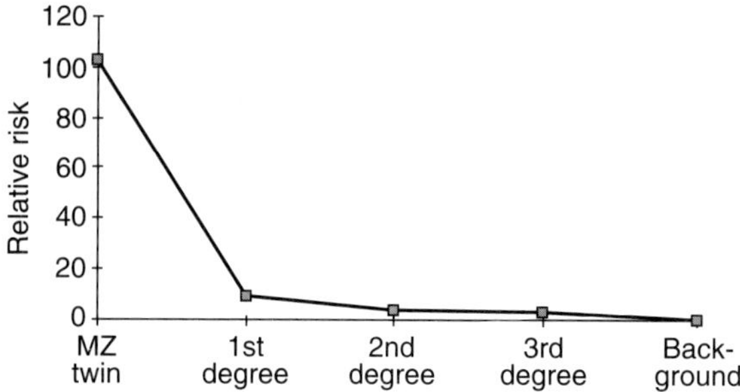

Figure 8.1 Age-adjusted recurrence risks with genetic distance from proband with multiple sclerosis (MZ: monozygous).

recurrence risk is known to vary from 0% to 66% depending on ethnic background and geography.[13,14]

The decrease in relative risk, from over 100 times that in the background population in monozygotic twins with increasing genetic distance from the proband (Fig. 8.1), provides the basis for application of recognized modelling of inheritance to observed patterns of recurrence. This has excluded simple Mendelian inheritance and is based on the observation that the risk to relatives falls by more than a factor of two for each degree of relationship, as would be expected for a single locus or additive model, it has been calculated that three to five genes are responsible for conferring susceptibility in MS assuming equal effect.

Concerns that the increased recurrence rate in relatives was an effect of transmissibility within the close confines of the family environment were addressed by an influential analysis of nonbiological relatives on patients with MS adopted at or soon after birth. Of 1201 nonbiological first-degree relatives of 238 adoptees, only 2 affected individuals were identified compared to the expected number of 51, a figure which did not differ significantly from the background disease frequency in the indigenous population.[15] This has provided convincing evidence that the phenomenon of familial aggregation is dominated by genetic factors. A further study of half siblings demonstrated a predictably intermediate result with 39 of 1395 full siblings, but only 18 of 1839 of the half siblings affected. There was a significant difference between the AAR of half siblings (1.32%) and full siblings (3.46%).[16]

The increased recurrence rate in sibling pairs raises a further interesting caveat to these studies. Doolittle et al.[17] reported a trend towards higher recurrence rates within pedigrees already known to contain concordant sibling pairs and noted an additional family history in 19 of 44 (43%) of cases, whereas the rate was 33% in a study of 166 such families in the UK. Further large population-based studies are needed to clarify this point; if confirmed, it may indicate either a heavier loading of shared susceptibility genes in certain families, perhaps with epistatic effects, or the involvement of different genes in these families, implying genetic heterogeneity. It would also suggest that advice to patients based on recurrence risk for the general population with MS are not appropriate in situations where two first-degree relatives are already affected. This is probably best illustrated by the observed rate of clinically affected offspring of concordant conjugal pairs,[18] which at nearly 6% is 10 times greater than for single affected parents and is undoubtedly the result of increased genetic loading. As in the twin studies, some clinically unaffected offspring with characteristic cranial MR appearances were also identified. The multiplicative rather than additive risk to these children also implicates a strong epistatic effect amongst susceptibility genes.

Molecular genetics

Until recently the avalanche of information provided by family studies has not been mirrored by similar advances in the understanding of molecular genetics. The allelic association with the products of the major histocompatibility complex (MHC) on chromosome 6p21 was reported over 20 years ago[19] and remains the only consistent genetic feature of the disease. Since then population studies have also demonstrated an association between the class II MHC alleles DR15 and DQ6 and their corresponding genotypes, DRB1*1501, DRB5*0101 and DQA1*0102, DQB2*0602.[20–23] Within the MHC region considerable linkage disequilibrium occurs, which has made it difficult to apportion susceptibility to any single gene from the many encoded within this region. At present some of the most promising candidates are genes for the cytokines tumor necrosis factor (TNF-α) and lymphotoxin (TNF-β) which are closely linked and arranged tandomly between the class I and class III loci.[24,25] Further investigation of non-MHC candidates using association and linkage studies has yielded putative candidate genes only in the VH2-5 immunoglobulin heavy chain and T-cell receptor β chain variable regions.[26,27] The proportional risk of each of these clearly does not explain the contribution suggested by family studies and implies the involvement of further genes or epistatic effects that remain to be characterized.

The disappointing results of the candidate gene approach led a number of investigators to tackle a screen of the whole human genome using identity by descent linkage analysis in affected sibling pairs. This method has several advantages over standard pedigree analysis in MS since it requires no assumption of the mode of inheritance, the degree of penetrance, or the disease status of other siblings. The main disadvantage is that each sibling pair contributes relatively little information because of the high chance of sharing genetic markers and many more families are needed to confirm or refute linkage than in a classical linkage study. Power calculations for this type of study are related to the informativeness of the marker (expressed as the polymorphic information content (PIC)),[28] the quality of genetic information available, the number of putative susceptibility loci[29] and the recombination fraction. Computations assuming a significance level of $p < 0.001$ suggest that even with a recombination fraction of 0.05, unequivocal assignment of parental haplotypes and power of only 0.90, the minimum number of sibling pairs required to demonstrate a susceptibility gene of major biological importance is around 75 and may be as high as 500 for a five-locus model with a recombination fraction of 0.05 attempting to gain a power of 99%.[30] Note that no contemporary studies have yet achieved these numbers.

Using methodology pioneered by the genetic analysis of type I diabetes, three genome screens for MS were published in the same edition of *Nature Genetics* in 1996.[31–33] All examined a preliminary cohort of sibling pairs for distortion in expected patterns of sharing of 261–443 anonymous markers at an average genetic distance of around 14cM, but note that the range of markers used by the studies was not consistent and the spread of markers through the genome was not even, so direct comparison of the studies is problematic. However, in this first stage the Canadian and British screen identified 20 and the French/American study 19 regions of preliminary interest with the highest lod score (the odds ratio, expressed as a logarithmic value, of the marker being linked to a susceptibility gene) of 4.24 at D5S406 in the Canadian study. In stage two these regions were examined further by the use of a second cohort of sibling pairs numbering between 23 and 114 and by the use of a denser marker map. This additional analysis and stricter inclusion criteria reduced the areas of interest further and most notable were 6p21 and 17q22 in the British screen, 6p for the French/American screen and 5p and 6p in the Canadian screen. Despite the encouraging epidemiological studies none of these studies identified a gene of major effect in the aetiology of MS and there was a surprising lack of conformity in identified areas of interest except, predictably, for the MHC region which produced the highest multipoint lod score of 3.6 in the French/American study and 19q. The highest maximum lod score (MLS) value in regions of agreement are shown in Table 8.3.

Since these studies use 'anonymous' markers they do not therefore confer risk unless they are known to be in linkage disequilibrium with a relevant gene. The failure of any of the screens to identify a substantial locus indicates that it is

Table 8.3 Stage 1 regions of agreement in genome screens

Region	Highest MLS value in the region		
	UK	American/ French	Canadian
1p	1.2	—	1
3q	—	1.4	1.1
5q	2.6	1.1	—
6p	0.8	2	0.2
6q	0.8	2.4	—
7p	1.8	—	0.9
7q	—	1.1	0.7
19q	1.6	1.6	0.7

very unlikely that such a gene exists; the probability that it would be missed in all three studies is very low. Indeed, exclusion maps of the human genome constructed from available data suggest that a gene of major effect has been excluded in 95%, a gene of moderate effect in 65%, but a gene of minor effect from none of the genome. However, all of the studies identified more low threshold lod scores than would be expected by chance alone, implying that at least some are probably genuine, but it will be important to ensure that these are causally related and do not simply represent survival genes by examining a control cohort. The results of a further genome screen using a smaller number of multiplex families from Scandinavia is also awaited.

QUALITATIVE RISK

Racial influences

Perhaps the most important genetic risk is racial, spreading disease frequency from almost zero in native Africans[34] to 300 per 100 000 population in the Orkney Islands off the northeast coast of Scotland.[35] Some investigators have linked this more closely to the distribution of Scandinavian ancestry associated with the travelling exploits of the Vikings and more recently of migration within the British Empire. Most descriptions of phenotype have been concerned with large populations of Caucasians in Western society, and a striking feature of these studies is the similarity of clinical features including age at onset, sex distribution, disease course, disease duration and diagnostic classification. Analysis of other ethnic groups, with a few exceptions, has been small. One of the most important initial observations on this subject was the modification of the clinical picture of MS in Japanese people by Shibaski et al. in 1981,[36] suggesting the dominant expression of opticospinal disease compared with British patients. This was confirmed in a larger nationwide study of MS in Japan.[37] A similar pattern of severe and dominant opticospinal involvement has subsequently been noted in Chinese Taiwanese people[38] and black Africans.[39]

More recently, immunogenetic and radiological investigations of these patients has revealed an association with the DR2-associated DRB1*1501 allele and DRB5*0101 allele, as well as radiological differences,[40] lending some support to the concept of aetiological heterogeneity in these groups, although the numbers used were small and remain to be confirmed in populations of similar ethnic backgrounds.

Mitochondrial genes

One of the most interesting phenotypic associations in MS is that of dominant visual failure in women and pathogenic mitochondrial mutations. In 1992 Harding et al.[41] reported eight female patients with Leber's hereditary optic neuropathy who went on to develop a MS-like illness with demyelination outside the visual system. These cases all had a mutation at position 11778 in their mitochondrial DNA. In a subsequent review of Leber's hereditary optic neuropathy, Riordan-Eva et al.[42] reported that 45% of 24 female patients with the 11778 mutation had an MS-like illness. Conversely, identification of patients who

Table 8.4 Studies of intrafamilial clinical concordance

Study	Relative	*n*	Age at onset	Year of onset	Disability	Course	Presenting symptom/ site	Sex
Doolittle et al. 1990[17]	Sibling pairs	48	+	–	na†	na	na	+
Sadovnick et al. 1990[48]	Various	47	+	–	–	–	–	+
Bulman et al. 1991[46]	Sibling pairs, Monozygous twins	106	+	–	na	na	na	+
Robertson et al. 1994[47]	Sibling pairs	177	–	–	–	+	–	+

+, Concordance.
–, No concordance.
†, na, data not available.

satisfied recognized criteria for MS who had dominant visual failure revealed that some also had pathogenic Leber's mutations. This syndrome has now also been reported in association with the 3460 mutation.[43]

Several groups have searched for pathological mitochondrial mutations in unrelated, randomly selected MS patients,[43–45] but without success. Other investigators have examined the frequency of the 11778 pathogenic Leber's mutation in Asian-type MS to explain the early and prominent optical involvement outlined above, but have found no difference to Caucasian populations. It seems unlikely, therefore, that a major susceptibility gene for MS is encoded within the mitochondrial genome, although this association probably represents the first gene known to modify the clinical course of MS.

Intrafamilial concordance

Over the past few years there have been several studies that have examined patterns of familial recurrence, but few that have examined patterns of clinical concordance. Classically concordant monozygotic twins would provide the optimum cohort to assess this question, but the numbers available in any one study do not exceed 11. The existing data do not show clear patterns of clinical concordance but there remains no systematic study addressing this issue. However, identification of patterns of clinical concordance within families would provide a useful insight into those features of phenotype that may be influenced by genetic factors and which are, therefore, potentially areas in which genotyping may offer prognostic value.

In the face of numerical limitations of twin studies investigators have looked for other, familial associations, especially in concordant sibling pairs. Three large contemporary analyses of the clinical features of sibling pairs have been published. All involve a formidable array of statistical interpretation with variable attempts to circumnavigate the selection bias that is inevitable in recruitment of these families and that tends to accentuate clinical similarities. Apart from age at onset, and possibly disease course, these studies demonstrate a general lack of correlation of clinical features among relatives (Table 8.4).

In a study of 48 sibling pairs with relapsing–remitting MS, Doolittle et al.[17] demonstrated that age at onset was within 5 years in 30 of 48 sibling pairs compared to only 16 of 48 controls—a phenomenon that was interpreted as supportive of a genetic effect. No analysis was undertaken for other clinical features. A larger analysis from the Canadian clinics[46] also approached the issue of year and age at onset, again finding a significant intraclass correlation in 99 non-twin sibling pairs ($p < 0.01$) which was more marked in seven concordant monozygotic twin pairs. No concordance was demonstrated for year at onset and it was concluded that the results support a genetic effect on age at onset with random environmental exposure and no evidence for a common environmental trigger.

The largest study from the UK[47] attempted to address various other aspects of clinical concordance apart from age and year at onset in 177 sibling pairs. No significant correlation for age at onset after correction for selection bias was observed, but a minor correlation for age at onset was found that was felt to be due to earlier recognition of symptoms in second affected siblings. There was no pair-wise concordance for presenting symptoms or disability at time of assessment. However, there was a strong correlation for disease course and to a lesser degree for gender. These results were interpreted as suggesting that the aetiology of MS involves random exposure to an as yet unidentified environmental trigger and that the clinical features of familial disease are indeed modified by inherited factors.

A further study by Sadovnick et al. examined clinical concordance in 47 various first-, second- and third-degree relative pairs,[48] and found no similarities for clinical course, lesion site or initial symptom, but again confirmed the later finding of the same group of correlation for age at onset in 15 sibling pairs. Finally, note that although no correlation for age at onset was demonstrated in the 12 parent–child pairs examined by this group, an analysis of affected offspring of concordant conjugal pairs, single affected parents and sporadic cases[18] demonstrated a trend for earlier age at onset in successive generations, which if confirmed would have interesting implications for genetic models of inheritance.

FUTURE STUDIES

Comparison of observed recurrence risks with identified molecular genetic risks suggests that there is still much to be explained and, despite recent advances, the best predictor of disease expression in unaffected individuals remains their relationship to an affected relative, and is the highest for monozygotic twins (Fig. 8.2). Most evidence now suggests that disease susceptibility is controlled by several genes, at least one of which is encoded within the MHC region on chromosome 6q; all may differ in their relative interaction and contribution, and they need not be spread evenly among populations at risk. Without the identification of a single susceptibility gene or cell systems to elucidate more precisely their role, it is clearly premature to think about genetic modification of phenotype. However, there is some encouraging epidemiological evidence that this may be possible and research areas that may be rewarding are disease course, age at onset and the relative excess of affected female sibling pairs, hinting at a contribution of sex independent of genes. Currently valuable information may be gleaned from a meta-analysis of the three genome screens and clinical and genetic stratification of the available data. The use of denser marker maps down to 1cM has so far proved of limited value, although this provides further confirmation of the relevance of some areas such as 17q in the UK study and its main benefit seems to be in extending the exclusion maps. Narrowing down the search in regions of interest is likely to require additional information provided by transmission disequilibrium testing (TDT).

Other epidemiological and family studies in which additional information would contribute to our understanding of this complex disease include the evaluation of recurrence risks in

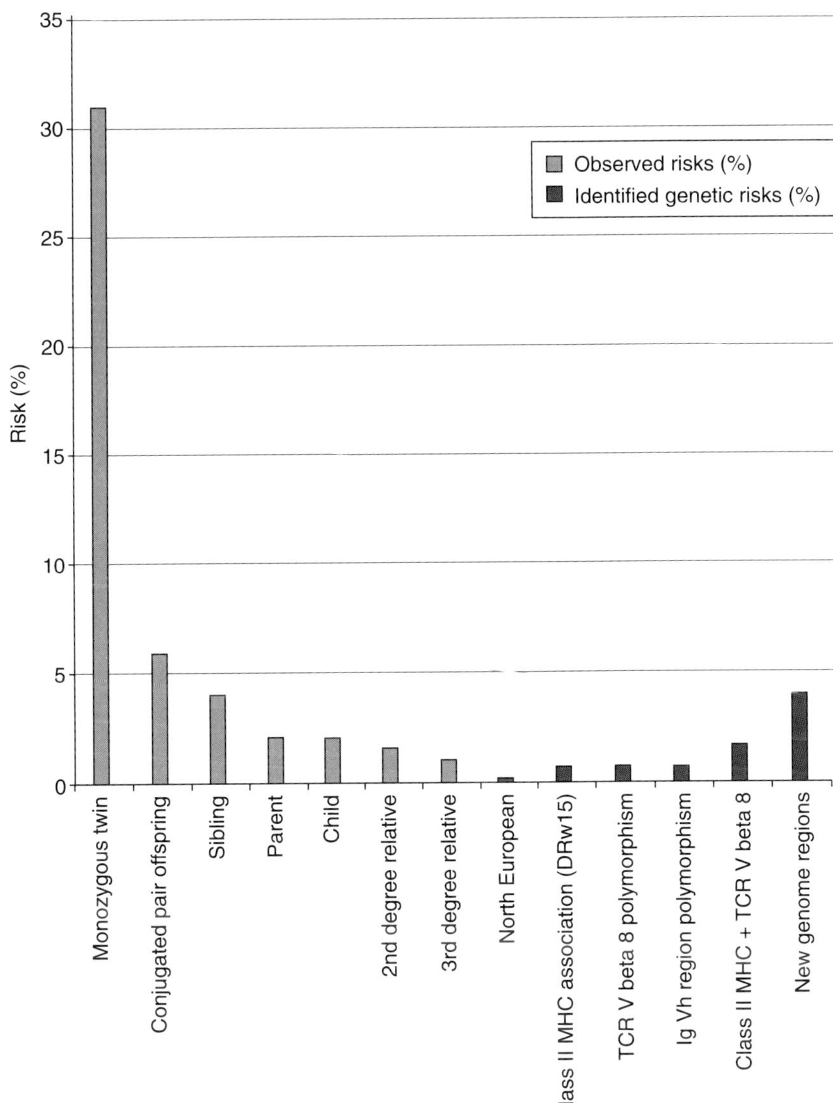

Figure 8.2 Comparison of identified molecular genetic and familial recurrence risks.

multiplex families to demonstrate whether risk is spread evenly over the population or concentrated in high-risk families, the variability of ethnic phenotype, clinical concordance in concordant monozygotic twins and age at onset in successive generations with MS.

The identification of a single gene unequivocally involved in disease susceptibility currently remains elusive, as does the identification of genes that have a major impact on disease course, but these goals remain attainable.

REFERENCES

1. Bobowick AR, Kurtzke JF, Brody JA et al. Twin study of multiple sclerosis: an epidemiological enquiry. *Neurology* 1978; **28**: 978–987.

2. Heltberg A, Holm NV. Concordance in twins and recurrence in sibships in multiple sclerosis. *Lancet* 1982; **i**: 1068.
3. Kinnunen E, Koskenvuo M, Kaprio J et al. Multiple sclerosis in a nationwide series of twins. *Neurology* 1987; **37**: 1627–1629.
4. Williams A, Eldridge R, MacFarland H et al. Multiple sclerosis in twins. *Neurology* 1980; **30**: 1139–1147.
5. Uitdehaag BMJ, Polman CH, Valk J et al. Magnetic resonance imaging studies in multiple sclerosis twins. *J Neurol Neurosurg Psychiatry* 1989; **52**: 1417–1419.
6. French Research Group on Multiple Sclerosis. Multiple sclerosis in 54 twinships: concordance is independent of zygosity. *Ann Neurol* 1992; **32**: 724–727.
7. Mumford CJ, Wood NW, Kellar-Wood H et al. The British Isles Survey of Multiple Sclerosis in Twins. *Neurology* 1994; **44**: 5–11.
8. Ebers GC, Bulman DE, Sadovnik AD et al. A population-based study of multiple sclerosis in twins. *N Engl J Med* 1986; **315**: 1638–1642.
9. Sadovnick AD, Armstrong H, Rice GPA et al. A population-based study of multiple sclerosis in twins: update. *Ann Neurol* 1993; **33**: 281–285.
10. Sadovnick AD, Baird PA, Ward RH. Multiple sclerosis: updated risks for relatives. *Am J Med Genet* 1988; **29**: 533–541.
11. Robertson N, Deans J, Fraser M et al. Recurrence risks for relatives of patients with multiple sclerosis. *Brain* 1996; **119**: 449–455.
12. Carton H, Vlietinck R, Debruyne J et al. Risks of multiple sclerosis in relatives of patients in Flanders, Belgium. *J Neurol Neurosurg Psychiatry* 1997; **62**: 329–333.
13. Binzer M, Forsgren L, Holmgren G et al. Familial clustering of multiple sclerosis in a northern Swedish rural district. *J Neurol Neurosurg Psychiatry* 1994; **57**: 497–499.
14. Yu YL, Woo E, Hawkins BR et al. Multiple sclerosis amongst Chinese in Hong Kong. *Brain* 1989; **112**: 1445–1467.
15. Ebers GC. A genetic basis for familial aggregation in multiple sclerosis. *Nature* 1995; **377**: 150–151.
16. Sadovnick AD, Ebers GC, Dyment DA et al. CCS. Evidence for genetic basis of multiple sclerosis. *Lancet* 1996; **347**: 1728–1730.
17. Doolittle TH, Myers RH, Lehrich JR et al. Multiple sclerosis sibling pairs: clustered onset and familial predisposition. *Neurology* 1990; **40**: 937–950.
18. Robertson NP, O'Riordan J, Chataway J et al. Offspring recurrence rates and clinical characteristics of conjugal multiple sclerosis. *Lancet* 1997; **349**: 1587–1590.
19. Jersild C, Svejgaard A, Fog J. HLA antigens and multiple sclerosis. *Lancet* 1972; **i**: 1240–1241.
20. Jersild C, Fog T, Hansen GS et al. Histocompatibility determinants in multiple sclerosis, with special reference to clinical course. *Lancet* 1973; **ii**: 1221–1225.
21. Olerup O, Hillert J. HLA class II-associated genetic susceptibility in multiple sclerosis: a critical evaluation. *Tissue Antigen* 1991; **38**: 1–15.
22. Spurkland A, Roniningen K, Vandvik B et al. HLA-DQA1 and HLA-DQB1 genes may jointly determine susceptibility to develop multiple sclerosis. *Hum Immun* 1991; **30**: 69–75.
23. Kellar-Wood HF, Holmans P, Clayton D et al. Multiple sclerosis and the HLA-D region—linkage and association studies. *J Neuroimmunol* 1995; **58**: 183–190.
24. Kirk CW, Droogan AG, Hawkins SA et al. Tumour necrosis factor microsatellites show association with multiple sclerosis. *J Neurol Sci* 1997; **147**: 21–25.
25. Epplen C, Jackel S, Santos EJM. Genetic predisposition to multiple sclerosis as revealed by immunoprinting. *Ann Neurol* 1997; **41**: 341–352.
26. Wood NW, Holmans P, Clayton P et al. The T-cell receptor-beta locus and susceptibility to multiple sclerosis. *Neurology* 1995; **45**: 1859–1863.
27. Wood NW, Kellar-Wood HF, Robertson NP et al. Susceptibility to multiple sclerosis and the immunoglobulin heavy chain variable region. *J Neurol* 1995; **242**: 677–682.
28. Risch N. Linkage strategies for genetically complex traits. III. The effect of marker polymorphism on the analysis of affected relative pairs. *Am J Hum Genet* 1990; **46**: 242–253.
29. Risch N. Linkage strategies for genetically complex traits. II. The power of affected relative pairs. *Am J Hum Genet* 1990; **46**: 229–241.
30. Robertson NP, Wood NW, Holmans P et al. Strategies for the identification of susceptibility genes in multiple sclerosis. *Int Multiple Sclerosis J* 1995; **2**: 1–7.
31. Sawcer S, Jones HB, Feakes R et al. A genome screen reveals susceptibility loci on chromosome 6p21 and 17q22. *Nature Genetics* 1996; **13**: 464–468.
32. The Multiple Sclerosis Genetics Group. A complete genomic screen for multiple sclerosis

underscores a role for the major histocompatibility complex. *Nature Genetics* 1996; **13**: 469–471.

33. Ebers GC, Kukay K, Bulman DE et al. A full genome search in multiple sclerosis. *Nature Genetics* 1996; **13**: 472–476.
34. Cochrane JC. Disseminated sclerosis in a non-European female. *South African Med J* 1947; **21**: 613–617.
35. Poskanzer DC, Prenny LB, Sheridan JL et al. Multiple sclerosis in the Orkney and Shetland Islands. 1: Epidemiology, clinical factors and methodology. *J Epidemiol Commun Health* 1980; **34**: 229–239.
36. Shibasaki H, MacDonald WI, Kuroiwa Y. Racial modification of clinical picture of multiple sclerosis: comparison between British and Japanese patients. *J Neurol Sci* 1981; **49**: 253–271.
37. Kuroiwa Y, Igata A, Itahara K et al. Nationwide survey of multiple sclerosis in Japan; clinical analysis of 1,084 cases. *Neurology* 1975; **25**: 845–851.
38. Hung T, Landsborough D, Hsi M. Multiple sclerosis amongst Chinese in Taiwan. *J Neurol Sci* 1976; **27**: 459–484.
39. Dean G, Bhigjee AIG, Bill PLA et al. Multiple sclerosis in black South Africans and Zimbabweans. *J Neurol Neurosurg Psychiatry* 1994; **57**: 1064–1069.
40. Kira J, Kanai T, Nishimura Y et al. Western versus Asian types of multiple sclerosis: Immunogenetically and clinically distinct disorders. *Ann Neurol* 1996; **40**: 569–574.
41. Harding AE, Sweeney MG, Miller DM et al. Occurrence of a multiple sclerosis-like illness in women who have a Leber's hereditary optic neuropathy mitochondrial DNA mutation. *Brain* 1992; **115**: 979–989.
42. Riordan-Eva P, Sanders M, Goven GG et al. The clinical features of Leber's hereditary optic neuropathy defined by the presence of a pathogenic mitochondrial mutation. *Brain* 1995; **118**: 319–337.
43. Kellar-Wood H, Robertson NP, Goven GG et al. Leber's optic neuropathy mitochondrial DNA mutations in multiple sclerosis. *Ann Neurol* 1994; **36**: 109–112.
44. Kalman B, Lublin FD, Alder H. Mitochondrial DNA mutations in multiple sclerosis. *Multiple Sclerosis* 1995; **1**: 32–36.
45. Nishimura M, Obayashi H, Ohta M et al. No association of the 11778 mitochondrial DNA mutation and multiple sclerosis in Japan. *Neurology* 1995; **45**: 1333–1334.
46. Bulman DE, Sadovnik AD, Ebers GC. Age of onset in sibling pairs concordant for multiple sclerosis. *Brain* 1991; **114**: 937–950.
47. Robertson NP, Fraser M, Deans J et al. Multiple sclerosis in sibling pairs. *Neurology* 1996; **47**: 347–352.
48. Sadovnick AD, Hashimoto LL, Hashimoto SA. Heterogeneity in multiple sclerosis: Comparison of clinical manifestations in relatives. *Can J Neurol Sci* 1990; **49**: 253–271.

9

Clinical predictive factors in multiple sclerosis

Christian Confavreux

INTRODUCTION

Predicting the outcome of multiple sclerosis (MS) is regaining interest at a time when MS is entering a therapeutic era; indeed, it is essential to identify the patients with a presumed bad prognosis who deserve early active treatment. Despite several works devoted to this topic, MS outcome still seems unpredictable. The disease course varies from periods of intense activity to utter clinical silence, apparently regardless of any logic, and the disease outcome is extremely diverse, as forms of MS range from benign to malignant. Lastly, it is even more difficult to predict disease outcome at disease onset, before assessment of the clinical activity of the disease in the patients has been possible. However, there are some evolutional laws emerging from this apparent chaos. This is what may be drawn from several works in the literature.[1–9]

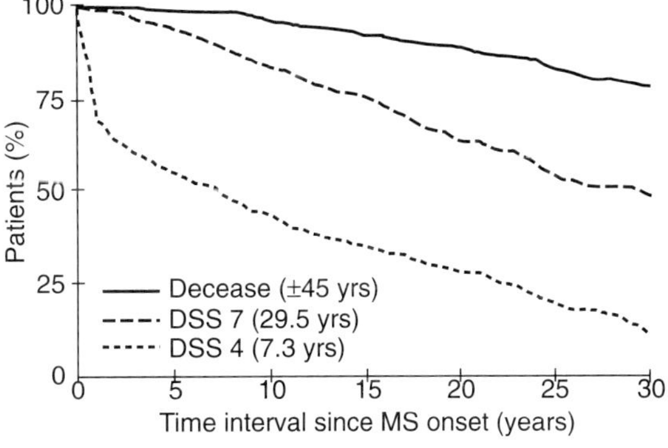

Figure 9.1 Residual disability and survival expectancy in MS. Actuarial method of Kaplan–Meier: proportion (%) of patients still free of DSS 4 (dotted curve), still free of DSS 7 (broken curve), and still alive (solid curve) according to time elapsed since the onset of MS. Lyon MS Database. All 1191 MS patients.

FIRST CERTAINTY: GENERAL EVOLUTION OF THE DISEASE

When considering a cohort of patients representative of the disease from a statistical point of view, the overall evolution is presently well defined. For instance, the inaugural study of our group[3] using the life-table analysis of Kaplan–Meier allowed us to show a 2-year interval between the first and the second relapses in the exacerbating–remitting forms of the disease. The residual disability assessed on Kurtzke's expanded disability status scale (EDSS), shows that 7 years on average elapse for patients to reach grade 4, and 29 years for grade 7. Survival is estimated at 45 years showing that MS does not affect overall survival; however, the patient spends 15 years or so in utter dependence (see Fig. 9.1). These data corroborate other studies of the literature using the same statistical method, notably the Canadian series,[4] which brought about additional information on the time interval to reach EDSS grade 6—15 years on average.

SECOND CERTAINTY: INTERINDIVIDUAL VARIABILITY

Patients should understand that these figures represent only an average. Though the information is representative and sufficient in diseases with a consistent and homogeneous outcome from one patient to another, like many cancers, this is completely different in MS. Indeed, there is a full range of evolution in MS, from benign forms without real sequelae after 20 years of evolution, to malignant forms that are rapidly disabling in a few months. There are even totally asymptomatic forms which are inadvertently discovered on brain magnetic resonance imaging (MRI) or anatomical verification and, in contrast lethal forms as described by Marburg. This notion is essential. Too often, people believe that MS condemns the patient to a wheelchair sooner or later. In fact, a proportion of patients lead a normal or almost normal life. In the large cohorts of the literature, benign forms represents 25–30% of the cases; epidemiological studies also confirm this rate, which goes unnoticed in hospital-based series.

THIRD CERTAINTY: A STEADY EVOLUTION FOR A GIVEN PATIENT

Though of acknowledged importance, the above notions offer only a relative interest when considering a given patient. At disease onset, the question that is raised regards the patient's future. Torben Fog's works in the late 1960s deserve to be quoted here.[5] This Danish neurologist had designed an original system of quantitative neurological examination and used it each time a patient came to visit. More than 70 patients were followed-up this way every 3 months for several years. For each patient, the successive scores were plotted on a diagram, with reference to the date of the examination on the x-axis. The result was all the more surprising since the disease is supposed to evolve by steps, i.e. by relapses, especially at onset. Indeed, for all his patients, Fog observed a very steady evolution of the scores of examination, in spite of minimal fluctuations. When making a regression analysis to identify the mathematical equation as close as possible to the real curve, the result was a linear curve in most cases. In some other cases, the result was a parabola or hyperbola, but with a very weak inflexion. In other words, when the patient is followed-up using this mathematical technique in a regular and frequent way, it is possible to establish the rate of worsening of the neurological disability. It is also quite possible to extrapolate and draw the curve beyond the last available score and, therefore, to predict the disease course.

Fog's work is well documented. Apart from very few exceptions, all his patients respected this steady pattern of evolution; and actually this conclusion is not that surprising. Isolated optic neuritis is a striking event at the functional level, but it represents minor changes in terms of objective examination and, by extension, of lesion load.

Fog's observations are of paramount importance. They suggest that the worsening of the neurological symptoms and, therefore, the central nervous system deterioration in patients with MS, most often follows a steady evolution for a given patient.

. . . AND THE NUMEROUS UNCERTAINTIES

Here are the three main certainties of the course of MS. Concretely, where does that lead to? The first two notions are essential to public health services, insurance companies and economists. They are useful also to physicians in sample size calculations for designing protocols of therapeutic trials, but they do not represent much to the patients. This is where Fog's work is meaningful. Unfortunately, Fog's determinist approach requires that the patient be seen on a regular and frequent basis for a time- and energy-consuming quantitative neurological examination. The period of observation must be long enough, and the patient, as well as the physician, must show obstinacy, rigour and reliability to this discipline over several months, and even years. If both protagonists match this portrait, after several years the curve of examination results will bring about a reliable extrapolation; thus, this technique allows a 'prognosis a posteriori' to be established.

As a consequence, other approaches have attempted to answer the question of the individual prognosis. For instance, probabilistic models allow us to study the influence of some factors upon the rate of installation of the different grades of disability, using for instance the model of life-table analysis. The factors usually studied are the ones easily identified at the onset of the disease, since it is then that the prognosis is asked for with the deepest interest. Other factors identified in the first stages of the disease have also been used, such as the time interval between the first two relapses or the interval to reach EDSS grade 4. Lately, the results of the initial MRI have also been considered. All the studies reveal corroborating information:[1–10]

(a) gender has no real impact on the prognosis; disease severity is comparable in male and female patients
(b) age at disease onset, the nature of the first symptoms, the form of onset either remittent or progressive, the time interval between the first two relapses and the interval to reach EDSS grade 4 of Kurtzke's scale are some factors which may have a predictive value on the course of the disease in the long run; an early onset, a semiology of optic neuritis or brainstem syndrome in the first place rather than a long tracts syndrome, an exacerbating–remitting rather than progressive course, a long interval between the first two relapses, a long interval to reach EDSS grade 4 of disability are as many factors which may predict a rather slow evolution of the disease
(c) considering the MRI data, the presence of lesions, a great number of lesions and a large lesion load indicate a greater short-term risk for a new relapse or for significant residual disability.[11–15]

All this information is true and has concrete applications. For instance, therapeutic trials carried out today in early MS exclude patients with a normal brain MRI. Indeed, the risk that such patients will suffer a new relapse or a residual disability in the short-term is too low. Unfortunately, these data are not really pertinent for a given patient. Even if the correlations are statistically significant, they are not powerful enough to allow a precise, accurate prognosis. Above all, although diverse, many factors are tightly interrelated. Indeed, age at disease onset, inaugural symptoms, disease course at onset and time interval to reach EDSS grade 4 are closely correlated. For instance, an early onset is most often associated to optic neuritis, an exacerbating–remitting form and a long interval to reach EDSS grade 4 of disability. Conversely, a late onset is most often associated with a primary progressive form, long tracts syndrome at onset and quick progress to grade 4 disability. The single outstanding factor for the previous group is the interval for the second relapse to occur in the exacerbating–remitting forms of the disease. This also applies to the MRI parameters: correlations with the prognosis are too weak to be of interest at the level of a single patient.

In conclusion, to establish the prognosis for a given patient with MS looks like a Gordian knot. Realistic approaches of the probabilistic kind bear little predictive value. The deterministic approaches, which are much more powerful, are none the less unrealistic in many respects. It seems that clinical markers will remain unreliable for predicting the outcome in MS. Other kinds of markers are to be assessed. It may be expected that new magnetic resonance techniques, by allowing a more precise analysis of axonal loss, demyelination and gliosis, could serve this purpose. However, they are still to be refined and validated.

ACKNOWLEDGEMENTS

Supported by grants from the Commission of the European Communities DG XII (Contracts No. BMH1-CT93-1529, No. CIPD-CT94-0227 and No. BMH4-CT96-0064), and by funds from the Ligue Française contre la Sclérose En Plaques (LFSEP) and the Association pour la Recherche sur la Sclérose en Plaques (ARSEP).

REFERENCES

1. Müller R. Studies on disseminated sclerosis. With special reference to symptomatology, course and prognosis. *Acta Med Scand* 1949; **133 (suppl 222)**:: 1–214.
2. McAlpine D, Lumsden CE, Acheson ED. *Multiple Sclerosis: A Reappraisal*. Edinburgh: Churchill Livingstone, 1972.
3. Confavreux C, Aimard G, Devic M. Course and prognosis of multiple sclerosis assessed by the computerized data processing of 349 patients. *Brain* 1980; **103**: 281–300.
4. Weinshenker BG, Bass B, Rice GPA et al. The natural history of multiple sclerosis: a geographically based study. 1. Clinical course and disability. *Brain* 1989; **112**: 133–146.
5. Fog T, Linneman F. The course of multiple sclerosis in 73 cases with computer designed curves. *Acta Neurol Scand* 1970; **46 (suppl 47)**: 1–175.
6. Patzold V, Pocklington PR. Course of multiple sclerosis. First results of a prospective study carried out of 102 MS patients from 1976–1980. *Acta Neurol Scand* 1982; **65**: 248–266.
7. Phadke JG. Clinical aspects of multiple sclerosis in north-east Scotland with particular reference to its course and prognosis. *Brain* 1990; **113**: 1597–1628.
8. Moreau T. *Pronostic de la Sclérose en Plaques. A propos de 1187 observations*. Thèse de Médecine, Université Claude Bernard, Lyon, 1992.
9. Runmarker B, Andersen O. Prognostic factors in a multiple sclerosis incidence cohort with twenty-five years of follow-up. *Brain* 1993; **116**: 117–134.
10. Weinshenker BG, Bass B, Rice GPA et al. The natural history of multiple sclerosis: a geographically based study. 2. Predictive value of the early clinical course. *Brain* 1989; **112**: 1419–1428.
11. Miller DH, Ormerod IEC, Rudge P et al. The early risk of multiple sclerosis following isolated acute syndromes of the brainstem and the spinal cord. *Ann Neurol* 1989; **26**: 635–639.
12. Lee KH, Hashimoto SA, Hooge JP et al. Magnetic resonance imaging of the head in the diagnosis of multiple sclerosis: a prospective 2-year follow-up with comparison of clinical evaluation, evoked potentials, oligoclonal banding, and CT. *Neurology* 1991; **41**: 657–660.
13. Miller DH, Morrissey SP, McDonald WI. The prognostic significance of brain MRI at presentation with a single clinical episode of suspected demyelination: a five-year follow-up study. *Neurology* 1992; **42 (suppl 3)**: 427 [abstract].
14. Filippi M, Horsfield MA, Morrissey SP et al. Quantitative brain MRI lesion load predicts the course of clinically isolated syndromes suggestive of multiple sclerosis. *Neurology* 1994; **44**: 635–641.
15. Paty DW, Koopmans RA, Ken Redekop W et al. Does the MRI activity rate predict the clinical course of MS? *Neurology* 1992; **42 (suppl 3)**: 427 [abstract].

10

Multiple sclerosis in children: a review

Mefkure Eraksoy

In this chapter, clinical and laboratory characteristics of childhood multiple sclerosis (MS) and its variants will be reviewed and the controversies surrounding childhood MS will be addressed.

INTRODUCTION

Children with MS have been reported since the end of the 1800s. However, there are few reliable reports concerning manifestations of MS before the age of 10.[1–3] Earlier reports described many patients in which several alternative diagnoses had been made, including acute disseminated encephalomyelitis (ADEM), leukodystrophy, and subacute sclerosing panencephalitis.[3,4] Observations from epidemiological studies conducted in regions where MS has a high incidence, and frequency of MS in individuals migrating from high risk areas to low risk areas, suggest that MS is an adulthood disease with an initial occurrence at 14–45 years of age.[5] Findings from epidemiological studies indicate there is general agreement that a disease course initiated by exposure to an infectious agent during prepuberty may, after a latency period, culminate in a disease process presenting with MS manifestations. Diagnostic criteria accepting the age of MS onset as 10–59 years have inevitably led to the neglect of disease occurrence below age 10.[6,7] Diagnosis of MS is rarely considered in young children on the part of a paediatricians and neurologists, who are unaware of the disease appearance before age 10. The onset may be so mild or recurrences so unimpressive that medical aid is not sought. A family may ignore the child's strange numbness, unsteadiness or slight weakness. A second attack may be similarly ignored and, if remission is followed by no further symptoms, the disorder may escape medical observation. Otherwise, an onset is so severe that the child visits a physician, but in this age group the correct diagnosis may be a problem, particularly when paraclinical findings are absent. Moreover, because relationships between MS and its variants (such as Schilder's myelinoclastic diffuse sclerosis (MDS), Devic's syndrome, and Marburg disease) and its atypical forms (such as acute encephalopathy) are not well recognized, and many patients may not receive appropriate attention or may be underdiagnosed. These patients, however, require follow-up—even for decades—for a precise diagnosis to be made.

Controversies on childhood MS can be listed as follows:

(a) actual incidence and more common mode of onset of MS below 10

(b) similarities and dissimilarities between childhood, juvenile and adult forms as regards clinical manifestations, its course and other clinical and laboratory characteristics
(c) relationships between MS and childhood infections and vaccinations.

INCIDENCE

Incidence of MS before age 16 has been reported as 1.2–6%.[8–12] An incidence of 1.5–7 per 1000 is estimated before age 10.[6,9–11, 14] Poser, in a study of 812 patients, reported only one patient with an onset of disease before age 10,[15] while Sheperd documented that none of the patients in his series ($n = 464$) presented with a history of MS manifestations before age 10.[16] The earliest age at onset of MS came from an autopsy report of a 10-month-old infant.[17] Other studies reported varying ages from 1.5 to 15 years.[3,4,9–12,18–27]

An analysis of childhood MS studies demonstrates a female preponderance.[3,9–12,23,28,29]

FAMILIAL CHARACTERISTICS

Familial occurrence is one of the cardinal epidemiological features of MS. Familial forms have been shown in several childhood MS series.[3,9,10–12] Risk of occurrence in childhood with MS-affected parents has been studied comprehensively.[30–32]

INFECTIONS AND VACCINATION

Infections occur frequently in childhood. Several studies have explored the possible role of infections and related vaccinations in future MS development but could not reach any firm conclusions.[33–35] Data from retrospective reviews of adult MS series have not been encouraging enough. However the demonstration in prospective series of the features of multiphasic diseases and the possibility of developing these diseases after para- and post-infectious encephalomyelopathies and isolated cranial nerve involvement in childhood may be of relevance.

INITIAL MANIFESTATIONS

Similar to most of the adult series, initial manifestations in childhood MS series are characterized by monosymptomatic onset or isolated syndromes. Optic neuritis and sensory and motor signs/symptoms, brainstem and spinal cord syndromes have been described as initial manifestations.[2–4,9–12,14,36] Initial presentation of childhood MS may resemble a clinical picture similar to that of an acute encephalopathy.[18,28,37–40] The higher incidence of seizures, encephalopathy and dementia seen in children in some series were not confirmed by other studies.[4,9–11,28,41–43]

Another atypical mode of presentation of childhood MS is that accompanied by one or two tumor-like, large, inflammatory demyelinating lesions confined more often to the centrum semiovale. Poser has shown that these symptoms are distinctive and rare in nature and represent an acute form of MS seen more often in children.[44] They are defined as Schilder's MDS.[44,45] The reliability and validity of these diagnostic criteria have been confirmed in juvenile and adult patients.[46,47] Kepes reported a total of 31 children and adults with large, focal, tumor-like cerebral demyelinating lesions.[48] Twenty-eight patients were free from new lesion development; however, three patients developed new lesions consistent with an MS course during 9–12 months of follow-up. The author proposed that these large, focal, tumor-like brain lesions may be a transitional pattern between MS and ADEM.[48] On the other hand, it is well-recognized that large, tumor-like demyelinating lesions may develop during the course of MS.[49–55] MS in an 11-year-old girl with an onset of a tumor-like lesion in the cerebellum exhibited a large demyelinating lesion.[56] Another significant observation is that Devic's syndrome was followed by Schilder's MDS in an adult patient.[57] Although Devic's neuromyelitis optica differs from classical MS with regard to clinical and laboratory findings, some of the childhood MS series included patients with opticospinal involvement mimicking Devic's syndrome with a relapsing–remitting course.[4,36,43,58–61] Recently, inflammatory demyelinating lesions in the spinal cord and cerebrum have been demonstrated on MRI examination of a 4-year-old boy who developed Devic's syndrome, and the need for a long-term follow-up to evaluate future MS risk has been emphasized.[62] Some atypical presentations and variants might represent transitional forms between MS, ADEM, MDS and Devic's syndrome, arising from both the development and interactions of the immune and central nervous systems.[4,48,63] The lack of definitive clinical signs and the presence of atypical radiological and histopathological findings of atypical MS forms and its variants may be misleading to clinicians, neuroradiologists and pathologists.[48,52,53] Appropriate recording of such cases and determining the abovementioned transitional forms may shed light on the inflammatory demyelinating course and the dynamics involved.

DIFFERENTIAL DIAGNOSIS

ADEM, adrenoleukodystrophy, other genetic metabolic diseases, subacute sclerosing panencephalitis and, more recently, mitochondrial encephalopathies, neuroborreliosis and collagen vascular diseases are important considerations for the clinical and histopathological differential diagnosis of childhood MS. With the introduction of new diagnostic techniques, such as magnetic resonance imaging (MRI) immunological evaluation of the cerebrospinal fluid (CSF), evoked potential tests, and metabolic screening tests, the differential diagnosis has been somewhat facilitated, and the number of reported patients is steadily increasing.[64–69]

DIAGNOSIS

Since no specific diagnostic test is available, diagnosis of childhood MS presents particular difficulty and additional challenge. Although criteria by Poser and coworkers do not take into consideration patients below age 10, it seems to be convenient, at least under current circumstances, to apply these criteria in reaching a diagnosis of MS during childhood.[70] To ensure a clinical diagnosis of MS at all ages a meticulous follow-up of patients is essential. Because of known difficulties in disease onset and differential diagnosis, paraclinical tests may help a correct diagnosis of MS in childhood.

CEREBROSPINAL FLUID FINDINGS

Pleocytosis of CSF is a well-recognized finding during acute exacerbations and initial episode of childhood MS. Intrathecal oligoclonal bands or CSF IgG elevation was only reported in a minority of the patients.[4,5,28,70] This is probably partly owing to various case reports from when adequate CSF techniques were not available. Some authors have reported that CSF in children with MS was less frequently positive than adults for oligoclonal IgG bands.[36,71]

NEUROIMAGING

Computerized tomography (CT) may often fail to demonstrate demyelinating lesions well enough to provide a diagnosis whereas the more sensitive MRI is an exclusively important diagnostic tool, particularly in the early stages. MRI appears to be the neuroimaging test of choice for making a diagnosis of childhood MS.[28,65–67,69,70] It reveals clinically silent lesions and demonstrates the multifocal distribution of lesions in the central nervous system, gadolinium-DTPA-enhanced MRI provides valuable information for dissemination in time. Imaging findings in children with MS are not significantly different from those in adults. The incidence of tumefacient plaques and posterior fossa plaques may be somewhat higher. Tumefacient plaques can sometimes be differentiated from tumors by the presence of other, more typical plaques, minimal or lack of mass effect, location adjacent to the ventricular surface, and enhancement limited to only one side of the lesion.[11,44,45,48,55,72] Magnetic resonance spectroscopy (MRS) findings of childhood

MS have been reported. Being a noninvasive technique, MRS seems to be useful in providing information about metabolic alterations of the MS plaques and prognosis of MS.[73]

EVOKED POTENTIALS

Although evoked potentials are useful in demonstrating silent MS lesions, they are not specific. Interpretation of evoked potentials obtained from a developing nervous system during childhood is difficult, and their role in routine examinations is controversial.[28,70]

NEUROPATHOLOGY

Confounding data has been provided by the many autopsy reports of childhood MS dating from the late 1800s, and more recent histological and cytological findings have also been drawn from case autopsies and biopsies. In some cases, findings were consistent with the classical forms of MS, while in others, although alternative diagnoses were excluded, available evidence was insufficient for an accurate diagnosis.[6,11,17,36,37,41,44,54,56,74–76] Well-classified clinical, laboratory and histopathological data collected through investigations performed using an appropriately designed protocol may give important diagnostic clues.

COURSE AND PROGNOSIS

There is limited data concerning the long-term prognosis of children with MS. Information obtained from large series shows that MS during childhood tends to exhibit a relapsing–remitting course and, compared to adult series, a primary progressive course is less likely. Childhood MS probably presents with a high rate of recovery from the initial attack, and exhibits a slow progression.[9–11] Poor progression has been reported in a few childhood MS series.[75,77]

THERAPY AND MANAGEMENT

There are no controlled clinical trials for the treatment of childhood MS. Many attacks may spontaneously improve in a short time, without leaving any sequela or requiring a specific treatment. A clinical picture of moderate severity affecting the quality of life can be treated with prednisolone 1–2 mg/kg per day, while severe forms can be treated with high doses of methylprednisolone.[40,78] In a progressive course, a combination of symptomatic treatment, psychological support, and physical therapy and rehabilitation is essential. The role of interferon beta therapy in the treatment of childhood MS should be evaluated only after elucidation of the natural course, the clinical and laboratory features, and the diagnostic criteria of the disease in this age group, and confirmation of its application to adult treatment modalities.

CONCLUSION

Current data suggest that classical MS seems to be rare below age 10. The disease is often initiated by visual loss, brainstem and sensory and/or motor manifestations. It has not yet been clarified, however, whether MS in children below age 10 has a mode of onset suggesting relapsing encephalomyelitis. A predilection of the diseases for girls is remarkable, particularly after puberty. In childhood, MS variants and atypical MS forms, which present a difficult diagnostic problem, may be encountered.

Imaging findings in childhood MS are not significantly different from those in adults except for some unusual tumefacient plaques. Although we do not know its sensitivity in childhood MS, MRI seems to be an important diagnostic tool.

Awareness of the disease in young children and multicentric studies focusing on the prospective long-term follow-up and evaluation of the patients based on a well-designed protocol may provide a better insight into the inflammatory demyelinating diseases of children and adults.

REFERENCES

1. Wechsler IS. Statistics of multiple sclerosis including a study of the infantile congenital, familial,

hereditary forms and the mental and psychic symptoms. *Arch Neurol Psychiatry* 1922; **8**: 59–75.
2. Carter HR, Multiple sclerosis in childhood. *Am J Dis Child* 1946; **71**: 138.
3. Bauer HJ, Hanefeld FA. *Multiple Sclerosis. Its Impact from Childhood to Old Age*. London: WB Saunders, 1993; 1-74.
4. Hauser SL, Bresman MJ, Reinherz EL, Weiner HL. Childhood multiple sclerosis: clinical features and demonstration of changes in T cell subsets with disease activity. *Ann Neurol* 1982; **11**: 463–467.
5. Sadovnick AD, Ebers GC. Epidemiology of multiple sclerosis: a critical overview. *Can J Neurol Sci* 1993; **20**: 17–29.
6. Mathews WB. Clinical aspects. In: Mathews WB, Compston DAS, Allen I, eds. *McAlpine's Multiple Sclerosis*, 2nd edn. Edinburgh: Churchill Livingstone, 1991; 41–251.
7. Poser CM, Paty DW, Scheinberg L et al. New diagnostic criteria for multiple sclerosis: guidelines for research protocols. *Ann Neurol* 1983; **3**: 227–231.
8. Müller R. Course and prognosis of disseminated sclerosis in relation to age of onset. *Arch Neurol* 1951; **66**: 561–570.
9. Duquette P, Murray TJ, Pleines J et al. Multiple sclerosis in childhood: clinical profile in 125 patients. *J Pediatr* 1987; **111**: 359–363.
10. Cole GF, Stuart CA. A long perspective on childhood multiple sclerosis. *Dev Med Child Neurol* 1995; **37**: 661–666.
11. Eraksoy M, Demir G, Özcan H et al. Multiple sclerosis in childhood: a prospective study. *J Neurol* 1996; **243 (suppl 2)**: S82 [abstract].
12. İdiman E, İdiman F, Baklan B et al. Multiple sclerosis in childhood: clinical and paraclinical characteristics. *Düşünen Adam* 1994; **4**: 42–46 [in Turkish].
13. Poskanzer DC, Schapira K, Miller H. Epidemiology of multiple sclerosis in the counties of Northumberland and Durham. *J Neurol Neurosurg Psychiatry* 1963 **26**: 368–376.
14. Gall JC, Hayles AB, Siekert RG et al. Multiple sclerosis in children, *Pediatrics* 1958; **21**: 703–709.
15. Poser S. *Multiple Sclerosis* Berlin: Springer, 1978.
16. Sheperd DI. Clinical features of multiple sclerosis in north-east Scotland. *Acta Neurol Scand* 1979; **60**: 218–230.
17. Shaw CM, Alvord EC Jr. Multiple sclerosis beginning in infancy. *J Child Neurology* 1987; **2**: 252–256.
18. Andler W, Roosen K. Multiple Sklerose im ersten Lebensjahrzehnt. *Klin Pädiatr* 1980; **192**: 365–369.
19. Brandt S, Gyldensted C, Offner H et al. Multiple sclerosis with onset in a two year old boy. *Neuropediatrics* 1981; **12**: 75–82.
20. Hanefeld FA, Bauer HJ, Christen HJ et al. Multiple sclerosis in childhood: report of 15 cases. *Brain Dev* 1991; **13**: 410–416.
21. Bejar JM, Ziegler DK. Onset of multiple sclerosis in a 24-month-old child. *Arch Neurol* 1984; **41**: 881–882.
22. DiMario FJ, Berman PH. Multiple sclerosis presenting at 4 years of age: clinical and MR correlations. *Clin Pediatr* 1987; **27**: 32–37.
23. Ebner F, Milner MM, Justich E. Multiple sclerosis in children: value of serial MR studies to monitor patients. *AJNR* 1990; **11**: 1023–1027.
24. Selcen D, Anlar B, Renda Y. Multiple sclerosis in children: report of 16 cases. *Eur Neurol* 1996; **36**: 79–84.
25. Scaioli V, Rumi V, Cimino C et al. Childhood multiple sclerosis (MS): multimodal evoked potentials and magnetic resonance imaging study. *Neuropediatrics* 1992; **23**: 192–195.
26. Scheider RD, Ong BH, Moran MJ et al. Multiple sclerosis in early childhood: case report with notes on frequency. *Clin Pediatr* 1969; **8**: 115–118.
27. Sindern E, Hass J, Stark E et al. Early onset MS under the age of 16: clinical and paraclinical features. *Acta Neurol Scand* 1992; **86**: 280–284.
28. Bye AME, Kendall B, Wilson J. Multiple sclerosis in childhood: a new look. *Dev Med Child Neurol* 1985; **27**: 215–222.
29. Ghezzi A, Deplano V, Faroni J et al. Multiple sclerosis in childhood: clinical features of 149 cases. *J Neurol* 1996; **6 (suppl 2)**: S71 [abstract].
30. Robertson N, Fraser M, Deans D et al. Age-adjusted recurrence risks for relatives of patients with multiple sclerosis. *Brain* 1996; **119**: 449–455.
31. Robertson NP, O'Riordan JI, Chataway J et al. Offspring recurrence rates and clinical characteristics of conjugal sclerosis. *Lancet* 1997; **349**: 1587–1590.
32. Sadovnick AD, Familial recurrence risks and inheritance of multiple sclerosis. *Curr Opin Neurol Neurosurg* 1993; **6**. 189 194.
33. Riikonen R. The role of infection and vaccination in the genesis of optic neuritis and multiple sclerosis in children. *Acta Neurol Scand* 1989; **80**: 425–431.
34. Alvord EC, Jahnke U, Fischer EH et al. The multiple causes of multiple sclerosis: the importance of age infections in childhood. *J Child Neurol* 1987; **2**: 313–321.

35. Hays P. Multiple sclerosis and delayed mumps. *Acta Neurol Scand* 1992; **85**: 200–203.
36. Glasier CM, Robbins MB, Davies PC et al. Clinical, neurodiagnostic and MR findings in children with spinal and brainstem multiple sclerosis. *AJNR* 1995; **16**: 87–95.
37. Picard EH, Richardson EP. Rapidly evolving neurologic illness in a six year-old girl. Case records of the Massachusetts General Hospital (Case 43–1965). *New Engl J Med* 1965; **273**: 760–767.
38. Boutin B, Esquivel E, Mayer M et al. Multiple sclerosis in children: report of clinical and paraclinical features of 19 cases. *Neuropediatrics* 1988; **19**: 118–123.
39. Bauer HJ, Hanefeld FA, Christen HJ. Multiple sclerosis in early childhood. *Lancet* 1990; **336**: 1190.
40. Mostafapour SP, Enzmann D, North W et al. Brainstem multiple sclerosis in an 11-year-old child presenting as acute disseminated encephalomyelitis. *J Child Neurol* 1995; **10**: 476–480.
41. Mattyus A, Vres E. Multiple sclerosis in childhood: longterm katamnestic investigations. *Acta Paediatr Hungarica* 1985; **26**: 193–204.
42. Septien L, Bourgeois M, Altaba A. La sclérose en plaques chez l'enfant. *Arch Fr Pediatr* 1991; **48**: 263–265.
43. Low NL, Carter S. Multiple sclerosis in children. *Pediatrics* 1956; **18**: 24–30.
44. Poser CM. Myelinoclastic diffuse sclerosis. In: Koetsier JC, ed. *Handbook of Clinical Neurology*. Amsterdam: Elsevier Science, 1985: 419–428.
45. Poser CM, Youtries F, Carpentier M, Aicardi J. Schilder's myelinoclastic diffuse sclerosis. *Pediatrics* 1986; **77**: 107–112.
46. Eblen F, Poremba M, Grodd W et al. Myelinoclastic diffuse sclerosis (Schilder's disease): clinicoradiologic correlations. *Neurology* 1991; **41**: 589–591.
47. Dresser LP, Tourian AY, Anthony DC. A case of myelinoclastic diffuse sclerosis in an adult. *Neurology* 1991; **41**: 316–318.
48. Kepes JJ. Large focal tumor-like demyelinating lesions of the brain: intermediate entity between multiple sclerosis and acute disseminated encephalomyelitis? A study of 31 patients. *Ann Neurol* 1993; **33**: 18–27.
49. Sagar HJ, Warlow CP, Sheldon PWE et al. Multiple sclerosis with clinical and radiological features of cerebral tumour. *J Neurol Neurosurg Psychiatry* 1982; **45**: 802–808.
50. Youl BD, Kermode AG, Thompson AJ. Destructive lesions in demyelinating disease. *J Neurol Neurosurg Psychiatry* 1991; **54**: 288–292.
51. Gutling E, Landis T. CT ring sign imitating tumor, disclosed as multiple sclerosis by MRI by MRI: a case report. *J Neurol Neurosurg Psychiatry* 1989; **52**: 903–906.
52. Giang DW, Poduri KR, Eskin TA. Multiple sclerosis masquerading as a mass lesion. *Neuroradiology* 1992; **34**: 150–154.
53. Peterson K, Rosenblum MK, Powers JM et al. Effect of brain irradiation on demyelinating lesions. *Neurology* 1993; **43**: 2105–2112.
54. Nobel E. Histologischer Befund in einem Falle von akuter multiplen Sklerose. *Wien med Wochenschr* 1912; **62**: 26–32.
55. Barkovich AJ. *Pediatric Neuroimaging*, 2nd edn. New York: Raven Press, 1995.
56. Rusin JA, Vezina LG, Chadduck WM et al. Tumoral multiple sclerosis of the cerebellum in a child. *AJNR* 1995; **16**: 1164–1166.
57. Hainfellner JA, Schmidbauer M, Schmutzhard E et al. Devic's neuromyelitis optica and Schilder's myelinoclastic diffuse sclerosis. *J Neurol Neurosurg Psychiatry* 1992; **55**: 1194–1196.
58. Mandler R, Davis A, Jeffery DR et al. Devic's neuromyelitis optica: a clinicopathological study of 8 patients. *Ann Neurol* 1993; **34**: 162–168.
59. O'Riordan JJ, Gallagher HL, Thompson AJ et al. Clinical, CSF and MRI findings in Devic's neuromyelitis optica. *J Neurol Neurosurg Psychiatry* 1996; **60**: 382–387.
60. Hogancamp WE, Weinshenker BG. The spectrum of Devic's syndrome. *Neurology* 1996; **46**: A254 (P03. 095) [abstract].
61. Eraksoy M, Kmay D, Gülsen-Parman Y. et al. Devic's neuromyelitis optica: clinical and laboratory findings. *J Neurol* 1997; **244 (suppl 3)**: S38 [abstract].
62. Davis R, Thiele E, Barnes P et al. Neuromyelitis optica in childhood: case report with sequential MRI findings. *J Child Neurol* 1996; **11**: 164–167.
63. Moscarello MA, Wood D, Ackerley C et al. Myelin in multiple sclerosis is developmentally immature. *J Clin Invest* 1994; **94**: 146–154.
64. Miller DH, Robb SA, Ormerod EC et al. Magnetic resonance imaging of inflammatory and demyelinating white matter disease of childhood. *Dev Med Child Neurol* 1990; **32**: 97–107.
65. Golden GS, Woody RC. The role of magnetic resonance imaging in the diagnosis of MS in childhood. *Neurology* 1987; **37**: 689–693.

66. Haas G, Schroth G, Krageloh-Man I et al. Magnetic resonance imaging of the brain of children with multiple sclerosis. *Dev Med Child Neurol* 1987; **29**: 586–591.
67. Osborn AG, Harnsberger HR, Smoker WRK, Boyer RS. Multiple sclerosis in adolescents: CT and MR findings. *AJNR* 1990; **11**: 489–494.
68. Van der Knapp MS, Valk J, Neeling N et al. Pattern recognition in magnetic resonance imaging of white matter disorders in children and young adults. *Neuroradiology* 1991; **33**: 478–493.
69. Ferreria Guilhoto LMF, Osorio CAM, Machado LR et al. Pediatric multiple sclerosis report of 14 cases. *Brain Dev* 1995; **17**: 9–12.
70. Van Lieshout HBM, Van Engelen BGM, Sanders EAC et al. Diagnosing multiple sclerosis in childhood. *Acta Neurol Scand* 1993; **88**: 339–343.
71. Haslam RH. Multiple sclerosis: experience at the Hospital for Sick Children. *Int Pediatr* 1987; **2**: 163–167.
72. Golden GS, Woody RC. The role of nuclear magnetic resonance imaging in the diagnosis of MS in childhood. *Neurology* 1987; **37**: 689–693.
73. Bruhn H, Frahm J, Merboldt KD et al. Multiple sclerosis in children, cerebral metabolic alterations monitored by localized proton magnetic resonance spectroscopy in vivo. *Ann Neurol* 1992; **32**: 140–150.
74. Salguero LF, Itabashi HH, Gutierrez NB. Childhood multiple sclerosis with psychiatric manifestations. *J Neurol Neurosurg Psychiatry* 1969; **32**: 572–579.
75. Izquierdo G, Lyon-Caen O, Marteau R et al. Early onset multiple sclerosis. Clinical study of 12 pathologically proven cases. *Acta Neurol Scand* 1986; **73**: 493–497.
76. Cole GF. Auchterlonie LA, Best PV. Very early multiple sclerosis. *Dev Med Child Neurol* 1995; **37**: 661–666.
77. Shermata W, Brown SB, Curless RR. Childhood multiple sclerosis: a report of 12 cases. *Ann Neurol* 1981; **10**: 304.
78. Hanefeld FA. Characteristics of childhood multiple sclerosis. *Int MS J* 1994; **3**: 91–97.

11

Survival in multiple sclerosis

Nils Koch-Henriksen and Henrik Brønnum-Hansen

INTRODUCTION

The natural history of multiple sclerosis (MS) is characterized by the occurrence of various clinical events or landmarks, which are used to determine the course of the disease, e.g. onset, transition to chronic progressive phase, loss of gait without aid, wheelchair, and, finally, death. However, the exact time at which these events occur is not easily detected and requires that the patients are observed regularly at close intervals. The ultimate outcome, death, is however exact and can be precisely ascertained. A short survival time may indicate early impairment and disability.

The survival time after onset of MS is highly variable with death occurring shortly after onset in very few cases, in the third to fourth decade after onset, or after a normal lifespan.

Several studies have shown that although MS is not a lethal disease, it has proved to be a disease of considerable excess mortality. Leibowitz et al.[1] followed 266 patients of whom 52 died, and found a mean survival time of 17.4 years. Kurtzke et al.[2] in their cohort of 527 US army veterans found a 20 year survival rate of 76% and a 25-year survival rate of 68.8%. In his Scottish patient series of 1055 cases Phadke[3] found a mean survival time of 24.5 years. With 136 deaths in a cohort of 598 patients from Western and southeastern Norway, Riise et al.[4] calculated the median survival time after diagnosis to be 27 years. Poser et al.[5] found an unusually long median survival time: 35–42 years in their 'epidemiologic series' from Göttingen. In a cohort of 206 MS patients from Olmsted County, Minnesota, followed for many decades, Wynn et al.[6] found a 25-year survival probability of 76%. Sadovnick et al.[7] in their Canadian study of 2348 patients found that the standardized mortality ratio was 2.0, and life expectancy was only shortened by 6–7 years. Miller et al.[8] included 107 cases in their regional survey in Wellington, New Zealand and found a 25-year survival probability of 60%. Finally, Midgård et al.[9] studied a cohort of 251 MS patients in Møre and Romsdal county in western Norway. They found that a 75% probability of survival was reached 15 years from onset in men and at 21 years from onset in women.

Since we published our first survival study[10] based on the Danish MS Registry, the registry has been updated twice, providing another 7 years of follow-up and adding more than 2000 cases to the previous analyses. This gain in precision and statistical power has encouraged us to repeat the survival analyses on this hitherto by far the largest population-based patient sample to look for predictors of mortality and to quantify their effects.

METHODS AND MATERIAL

Sources of data

This study was based on the nationwide Danish MS Registry and the National Registry of Causes of Death. The MS Registry was established based on Hyllested's 1949 prevalence survey[11] and since 1948 has collected information on virtually all new cases of MS in Denmark, with an eventual completeness estimated at more than 90% for diagnosed cases.[12] Discharge letters or case records on all notified cases are currently reviewed by a neurologist and classified or reclassified according to the diagnostic criteria of Allison and Millar.[13]

Data on patients complying with the diagnostic criteria were transferred to the study database. Year of onset was assessed retrospectively based on the clinical records as the first year in which a symptom attributable to MS occurred. Actuarial life tables were constructed with onset of MS as zero time and death as the endpoint, and surviving patients were censored at time of follow-up or emigration.

For each year from onset to follow-up in each patient, entries were made into Danish vital statistic tables for year-to-year survival probability to compute expected numbers of deaths allowing computation of excess death rate (i.e. observed minus expected number of deaths per 1000 person-years of observation); 95% confidence limits of excess death rate were calculated assuming numbers of deaths to be Poisson variables. We used the corrected relative survival ratio (survival probability in the specific cohort of patients divided by the survival probability in the matched population) to visualize differences between groups (e.g. see Fig 11.3). The effects of the initial symptom and sex on survival were estimated using proportional hazards regression models[14] that included sex, age at onset, and initial symptomatology. We used the statistical program SPSS® for the Cox proportional hazard regression analyses and a program developed by the authors to incorporate population vital statistics and compute the excess death rates and the corrected relative survival ratios.

Inclusion of patients

The total case series

In the part of the study in which average age at death and mean duration of the disease were estimated retrospectively, we included all patients who were prevalent in 1948 or had onset of MS in 1948–1993 and had died within 1948–1993, amounting to 6265 patients (2896 men and 3369 women). When excluding cases classified as 'possible MS' the number was 5652 (2589 men and 3063 women).

The incidence case series

In the cohort-based part of the study, in which life tables, survival probability, excess death rates and hazard ratios were computed, we included only patients with onset within 1948–1993. The number of patients in this series was 8842 (3638 men and 5204 women). When excluding possible cases, the number was 7504 (3090 men and 4414 women).

RESULTS

In the total case series, the average age at death was 58.7 years and the mean disease duration at time of death was 24.8 years. Excluding possible cases made virtually no difference (58.2 years and 24.6 years, respectively). Figure 11.1 shows a plot of age at death against age at onset. Apart from the fact that death logically occurred later than onset, age at death seemed to be virtually independent of age at onset.

Using the incidence case series, we calculated the actuarial survival function. The calculation was performed with all cases before and after

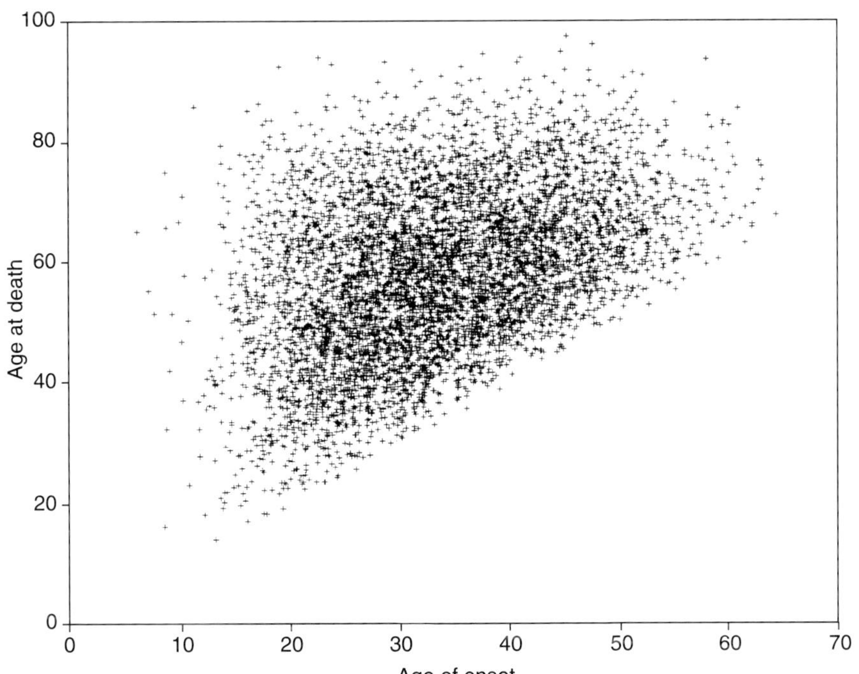

Figure 11.1 Scatterplot of age at death by age at onset.

excluding possible cases. Fig. 11.2 shows for each sex the actuarial survival curve in all patients and the survival probability of a synthetic cohort from the background population, matched to the patients by sex, age and calendar year of onset. It can be seen from the survival curves that life expectancy is 11–13 years shorter for the MS patients than for a matched population. The overally excess death rate was 11.2, and the median survival time was 30.7 years (versus 44

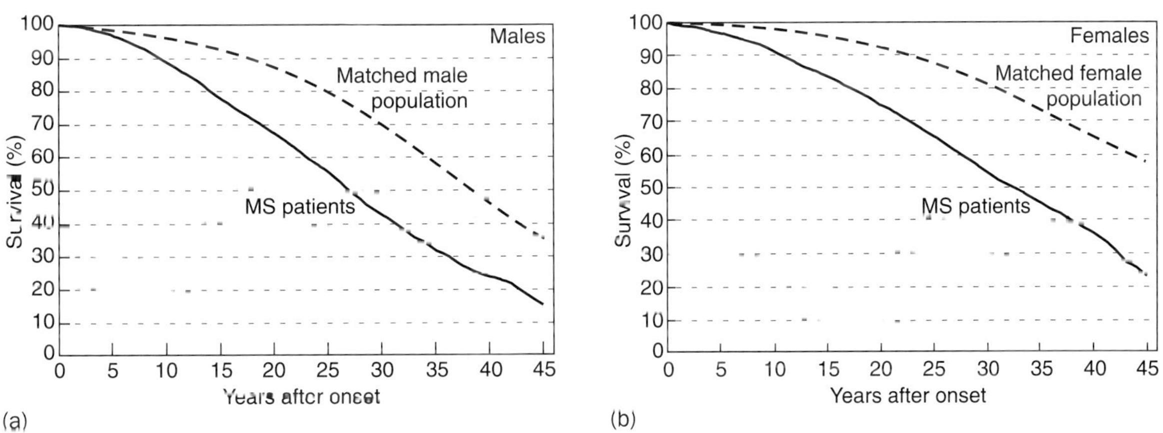

Figure 11.2 Actuarial life table of male and female cases with onset of MS in 1948–1993 with matched population survival probability.

Table 11.1 Key survival parameters in clinically definite, probable and possible cases of MS, by sex and age at onset

Age at onset	Sex	*N*	No. of observed deaths	No. of expected deaths	Person-years	Median survival time	Excess death rate	95% confidence interval
	Men	189	55	9.6	4632	>45	9.8	6.9–13.4
<20	Women	334	66	9.0	7972	>45	7.2	5.3–9.5
	All	523	121	18.6	12760	>45	8.2	6.5–10.0
	Men	1021	369	77.8	21781	32.8	13.4	11.7–15.2
20–29	Women	1626	417	80.2	35605	41.2	9.5	8.4–10.6
	All	2647	786	157.9	57386	38.7	10.9	10.0–11.9
	Men	1267	537	173.8	25192	28.5	14.4	12.7–16.3
30–39	Women	1698	585	154.2	33668	32.3	12.8	11.4–14.3
	All	2965	1122	328.1	58860	30.9	13.5	12.4–14.6
	Men	894	471	196.3	15601	23.1	17.6	14.9–20.5
40–49	Women	1138	494	173.0	20183	26.5	15.9	13.8–18.2
	All	2032	965	369.4	35784	24.7	16.7	15.0–18.4
	Men	267	152	87.6	3773	17.0	17.1	10.9–24.0
50+	Women	408	184	79.9	5659	20.1	18.4	13.9–23.5
	All	675	336	167.4	9432	19.1	17.9	14.2–21.9
All ages	Men	3638	1584	545.2	70978	28.0	14.6	13.6–15.8
	Women	5204	1746	496.3	103041	33.3	12.1	11.3–12.9
	All	8842	3330	1041.4	174019	30.7	13.2	15.8–13.8

years in a matched population). Details on the analyses including excess death rates for all cases including possible MS are shown in Table 11.1.

Survival and sex

In the background population women have a longer life expectancy than men. This is also true for MS patients. The median survival time for male patients was 29 years as opposed to 34.3 years for female patients. When excluding possible cases the median survival time was 28.5 years for men and 33.4 years for women. The excess mortality in terms of the excess death rate was significantly higher for men than for women (see Table 11.1). In the first 5 years after onset the excess mortality was low for people of each sex and even lower for men than for women. Subsequent to onset excess mortality rose markedly and after 10 years of onset it was significantly higher for men than for women. A Poisson regression model shows that the effects of sex and period after onset and their interaction were highly significant. Thus, the assumption of proportionality of hazards between men and women was not fulfilled. For this reason, the Cox proportional hazard regression analyses was made for each sex separately.

population) by time of onset for all patients including possible cases for both sexes separately. Patients with low age at onset had a better relative survival ratio and a lower excess death rate irrespective of whether or not possible cases were included.

Survival and age at onset

For all people the remaining life expectancy at any given point of time is determined by age. Accordingly, the age-dependent survival figures of the background population must be taken into account when comparing prognosis between MS patients with high and low age at onset. The excess death rate is suitable for comparing excess mortality in groups with different background mortality.

The cases were divided into five age-at-onset groups: 0–19, 20–29, 30–39, 40–49 and 50 years or more. Excess death rate increased from 8.2 with age at onset below 20 years to 17.9 with age at onset of > 50 years. In Table 11.1 we have listed the excess death rates in the five age-at-onset groups for both sexes, possible cases included. Figure 11.3 shows the relative survival ratio (survival probability for patients divided by survival probability in a matched

Interaction between sex and age at onset

The difference in prognosis between men and women was most evident with low age at onset. Thus, the excess death rate in patients in whom MS began in the age interval 20–29 years was 9.5 in women and 13.4 in men. At higher ages the difference levelled out, and with age at onset 50 years or more there was even a shift towards a lower excess death rate for men than for women, and the excess death rate for the oldest group of men was of the same magnitude as for men with onset in the age interval 40–49 years (Table 11.1). When excluding possible cases, the rates for men behaved in the same way as for women with increasing excess death rates through the age-at-onset intervals. Figure 11.3 shows that the effect of age at onset on the relative survival ratio is more clear in women than in men.

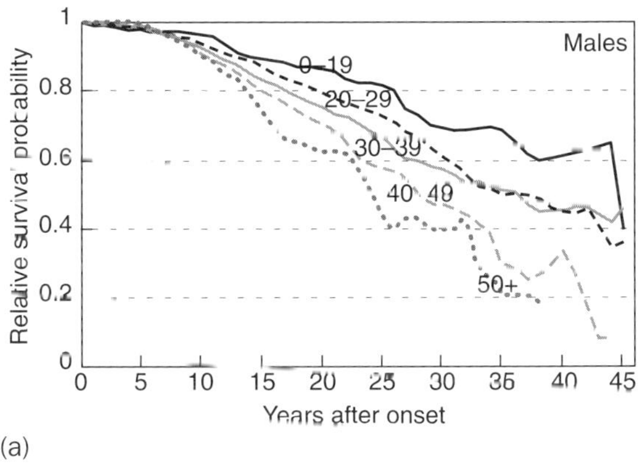

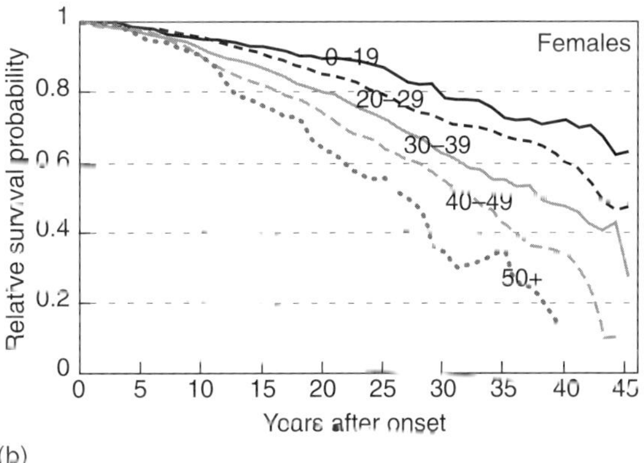

Figure 11.3 Corrected relative survival ratio by age at onset in male and female patients.

Table 11.2 Prognostic value of initial symptom analysed by a proportional hazards regression model. Estimated hazard ratios with optic neuritis as baseline. Model adjusted for age and year at onset. *N* = 3152 for men, 4438 for women

	Clinically definite/probable/possible MS			
	Men		Women	
Presenting symptom	Hazard ratio	95% CI†	Hazard ratio	95% CI
Optic neuritis	1.00	–	1.00	–
Diplopia	1.00	0.80–1.24	1.12	0.88–1.42
Pyramidal	1.01	0.85–1.19	1.18	1.00–1.38
Cerebellar	1.28*	1.07–1.53	1.79*	1.52–2.12
Sensory	0.91	0.77–1.07	1.18*	1.01–1.37

*$p < 0.05$.
†CI = confidence interval.

Survival and presenting symptom

The prognostic significance of the initial symptom for survival was evaluated by a proportional hazard regression model. The effects of age at onset, year of onset, and sex are included in the model. Of the 8842 patients with onset in the interval 1948–1993, 1252 were omitted from this analysis because some categories of presenting symptom, used in the database up to 1964, could not be recorded according to the improved classification used after that time.

Of the 7590 patients included in this analysis 1487 (19.6%) had optic neuritis, 595 (7.8%) had diplopia, 1930 (25.4%) had upper motor neuron symptoms, 996 (13.1%) had cerebellar symptoms, and 2582 (34.0%) had sensory symptoms at onset.

The excess death rate was lowest for optic neuritis: 10.7 (95% confidence interval 9.4–12.1) and highest for cerebellar symptoms at onset: 21.3 (95% confidence interval 19.0–23.7). For the sensory symptoms, diplopia, and upper motor neuron symptoms at onset, the excess death rates were close: 11.4, 12.1 and 12.8, respectively.

Table 11.2 shows the proportional hazard ratios adjusted to the hazard of optic neuritis at onset. Only cerebellar onset in both sexes and sensory onset in females were statistically significantly worse than optic neuritis. Along with the excess death rates, the hazard ratios underscore that cerebellar onset carried a much poorer prognosis than the other onset symptoms.

Calendar-year effect

As survival has improved in the general population during the study period, it was expected that survival from time of onset in MS would also improve. We calculated 10-year survival parameters for three onset cohorts of MS patients: 1954–1963, 1964–1973, 1974–1983. To avoid bias from delay of diagnosis and notification relative to onset, we omitted cases with a lapse of time of more than 10 years between onset and diagnosis. The 10-year survival appears to have improved for both sexes. This improvement in the survival

Table 11.3 Time trends of 10-year survival and excess death rates from MS per 1000 per year

Period	Sex	*N*	No. of observed deaths	No. of expected deaths	Person-years	10-year survival probability	Popul. 10-year survival probability	Excess death rate	95% confidence interval
1954–	Men	699	93	25.6	7417	0.869	0.964	9.1	6.7–11.9
1963	Women	963	124	18.4	9847	0.869	0.980	10.7	8.6–13.2
	All	1635	217	44.0	17264	0.869	0.973	10.0	8.4–11.8
1964–	Men	641	80	23.4	6804	0.878	0.964	8.3	5.9–11.2
1973	Women	843	78	19.6	8975	0.912	0.977	6.5	4.7–8.7
	All	1484	158	43.1	15779	0.897	0.971	7.3	5.8–9.0
1974–	Men	783	69	31.2	8351	0.914	0.961	4.5	2.7–6.7
1983	Women	1184	91	29.6	12652	0.923	0.976	4.9	3.5–6.5
	All	1967	160	60.8	21006	0.919	0.970	4.7	3.6–6.0

of MS patients with time is not due only to lower mortality in the general population, since a comparison of the three onset cohorts showed a significant decrease in the excess death rates per 1000 per year (Table 11.3).

DISCUSSION

Studies on the survival of MS patients have had widely variable study design, patient sample type (prevalent, incident or mixed), methods of ascertainment, completeness of follow-up, and sample size. Few studies have involved prospective analyses of incident cases.[2,4,6,9,10,15] The only prospective analyses of survival in population-based cohorts are, to our knowledge, those from the Mayo Clinic,[6] the two studies from Norway[4,9] and from Denmark.[10] Our prospective study involved follow-up of the largest unselected cohort of MS patients published to date with complete follow-up of virtually all patients in one country over the course of 45 years. Thus, only minor sources of bias are present, which could affect the results to a modest and estimable degree. The starting point of the survival analysis is the time of onset, but the Danish MS Registry ascertains patients after the time of diagnosis, which may be separated from the onset by several years. The summary probability of being ascertained by the Registry was 67% within 5 years of onset and 85% within 10 years of onset; for 3% of the patients more than 20 years had lapsed between onset and ascertainment. Most MS patients not diagnosed and ascertained by follow-up are expected to be alive; the exceptions would be a small but unknown number of latent MS cases who have died from competing causes before a diagnosis was made. In our previous survival study[10] we tried to include the estimated number of cases missing due to delayed diagnosis, and assumed that these patients were all alive at follow-up. The resulting drop in the excess death rate was only about 1 per 1000 person-years.

We did not distinguish between death from natural causes and death from suicide, as there were less than 60 suicides in the entire onset cohort. Neither did we distinguish between deaths attributed to MS and to other natural causes of death.

To determine whether cases classified as possible MS could be included in the analyses without reservation, we employed a proportional hazard regression model into which we had included age at onset. We estimated the hazard of dying with possible MS at 0.65 relative to the hazard of dying with clinically definite/probable MS; the 95% confidence interval of the hazard ratio was 0.58–0.72. Thus, the prognosis differed significantly among the two groups. However, as possible cases comprised only 15.1% of all cases, and excluding/including them had little effect on the overall results, we decided to present most of the data on all patients including possible cases. The group of possible cases probably contains some non-MS patients. On the other hand, by omitting possible MS, some cases of true MS—but with few lesions—may be lost for the analyses, which may distort the results slightly in the direction of a worse prognosis.

The crude survival estimates in this study are of the same magnitude as those in several other survival studies.[1–9] The differences may be owing to small sample sizes and different sampling methods. In a study form Sahlgrens Hospital, Gothenburg, Sweden,[16] a life-table analysis indicated a 25-year survival probability of about 81%. It appears that the authors censored patients who died from competing causes, as one of their endpoints was reaching an expanded disability status scale (EDSS) of 10. In the Canadian study[7] the survival seemed better than in most other studies. One reason for this deviation may be that death/living status could not be completely ascertained by follow-up, although the authors claimed only a few patients lost to follow-up, or that their population mortality estimates, based on insurance companies, may have overestimated the population mortality.

Several studies have shown a better prognosis or survival in females than in males.[6,9,16,17] The cause of this sex difference is unknown. It contrasts with the fact that MS is more common in females than in males. However life expectancy in the female population is greater than in the male population, and for that reason, a longer survival in female MS patients is also expected. This study shows a significantly higher excess death rate in male than in female patients; hence, the sex difference could not be explained by the sex differences of population mortality. Moreover, the probability of survival in MS patients divided by the probability of survival in a population matched for age, sex and calendar year (the relative survival ratio) is also notably higher in the female patients.

Most studies have shown a better survival with low age at onset.[1,4,8,9,18–20] Figure 11.1 readily explains that people with low age at onset have a longer time available in which they are at risk of dying, whereas people with onset of MS at a relatively high age have a much shorter time during which death will probably occur, thus resulting in a shorter survival time. In a study from Göttingen[5] the authors indicated that female sex and low age at onset were followed by a better survival, but using population vital statistics they showed that the favourable survival could be attributed to sex and age per se rather than to the disease itself. It has, however, also been shown that the state of DSS 6 (unable to walk without aids) is reached in a shorter time for patients with high age at onset.[18,19] Again we have to turn to the population vital statistics to decide whether patients with onset of MS at an older age have a higher mortality compared with that expected, than younger patients. The present analysis shows unequivocally that patients with high age at onset have a higher excess mortality in terms of excess death rates, and their relative survival ratio was lower.

In subpopulations with very different underlying mortality, the usual term, standardized mortality ratio (observed number of deaths divided by expected number of deaths), can directly misleading; if the denominator in the expression—the expected number of deaths in a matched normal population—is very low, as in a cohort of, for example, young females, the standardized mortality ratio will be disproportionately high, in fact causing an apparent reversal of the excess mortality among patients with low and high age at onset. For that reason the use of standardized mortality ratios was abandoned in this study.

Some onset symptoms are predictors of disability and mortality. Consistently, cerebellar symptoms or motor symptoms of the limbs at onset have been linked to a poor prognosis,[3,4,8,15,18–20] whereas sensory symptoms[9,20] and optic neuritis at onset[3] have been linked to a more favourable prognosis. In the present study we found that survival following cerebellar onset was significantly shorter when compared with survival following the other onset symptoms. The association resisted inclusion of age at onset and year of onset into the Cox proportional hazard model and was marked for both sexes. The biological background for the bad prognosis with cerebellar onset is not clear. As cerebellar onset was only found in 13% of the cases, it could be argued that cerebellar structures are more resistant against the disease process than other parts of the CNS, and, hence, that cerebellar involvement is evidence of more widespread and diffuse involvement following a more aggressive disease. Another explanation may be that even modest lesions of cerebellar structures causes marked physical disability resulting in higher EDSS scores and higher risk of complicating lethal somatic diseases.

Unfortunately, the Danish MS Registry does not keep information on disease course in its database, so we have not been able to confirm the assumption that a gradual onset is associated with a worse prognosis, which has been demonstrated convincingly in many studies.

We found that the prognosis in terms of 10-year survival and 10-year excess death rate was better in patients with onset during 1974 1983 compared with earlier onset cohorts, which is in contrast to the study of Midgård et al.[9] who found that the prognosis in recent onset cohorts had worsened. Patients with onset a few years before follow-up may, because of delay of diagnosis and ascertainment, be incompletely registered, and the most benign cases in particular may escape detection until after follow-up. This bias causes an artificial trend towards more malignant disease in cases with onset in recent years and could be the cause of the trend in the Norwegian data. In our analyses we omitted cases with more than 10 years delay of ascertainment from all onset cohorts to balance out this bias. We believe that the improved survival is the result of better ascertainment of benign cases owing to better knowledge about MS among patients and doctors and to generally better health care, keeping patients with advanced MS free from complicating diseases for a longer time.

Along with the disability, the impairment and the handicap that follows MS, the considerable excess mortality stresses the need for an effective treatment. However, some years will elapse before the effects of the new immune-modulating treatments can be detected in survival analyses.

ACKNOWLEDGEMENTS

The DMSG is funded by the Danish Multiple Sclerosis Society. The authors wish to thank the secretary at the Danish Multiple Sclerosis Registry Mrs Helle Birk Jensen for keeping the case files, Lise Stener Eriksen of the Danish Institute for Clinical Epidemiology (DICE) for maintaining the database, and chief statistician Mrs Mette Madsen, DICE, for helpful advice and suggestions.

REFERENCES

1. Leibowitz U, Kahana E, ALter M. Survival and death in multiple sclerosis. *Brain* 1969; **92**: 115–130.
2. Kurtzke JF, Beebe GW, Nagler B et al. Studies on the natural history of multiple sclerosis. V. Long term survival in young men. *Arch Neurol* 1970; **22**: 215–225.
3. Phadke JG. Survival pattern and cause of death in patients with multiple sclerosis: results from an epidemiological survey in north east Scotland. *J Neurol Neurosurg Psychiatry* 1988; **243**: 181–182.
4. Riise T, Grønning M, Aarli JA et al. Prognostic factors for life expectancy in multiple sclerosis analysed by Cox-models. *J Clin Epidemiol* 1988; **41**: 1031–1036.
5. Poser S, Kurtzke JF, Poser W et al. Survival in multiple sclerosis. *J Clin Epidemiol* 1989; **42**: 159–168.

6. Wynn DR, Rodriguez M, O'Fallon WM et al. A reappraisal of the epidemiology of multiple sclerosis Olmsted County, Minnesota. *Neurology* 1990; **40**: 780–786.
7. Sadovnick AD, Ebers GC, Wilson RW et al. Life expectancy in patients attending multiple sclerosis clinics. *Neurology* 1992; **42**: 991–994.
8. Miller DH, Hornabrook RW, Purdie G. The natural history of multiple sclerosis: a regional study with some longitudinal data. *J Neurol Neurosurg Psychiatry* 1992; **55**: 341–346.
9. Midgård R, Albrektsen G, Riise T et al. Prognostic factors for survival in multiple sclerosis: a longitudinal, population based study in More and Romsdal, Norway. *J Neurol Neurosurg Psychiatry* 1995; **58**: 417–421.
10. Brønnum-Hansen H, Koch-Henriksen N, Hyllested K. Survival of patients with multiple sclerosis in Denmark: a nationwide, long-term epidemiologic survey. *Neurology* 1994; **44**: 1901–1907.
11. Hyllested K. *Disseminated Sclerosis in Denmark: Prevalence and Geographical Distribution.* Copenhagen: J. Jørgensen, 1956.
12. Koch-Henriksen N, Hyllested K. Epidemiology of multiple sclerosis: incidence and prevalence rates in Denmark 1948–64 based on the Danish Multiple Sclerosis Registry. *Acta Neurol Scand* 1988; **78**: 369–380.
13. Allison RS, Millar JDH. Prevalence and familial incidence of disseminated sclerosis. *Ulster Med J* 1954; **23 (suppl)**: 5–49.
14. Cox DR. Regression models and life tables. *J R Stat Soc Ser B* 1972; **34**: 187–220.
15. McAlpine D. Benign form of multiple sclerosis: a study based on 241 cases seen within 3 years of onset and followed up to the tenth year or more of the disease. *Brain* 1961; **84**: 186–203.
16. Runmarker B, Anderson O. Prognostic factors in a multiple sclerosis incidence cohort with twenty-five years of follow-up. *Brain* 1993; **116**: 117–134.
17. Hyllested K. Lethality, duration, and mortality of disseminated sclerosis in Denmark. *Acta Psychr Neurol Scand* 1961; **36**: 553–564.
18. Weinshenker BG, Rice GP, Noseworthy JH et al. The natural history of multiple sclerosis: a geographically based study. 3. Multivariate analysis of predictive factors and models of outcome. *Brain* 1991; **114**: 1045–1056.
19. Riise T, Grønning M, Fernandez O et al. Early prognostic factors for disability in multiple sclerosis, a European multicenter study. *Acta Neurol Scand* 1992; **85**: 212–218.
20. Visscher BR, Liu K-S, Clark VA et al. Onset symptoms as predictors of mortality and disability in multiple sclerosis. *Acta Neurol Scand* 1984; **70**: 321–328.

12

Adhesion molecules in multiple sclerosis: a review

Juan J Archelos and Hans-Peter Hartung

INTRODUCTION

Multiple sclerosis (MS) remains a major challenge to basic and clinical research. Some of the pivotal immune mechanisms operating in this chronic inflammatory disease have recently been characterized. Development of a more satisfactory treatment requires a better understanding of the pathogenesis and especially of the immunopathology of MS. Cell surface anchored adhesion molecules are of fundamental importance in the immune response during autoimmune disease. Circulating forms of adhesion molecules may help to monitor disease activity. A variety of new therapeutic approaches targeting crucial adhesion molecules have emerged in the last years and they open new avenues to improve the outcome of this disabling disease.[1]

THE FUNDAMENTAL ROLE OF THE IMMUNE SYSTEM IN MS PATHOGENESIS

The histopathology of the lesion in multiple sclerosis (MS), although most likely heterogeneous, is characterized by multifocal perivenular infiltration of the white matter by lymphocytes and monocytes/macrophages in the central nervous system (CNS), and a selective destruction of myelin and myelin-forming oligodendrocytes sparing—at least initially—the axons.[2–4] The main cellular components involved in MS lesion genesis are: T cells, macrophages which remove the myelin sheath from axons resulting in severe functional impairment; and B cells. The combined actions of the cellular and humoral immune components and the failure to detect a specific infectious agent supported the notion that MS could be an autoimmune disease.[5] An autoimmune hypothesis that postulates a fundamental immune dysregulation where autoreactive myelin protein-specific T cells orchestrate an aberrant immune response to antigens in the CNS was initially developed on the basis of clinical, histological and—more recently—immunological similarities observed in experimental autoimmune encephalomyelitis (EAE), an animal model of MS. Acute and chronic disease variants of this T-cell-driven autoimmune disorder of the CNS have been established in rodents (mouse strains: SJL/J, PL/J, Biozzi; rat strains: Lewis, DA; guinea pig strains: 13, Hartley; rabbits)[6] and non-human primates.[7,8] Depending on the species and the agent used to elicit EAE, distinct histological and clinical features result, that resemble MS to a variable degree. Generally, these animal models are induced by sensitization with a myelin antigen such as myelin basic protein

(MBP), proteolipid protein (PLP), myelin/oligodendrocyte glycoprotein (MOG), or S-100—an intracellular protein present in astrocytes among other cell types—or by injection of myelin-specific CD4+ T cells that have been activated in vitro. The histopathological hallmarks of EAE are mononuclear infiltration and a variable degree of demyelination depending on the model used.[9] EAE lacks the clinical complexity of MS but lends itself to the study of the basic mechanisms involved in the immune attack on the CNS.

Additional evidence to support an autoimmune origin of MS stems from the detection of myelin-reactive T lymphocytes in the blood and cerebrospinal fluid (CSF) of MS patients. However, autoreactive T cells form part of the normal T-cell repertoire in healthy donors[10] and strong T-cell immunosuppressive treatments such as cyclophosphamide, or even total lymphoid irradiation, which are highly effective in EAE have only a modest or no proven effect in MS.[11] Despite an extensive search over the past decades for autoantigens that elicit a self-reactive immune response in MS, none of the candidates—most of them myelin proteins encephalitogenic in EAE such as MBP, PLP, MOG, and myelin-associated glycoprotein (MAG)—have been definitely proved to be causative. An alternative hypothesis favours a primarily viral aetiology. This hypothesis holds that the CNS becomes infected by a neurotropic virus. In response, the immune system engenders T cells that infiltrate the brain and target foreign viral antigens. The neural tissue is damaged either directly by cytotoxic T cells or through a bystander effect of the ongoing inflammatory response. To date however, no causative virus has been identified. Whatever the putative cause, there is overall agreement that the pathogenesis of MS is immune mediated.

THE IMMUNE RESPONSE IN EAE

In EAE the immune response can be dissected into different phases. First, animals are injected with known myelin autoantigens. In response to this, 'naive' T cells exit the peripheral circulation across specialized postcapillary endothelium in the peripheral lymph nodes draining the injection site, so-called high endothelial venules (HEV). There they are activated in response to antigen presented to them by professional antigen-presenting cells (APCs) such as macrophages or dendritic cells. This first step of T-cell priming by antigen presentation is called the induction phase of the immune response. The activated T cells then leave the lymph node via the efferent lymphatics into the peripheral blood, attach to the venular endothelium in the CNS and migrate across the blood–brain barrier (BBB). This transendothelial migration gives rise to the effector phase of the immune response in EAE. In the CNS the autoantigen is presented by microglia—the resident macrophages of the brain—to T cells. The reactivated and clonally expanded CD4+ T cells amplify the immune response by recruiting further T cells and macrophages via chemokines and cytokines, finally resulting in mononuclear-cell infiltration. This influx also allows the passage of circulating autoantibodies which are thought to synergize with T cells to initiate demyelination. In the adoptive-transfer variants of EAE (AT-EAE), T cells recovered from the lymph nodes of diseased animals are primed, expanded and activated in vitro and then injected intravenously into the recipient animal. Hence, AT-EAE lacks the induction phase in vivo and has a more precipitous disease onset.

ADHESION MOLECULES AND THE IMMUNE RESPONSE

Adhesion molecules: structural and functional features

On a molecular level adhesion molecules (AM) are critically involved in all steps of the immune response.[12–15] Initially, AM were defined operationally as cell-surface structures mediating cell–cell and cell–extracellular matrix (ECM) interactions.

Based on their structure three main classes of AM can be distinguished:

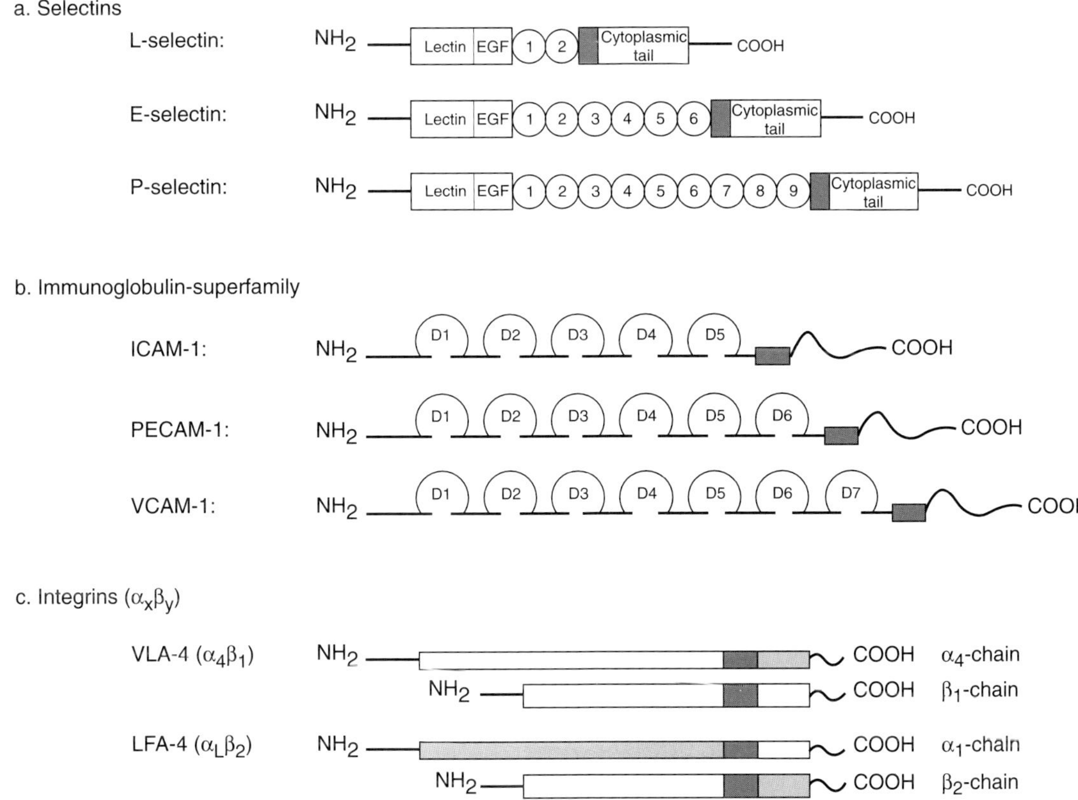

Figure 12.1 Structural characteristics of adhesion molecules. (a) Selectins have a common modular structure consisting of an N-terminal lectin domain, an epidermal growth factor (EGF)-like region, 2–9 short consensus-repeats homologous to a complement-binding domain, a transmembrane region and a short cytoplasmic tail. Despite their structural similarities, the three selectins have distinct patterns of expression. The lectin domain is directly involved in binding to carbohydrate ligands on a variety of molecules inducing mucins. Selectins have a low intrinsic binding affinity but a high avidity for their ligands. The activity of selectins is mainly regulated by modulation of their expression. (b) Cell adhesion molecules of the immunoglobulin superfamily such as ICAM-1, PECAM-1 and VCAM-1 are all transmembrane molecules characterized by an extracellular region composed of immunoglobulin (Ig)-like domains. This stable Ig-backbone interacts with other members of the Ig family and with integrins. Binding of members of the Ig superfamily to their counterreceptors is mainly regulated at the expression level. (c) Integrins, such as VLA-4 and LFA-1 are transmembrane, noncovalently linked heterodimers formed by two variable chains with a common structure $\alpha_x\beta_y$. The α and β chains do not associate randomly. Integrins bind to members of the Ig-superfamily and to a variety of adhesive glycoproteins on cells and in the extracellular matrix. Integrins mediate high-strength interactions with ligands and their affinity is mainly regulated by conformational changes in the heterodimer. For abbreviations, see legend to Table 12.1.

1. members of the immunoglobulin superfamily
2. integrins
3. selectins (Fig. 12.1).

Table 1 gives an overview of the best characterized members of each group and their ligands.

Table 12.1 Adhesion molecules involved in antigen presentation and transendothelial migration during T-cell-mediated disease

Adhesion molecule[a] (alternative name)	Cellular expression[b]	Ligands	Main function[c]
Immunoglobulin superfamily:			
ICAM-1 (CD54):5 Ig domains	E, T, B, Ma, Mi, A	LFA-1, MAC-1, CD43	CS, TM of T
VCAM-1 (CD106):7 Ig domains	E, Ma, Pe	VLA-4, $\alpha_4\beta_7$	TM of T, Ma
PECAM-1 (CD31):6 Ig domains	E, T (naive), Ma, NK	PECAM-1, $\alpha_v\beta_3$	TM of T, NK, Ma
LFA-2 (CD2):2 Ig domains	T, NK	LFA-3	CS
LFA-3 (CD58):2 Ig domains	E, T, B, Ma, Mi	LFA-2	CS
CD28:1 Ig domain (dimer)	T (resting, activated)	B7-1, B7-2	CS
CTLA-4 (CD152):1 Ig domain	T (activated)	B7-1, B7-2	CS of CTL
B7-1 (CD80):2 Ig domains	T, B, Ma, Mi, A	CTLA-4, CD28	CS, IR
B7-2 (CD86):2 Ig domains	T, B, Ma, Mi, A	CTLA-4, CD28	CS, IR
Integrins:			
VLA-4 ($\alpha_4\beta_1$) (CD49d/CD29)	T, B, Ma	VCAM-1, FN, VLA-4, $\alpha_4\beta_7$	TM of T, Ma
LPAM-1 ($\alpha_4\beta_7$) (CD49d/CD104)	T (memory)	VCAM-1, FN, MAdCAM-1	TM of T (memory)
LFA-1 ($\alpha_L\beta_2$) (CD11a/CD18)	Ma, Mi	ICAM-1, -2, -3	CS, TM or T, Ma
MAC-1 ($\alpha_M\beta_2$) (CD11b/CD18)	Ma, Mi, NK	ICAM-1, FN, C3bi	TM of Ma
Selectins:			
E-selectin (CD62E)	E	sLewis^x, ESL-1	R of T
L-selectin (CD62L)	T, B, Ma	sLewis^x, mucins*	R of T, Ma, RC
P-selectin (CD62P)	E	sLewis^x, PSGL-1	R of Ma
Other:			
CD40	B, Ma, E	CD154 (CD40L)	CS
CD40L (CD154)	T (activated), Ma	CD40	CS
CD44	T, B, Ma, A O	ECM	TM of T
MAdCAM-1	HEV	VLA-4, LPAM-1	HR

Only cellular distributions and functions of adhesion molecules with potential relevance for the pathogenesis of multiple sclerosis are given.

[a]*Abbreviations:* C3bi: complement factor 3bi; CTLA-4: cytotoxic T lymphocyte antigen-4; ECM: hyaluronate, collagen, fibronectin, laminin; ESL-1: E-selectin ligand-1; FN: fibronectin; GlyCAM-1: glycosylation-dependent cell adhesion molecule-1; HEV: high endothelial venules; ICAM-1: intercellular cell adhesion molecule-1; LFA-1: lymphocyte function-associated molecule-1; LPAM-1: lymphocyte Peyer's patch adhesion molecule-1; MAC-1: macrophage glycoprotein associated with complement receptor function-1; MAdCAM-1: mucosal addressin cell adhesion molecule-1; PECAM-1: platelet/endothelial cell adhesion molecule-1; PSGL-1: P-selectin glycoprotein ligand-1; VCAM-1: vascular cell adhesion molecule-1; VLA-4: very late antigen-4; *Mucins: serine- and threonine-rich proteins that are heavily glycosylated and have an extended structure (CD34, MAdCAM-1, GlyCAM-1, PSGL-1).

[b]*Abbreviations:* A: astrocytes; B: B cells; E: endothelial cells; Ma: macrophages, monocytes; Mi: microglia; NK: natural killer cells; Pe: pericytes, O: oligodendrocytes, T: T cells (naive or memory).

[c]*Abbreviations:* CS: costimulatory T cell activation during antigen presentation, TM: transendothelial migration, R: rolling on endothelium, HR: homing to lymph nodes and lymphocyte recirculation, IR: immunoregulative action on T cells.

Adhesion molecules are crucial in the immune response

The functions of the AM have been elucidated by extensive in vitro and in vivo research over recent years.[13,16] Their involvement in different pathophysiological settings has been probed in animal models either indirectly by blocking the action of AM with specific monoclonal antibodies (mAbs) or more directly by producing 'knock-out' mice in which the corresponding gene for a particular AM is rendered inactive. Several well-defined alterations of the cellular and humoral immune response have already been described in 'knock-outs' for intercellular cell adhesion molecule-1 (ICAM-1, CD54),[17] selectins (CD62)[18–21] and cytotoxic T lymphocyte antigen-4 (CTLA-4, CD152).[22]

Antigen presentation

Antigen presentation is essential for the physiological activation and subsequent maturation of T cells. Two external signals provided by APCs are required for this activation of T cells (Fig. 12.2): one is the antigen-specific signal provided by the interaction between the T-cell antigen receptor and immunogenic peptide presented in the context of major histocompatibility complex (MHC) molecules on APCs. The second signal is antigen-independent, but is essentially required for effective T-cell activation and is mediated by AM on both T cells and APCs; these are called accessory or costimulatory molecules. Important pairs of interacting molecules are ICAM-1/lymphocyte function-associated molecule-1 (LFA-1, CD11a/CD18), CD2/LFA-3 (CD58) and, possibly the most important costimulatory pathway, CD28/B7-1/2 (CD80/CD86), CD40/CD154 (CD40L) and CTLA-4/B7-1/2 (Fig. 12.2).[23–26]

Transendothelial migration

Systemic autoreactivity only results in local autoaggression when activated T cells penetrate an intact BBB, whose first and strongest component is the endothelial lining. Blockade of the egress of T cells from blood vessels could prevent inflammation and subsequent demyelination in the CNS.

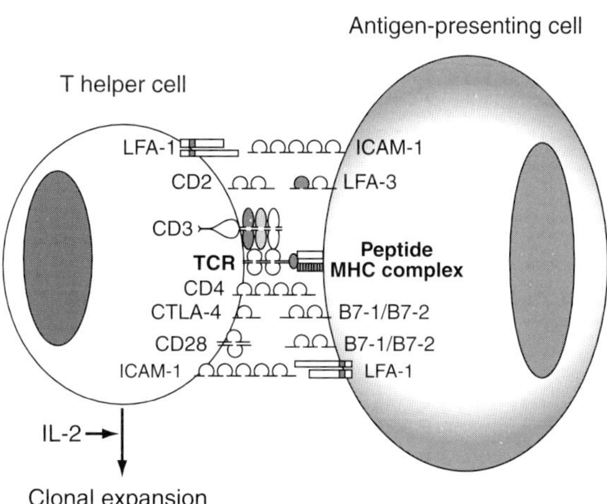

Figure 12.2 Pivotal role of adhesion molecules as costimulatory molecules in antigen recognition. Receptor–ligand pairs of adhesion molecules such as ICAM-1–LFA-1, B7-CD28/CTLA-4 or CD2–LFA-3 provide essential costimulatory signals for T cells. The specificity of T-cell stimulation resides in a unique recognition complex of an antigen-derived defined peptide associated with major histocompatibility complex (MHC) expressed by antigen presenting cells and the corresponding T-cell receptor that recognizes this complex. As a result of these interactions the T cells are driven by interleukin 2 (IL-2) into clonal expansion. For abbreviations, see legend to Table 12.1.

A cascade of sequentially interacting pairs of AM seems to be responsible for the crucial transendothelial migration of T cells into the target organ (Fig. 12.3).[13,15,27]

In vitro, T cells predominantly use ICAM-1/LFA-1 pathways if exposed to unstimulated endothelium. By contrast, very late antigen-4 (VLA-4) vascular cell adhesion molecule 1 (VCAM-1) is crucial for their transmigration through stimulated endothelium.[28] CD44—a transmembrane glycoprotein expressed on T cells, macrophages and other non-haematopoietic cells such as astrocytes—is involved in T-cell migration into inflamed sites in several animal models, although its exact role in T-cell recruitment to the CNS remains to be defined.[29]

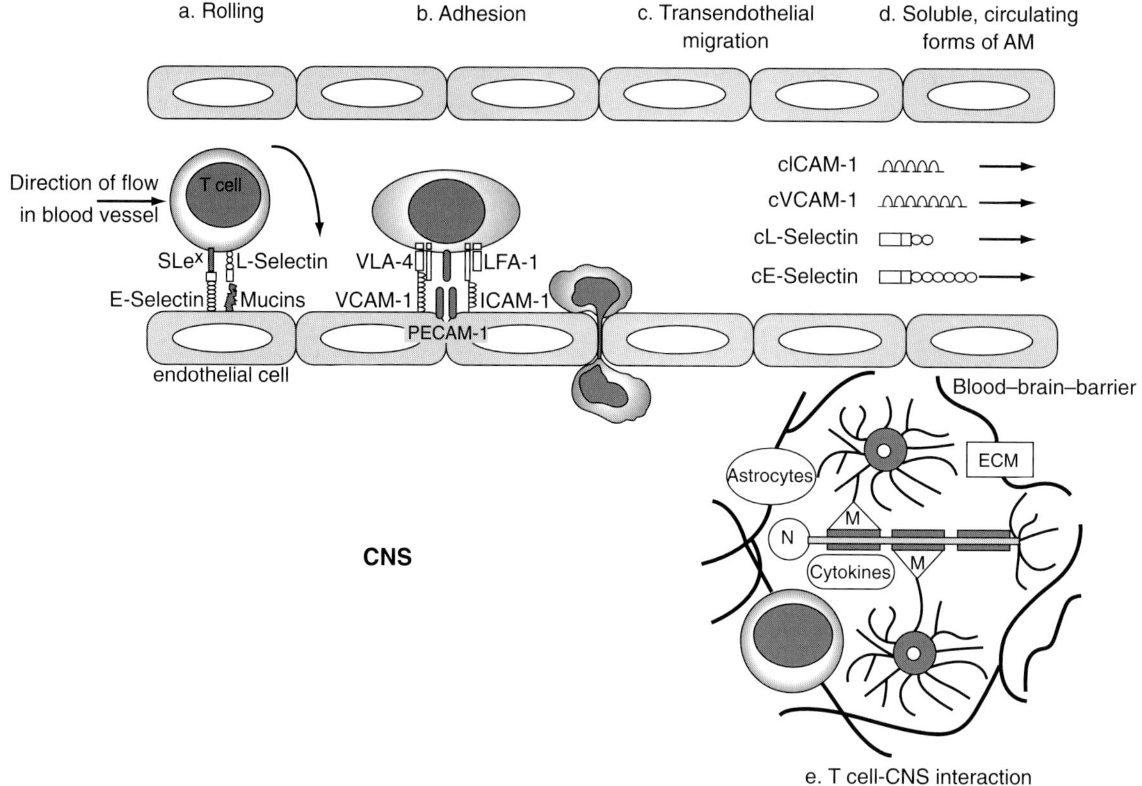

Figure 12.3 Transendothelial migration of T lymphocytes across the blood–brain barrier in experimental autoimmune encephalomyelitis is mediated by adhesion molecules. (a) Through the action of selectins T cells establish a loose reversible contact ('tethering') with endothelial cells via selectins and their ligands. This reduces the velocity of the lymphocytes travelling in the blood. (b) This initial rolling is followed by a firm irreversible adhesion mediated by integrins (VLA-4, LFA-1) on T cells and their immunoglobulin-like receptors on endothelium (VCAM-1, ICAM-1). Chemokines[163,164] released locally increase integrin adhesiveness and induce directed movement across the endothelial lining in T cells and monocytes. (c) The subsequent transendothelial migration of T cells through the blood–brain barrier is thought to be mediated mainly by VLA-4–VCAM-1 and, more recently characterized by the homophilic interaction (i.e. binding of a molecule to another identical molecule) of PECAM-1 which is concentrated at the intercellular junctions between endothelial cells. (d) The extracellular domain of some of the adhesion molecules is shed from the cell surface after T-cell–endothelial-cell interaction, and soluble forms circulate in the blood and cerebrospinal fluid in forms such as circulating ICAM-1 (cICAM-1), cVCAM-1, cL-selectin or cE-selectin. Physiological levels of circulating forms of AM (cAM) increase with pathology.[91] (e) T cells that have migrated into the CNS interact with local cellular (A: astrocytes, O: oligodendrocytes, N: neurons, microglia, M: myelin) and acellular components (ECM, cytokines) of the CNS.[165] The nature of this complex interaction determines the outcome of the immune response in the target tissue. If the inflammatory process abates or the damage is resolved the immune response is terminated by emigration of immune cells back into the lymphatic system or by the induction of programmed cell death (apoptosis) in T cells. For abbreviations, see legend to Table 12.1.

It is noteworthy that the kinetics of endothelial AM expression are not regulated uniformly. ICAM-1, VCAM-1 and E-selectin are expressed at low baseline levels and strongly upregulated upon cytokine stimulation. In contrast, endothelial PECAM-1 and mucins exhibit a high level of constitutive expression and are upregulated much less upon cytokine challenge.[12]

Summarizing in vitro and in vivo experimentation, the following role of membrane-anchored AM in the immune response emerges: integrins and members of the immunoglobulin superfamily are involved in both antigen presentation and in the migration of T cells and monocytes/macrophages across vessel walls. Selectins are necessary for T-cell recirculation and for transendothelial migration (Table 12.1).

AUTOIMMUNE INFLAMMATION IN THE CNS—SPECIAL CONSIDERATIONS

Influx of nonspecific T cells

Some unique features of the anatomic compartment CNS dictate how the immune system impacts on this organ. In the last decade it was well established that only activated T cells, regardless of their specificity, can cross the intact BBB. If T cells encounter their antigen presented by APCs they will be further activated. Otherwise they will leave the CNS compartment within a few hours. In EAE, T cells specific for an encephalitogenic protein will be activated, and released cytokines and chemokines will prompt an influx of secondarily attracted 'nonspecific' circulating T cells. In the murine EAE these T cells represent a majority (over 90%) of the total T-cell population in the lesion.[30–32]

Epitope spreading

A second peculiar important phenomenon observed in EAE and possibly also occurring in MS is epitope spreading. This process implies that, for example, after induction of EAE in rats or mice, the recipient animal mounts a specific cellular and humoral immune response against the peptide used for immunization. After a few weeks T cells and antibodies recognizing other epitopes of the same protein, or of other myelin proteins not used for immunization, are present in the circulation. This intra- and intermolecular spreading of the immune response to other initially unrelated proteins of the CNS is called epitope spreading.[33,34] Epitope spreading has been demonstrated for PLP and MBP in a variety of EAE models.[35–41]

With regard to MS, the possible presence of a majority of 'nonspecific' T cells in the lesion and an immune response possibly diversified and amplified by epitope spreading, makes it necessary to develop treatment strategies that do not depend on a certain autoantigen. One such strategy could target the recruitment of any T cell to the CNS compartment. From this theoretical point of view transendothelial migration of T cells into the CNS is of paramount importance for experimental anti-AM therapy.

ADHESION MOLECULES IN EAE

Expression of adhesion molecules in EAE

In naive EAE-susceptible mice, ICAM-1, VCAM-1 and PCAM-1 are present at low constitutive levels on endothelial cells of large venules in the spinal cord and brain. Mucosal addressin cell adhesion molecule-1 (MAdCAM-1), P- and E-selectin are not detected in the CNS of these animals.[42–44]

In the acute phase of EAE both ICAM-1 and VCAM-1 are upregulated on lesion- and nonlesion-associated blood vessels, PECAM-1 seems to be redistributed and enriched at the endothelial tight junctions without an increase of expression, and MAdCAM-1, P- and E-selectin are not found at any stage of the disease.[45–48] Clinical relapses and parenchymal infiltration are paralleled by an upregulation of ICAM-1 and VCAM-1 on blood vessels.[49–51]

The AM profile of the perivascular inflammatory cells has been studied in situ and ex vivo in the rodent EAE models. In situ, most mononuclear cells in the lesion have the phenotype: VLA-4^{high}, ICAM-1^{high}, LFA-1^{high}, CD44^{high}, Mac-1^{high}, L-selectin^{low}, LPAM-1^{low} ($\alpha4\beta7$), PECAM-1$^{low/-}$.[42,45,46]

Ex vivo, infiltrating T cells are: VLA-4^{high}, ICAM-1^{high}, LFA-1^{high}, CD44^{high}, Mac-1^{low}, L-selectin$^{low/-}$, LPAM-1^{low}, and infiltrating macrophages: VLA-4^{high}, ICAM-1^{high}, LFA-1^{high}, CD44^{high}, Mac-1^{high}, LPAM-1^{low}, PECAM-1$^{low/-}$.[52–55]

The presence of a variety of AM on mononuclear cells in EAE and their upregulation on endothelial cells during active disease suggests a pathophysiological role of AM in the initiation of CNS inflammation.

Treatment of EAE with antibodies to AM

To obtain more suggestive evidence for a pathogenic role of AM in EAE, therapeutic manipulation of EAE with mAbs has been undertaken. Antibodies to AM involved in antigen presentation and transendothelial migration prevented clinical disease and reduced mononuclear infiltration and demyelination (Fig. 12.4). The mechanisms underlying suppression of EAE achieved with such intervention vary considerably depending on which AM is targeted. Thus, antibodies directed to ICAM-1, LFA-1, CD2 and CTLA-4/CD28 and B7-1, B1-2 primarily inhibit the process of antigen presentation that takes place in the lymph node draining the immunization site during the induction phase of EAE or in the ENS where local antigen presentation amplifies the incipient immune reaction. By contrast, antibodies to VLA-4, VCAM-1, LFA-1, Mac-1 or L-selectin interfere with transendothelial migration of lymphocytes and monocytes in EAE (Table 12.2; Archelos and Hartung, unpublished). Antibodies to Mac-1 involved in transendothelial migration of monocytes and to the chemoattractant macrophage inflammatory protein-1α (MIP-1α)[56] activating integrin-dependent adhesion of T cells to endothelium, markedly diminished severity of murine EAE (Table 12.2).

In rodent models of EAE not all antibodies masking a specific AM are equipotent: some prevent clinical signs completely while others retard disease; even worsening of EAE with anti-adhesion monoclonal treatment was observed.[57,58] It is difficult to interpret these conflicting results. A single AM member can exhibit many different functions; each one could be 'localized' to different domains of the molecule. Some domains of AM act as functional receptors for common viruses such as rhinoviruses (on ICAM-1),[59] echovirus (on VLA-2, $\alpha_2\beta_1$, CD49b/CD29)[60] or for bacterial molecules involved in host cell entry (invasins) such as those from *Yersinia pseudotuberculosis* (on the β_1-chain of integrins such as in VLA-4).[61] ICAM-1, LFA-1 and PECAM-1 are the best characterized AM on T cells exhibiting different domain-dependent functions in one molecule. Depending on the epitope of AM recognized, antibodies to LFA-1 can provide either stimulatory or inhibitory signals to T cells, or even mimic the binding of a ligand with subsequent conformational change of this integrin resulting in activation.[62,63] For PECAM-1, domains 1 and 2 seem to be responsible for transendothelial migration of monocytes in response to chemokines, and domain 6 appears to mediate the migration of macrophages in the ECM once these have left the vessel.[64–67] Severe side-effects of antibodies to AM have been described. Antibodies to ICAM-1 induced focal spleen and liver necrosis, a generalized state of immunosuppression,[68] and cerebral bleeding,[69] whereas antibodies to L-selectin precipitated a severe lymphopenia in the Lewis rat EAE model (Archelos and Hartung, unpublished).

Potentially opposing actions and even severe side-effects noted with these antibodies underscore the complexity of the biological role of cell-adhesion molecules and emphasize the need for careful experimentation in appropriate animal models before initiating clinical trials of antibodies to AM in MS. To understand the multitude of individual functions and to be able to target the most appropriate ones with high specificity, further studies are needed using antibodies with well-characterized specificity or even engineered to react with defined epitopes/domains.

Based on the studies published to date the α_4 chain of VLA-4, CTLA-4, and ICAM-1 appear to be the most promising targets for intervention.

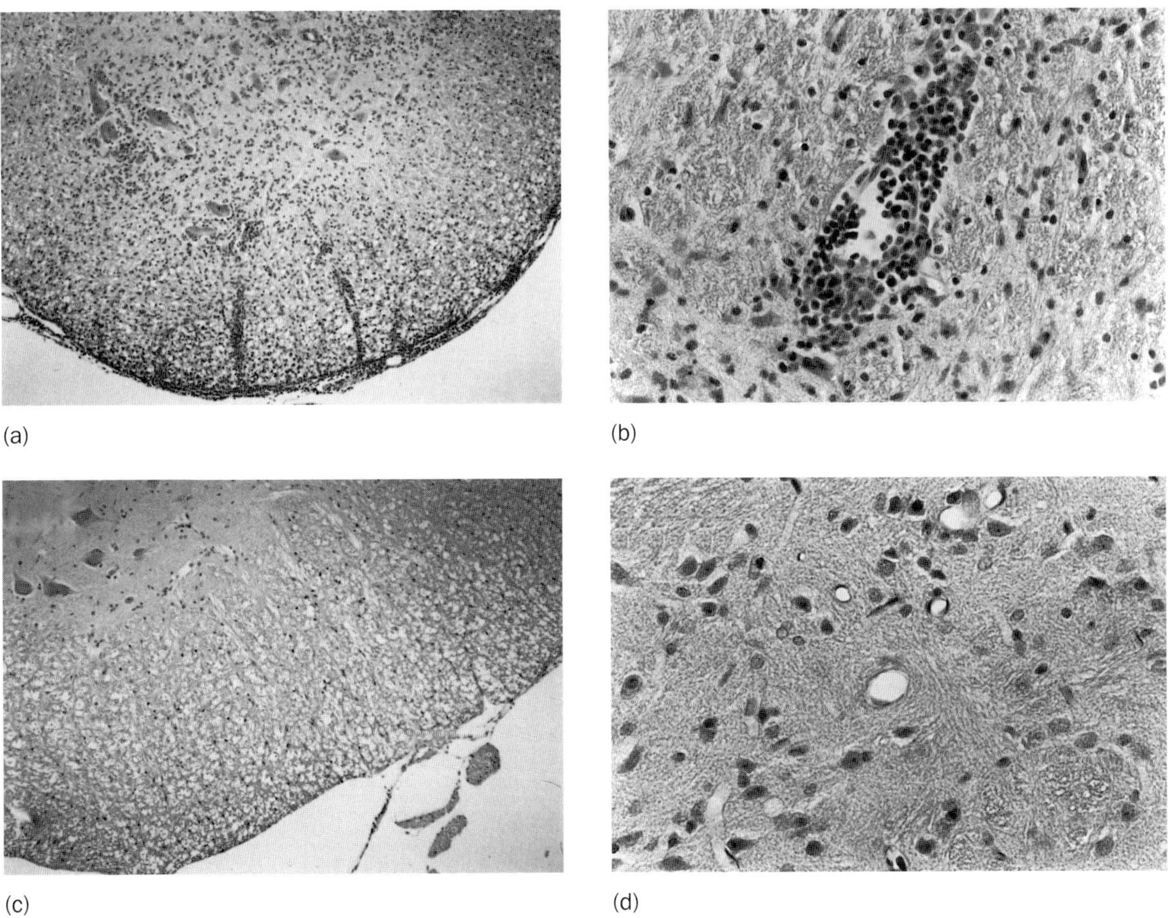

Figure 12.4 Inhibition of spinal cord inflammation during experimental autoimmune encephalomyelitis by anti-adhesion molecule therapy. Experimental autoimmune encephalomyelitis (EAE) was induced in Lewis rats by systemic sensitization of the animals using the encephalitogenic myelin basic protein (MBP, 40 μg/rat) with Freund's adjuvant. Animals were treated either with saline as a control (a,b) or a monoclonal antibody to ICAM-1 (1 mg/rat every other day, injected intraperitoneally) (c,d). Lumbar spinal cord sections (a–d) were stained with haematoxylin and eosin. A substantial mononuclear cell infiltration was present in the parenchyma and in the meningeal layer (a) and around the venules (b) in the sham-treated animal. In contrast, treatment with antibody to ICAM-1 inhibited mononuclear cell infiltration (c, d). In parallel to the histological findings, a marked inhibition of clinical disease was observed.

Disease activity and MRI and EAE

In EAE disease, activity has been monitored and quantified by using a semiquantitative clinical score and by immunohistochemistry. Recent technical improvements offer the possibility to monitor disease activity by MRI.[70–72] Similar to the situation in MS, gadolinium (Gd)-enhancing lesions detect a breakdown of the BBB in EAE and Gd+ lesions correlate with mononuclear cell infiltrations in situ.[73–76]

Table 12.2 Anti-adhesion molecule therapy in EAE

Adhesion molecule	Antibody therapy	Animal model	Effect on EAE	Reference
A. VLA-4/VCAM-1-pathway:				
VLA-4	HP2/1, α-human-VLA-4, ip.	AT-EAE Lewis rat	Suppression	165
VLA-4	PS/2, rat-α-mouse VLA-4, iv.	AT-EAE PL/JxSJL mouse	Suppression	167
VLA-4	AN100226, mouse-α-human VLA-4, ic.	Active EAE Hartley gp	Suppression and reversal	168
VLA-4	GG5/3, mouse-α-human α4, sc.	Active EAE Hartley gp	Suppression and reversal	169
VLA-4	PS/2, rat-α-mouse VLA-4, iv.	Active and AT-EAE SJL/J mouse	Suppression	46
VLA-4	PS/2, rat-α-mouse VLA-4, ip.	Active EAE* Balb/c mouse	Suppression	69
VCAM-1	MK1, iv.	AT-EAE PL/JxSJL mouse	Suppression	167
B. ICAM-1/LFA-1- and ICAM-1/Mac-1-pathways:				
ICAM-1	IA29, mouse-α-rat ICAM-1, ip.	Active-EAE Lewis rat	Suppression	68
ICAM-1	IA29, mouse-α-rat ICAM-1, ip.	AT-EAE Lewis rat	No effect	68
ICAM-1	YN1/1.7.4, rat-α-mouse ICAM-1, iv.	AT-EAE PL/JxSJL mouse	Suppression	167
ICAM-1	YN1/1.7.4, rat-α-mouse ICAM-1, ip.	AT-EAE SJL/J mouse	Suppression (trend)	57
ICAM-1	IA29, mouse-α-rat ICAM-1, ip.	AT-EAE Lewis rat	Suppression	170
ICAM-1	IA29, mouse-α-rat ICAM-1, ip.	Active-EAE Lewis rat	No effect	170
ICAM-1	IA29, mouse-α-rat ICAM-1, ic.	AT-EAE Lewis rat	Suppression	70
ICAM-1	YN1/1.7.4, rat-α-mouse ICAM-1, ip.	Active EAE* Balb/c mouse	Suppression	69
LFA-1	M17/5.2, rat-α-mouse LFA-1, ip.	AT-EAE SJL/J mouse	Exacerbation	57
LFA-1	M17/4.2, rat-α-mouse LFA-1, ip.	AT-EAE SJL/J mouse	Exacerbation	58
LFA-1	M17/5.2, rat-α-mouse LFA-1, ip.	AT-EAE PL/JxSJL mouse	Suppression	171
LFA-1	WT-1, mouse-α-rat LFA-1, ip.	Active-EAE Lewis rat	Suppression	172
ICAM-1 + LFA-1	IA29 and WT-1 combined, icv.	Active and AT-EAE Lewis rat	Suppression	173
Mac-1	ED7, ED8, mouse-α-rat Mac-1	EAE Lewis rat	Suppression	174
Mac-1	OX42, mouse-α-rat Mac-1	EAE Lewis rat	No effect	174
Mac-1	5C6, rat-α-mouse Mac-1, ip.	AT-EAE PL/JxSJL mouse	Suppression	171
Mac-1	5C6, rat-α-mouse Mac-1, ip.	Active EAE* Balb/c mouse	No effect	69

Adhesion molecule	Antibody therapy	Animal model	Effect on EAE	Reference
C. Selectin-pathways:				
L-selectin	MEL-14, rat-α-mouse L-selectin, ip.	Active EAE SWXJ mouse	No effect	45
L-selectin	HRL3, hamster-α-rat L-selectin, ip.	Active EAE Lewis rat	Suppression	175
E-selectin	UZ4, rat-α-mouse E-selectin, iv.	Active and AT-EAE SJL/J mouse	No effect	46
P-selectin	RB40.34.4, rat-α-mouse P-selectin, iv.	Active and AT-EAE SJL/L mouse	No effect	46
D. CTLA-4/B7-pathway:				
B7-1	16-10A1, rat-α-mouse CD80, ip.	Active and AT-EAE PL/JxSJL mouse	Suppression	176
B7-1	1G10, rat-α-mouse CD80, ip.	Active EAE SJL/J mouse	Suppression	25
B7-1	16-10A1, IG10, rat-α-mouse CD80	Active EAE SJL/J mouse	Exacerbation	39
B7-2	2G10, GL-1, rat-α-mouse CD86, ip.	Active EAE SJL/J mouse	Exacerbation	25
B7-2	GL-1, rat-α-mouse CD86, ip.	Active and AT-EAE PL/JxSJL mouse	Suppression	176
B7-1 and B7-2	16-10A1 and GL-1, combined, ip.	Active EAE PL/JxSJL mouse	Exacerbation	177
CTLA-4	UC10/4F10, hamster-α-mouse CTLA-4	Active and AT-EAE SJL/J mouse	Exacerbation	24
CTLA-4	UC10/4F10, hamster-α-mouse CTLA-4	Active EAE PL/JxSJL mouse	Exacerbation	177
CTLA-4	Hamster-α-mouse CTLA-4, ip.	Active EAE PL/JxSJL mouse	Exacerbation	178
E. Other adhesion molecules:				
PECAM-1	TLD 3A12, mouse-α-rat PECAM-1, iv.	AT-EAE Lewis rat	No effect	48
LFA-2	OX34, mouse-α-rat CD2, iv.	Active and AT-EAE Lewis rat	Suppression and reversal	179
CD40L	hamster-α-CD40L, ip.	Active EAE SJL mouse	Suppression	180

Several studies on the impact of antiadhesion molecule treatment on EAE have been published. The table gives an overview about the targeted adhesion molecule (AM), the type of monoclonal antibody used to block AM function, the EAE animal model investigated and the treatment effect.

Abbreviations: *, virus-facilitated; AT, adoptive transfer; gp, guinea pig; ic., intracardiac; ip., intraperitoneal; iv., intravenous; icv., intracerebroventricular; sc., subcutaneous. For CD nomenclature see Table 12.1.
We apologize, if an important study has not been included in Tables 12.2 and 12.3.

Circulating adhesion molecules in EAE

We are not aware of published data on circulating adhesion molecules (cAM) in EAE. The lack of commercially available reagents and the feasibility to measure these parameters in MS may explain this. Levels of cAM may vary considerably between species: e.g. cL-selectin levels are much lower in Lewis rats than in humans, and correlate with clinical severity of active EAE (Archelos and Hartung, unpublished observation).

ADHESION MOLECULES AND MS

Do the mechanisms of antigen presentation and transendothelial migration studied in EAE by antibody blockade also govern the immune response in MS? Most of the studies of the role of AM during MS have relied on immunohistochemical analysis of the expression of AM during the different stages of disease on autopsy CNS material or on blood or CSF-derived lymphocytes from patients with MS. In addition, cAM have been measured in blood and CSF in MS patients.

Adhesion molecule expression in the CNS

In the acute and chronic active lesion, ICAM-1, VCAM-1 and E-selectin are upregulated on endothelial cells. In situ, infiltrating T cells express CD44, LFA-1, VLA-4, ICAM-3, LFA-3, CD40L, B7-1 and monocytes in addition to CD40 and B7-2. In the MS lesion, resident cells of the CNS such as astrocytes stain for ICAM-1, LFA-3, CD44, and microglia is positive for LFA-1 and B7[77–83] suggesting a contributory role of these resident cells in the initiation, maintenance and termination of the inflammatory response in the CNS. It is noteworthy that ICAM-1/LFA-1 expression is present at relatively high levels in plaques of all ages. In contrast, VCAM-1/VLA-4 was lowest in acute lesions and increased in chronic lesions.

AM expression in T cells

Blood

Blood-derived T cells of MS patients have increased levels of LFA-1, ICAM-1, LFA-3, CD2, CD44 on their surface but a decreased expression of VLA-4 and VLA-5.[84] Others have not found such an expression pattern in MS.[85] Adhesion of T cells to normal and MS-patient-derived endothelial cells is enhanced.

AM expression patterns on peripheral T cells have been analyzed in a longitudinal study: levels of CD28, VLA-4 and LFA-1 did not change significantly over 6 months, although patients showed disease activity in MRI.[84] Treatment with interferon β-1a (IFN-β1a) downregulates VLA-4 expression, but not LFA-1, ICAM-1, L-selectin, or CD44.[86] Treatment with methylprednisolone transiently reduces LFA-1 expression on T cells,[87] had no effect on L-selectin and VLA-4 on T cells, but significantly altered the expression pattern of L-selectin, Mac-1 and VLA-4 on circulating monocytes.[85]

Cerebrospinal fluid

T cells isolated from CSF show an increased expression of LFA-1, ICAM-1, VLA-3, VLA-4, VLA-5, VLA-6, LFA-3, CD2, B7-1, and CD44.[88,89]

Circulating adhesion molecules in MS

AM are not only present as anchored transmembrane molecules but after interaction with the corresponding ligand, some are also cleaved or shed and circulate as soluble forms in body fluids.[90,91] Areas of interest are the cellular origin of the circulating forms, the agents inducing cleavage and shedding, and the physiological function of cAM. In addition, in MS an easy-to-measure disease activity marker is much needed. cAM could be promising candidates.

In MS circulating forms of ICAM-1, ICAM-3,[92] VCAM-1, E-selectin, and L-selectin, have been studied (Table 12.3). Other forms such as cCD44, cP-selectin, circulating glycosylation-dependent cell adhesion molecule-1 (cGlyCAM-1), have not been examined so far.

Circulating ICAM-1 (cICAM-1)

cICAM-1 is present in serum of healthy individuals.[90] Cell sources of relevance in MS are activated endothelial cells, lymphocytes and monocytes. Measurements of cICAM-1 in serum of patients with relapsing–remitting MS (RRMS) revealed elevated, normal and in one study reduced levels (Table 12.3). A consistent finding was the presence of significant higher cICAM-1 concentrations in patients with clinically active disease as determined by the occurrence of recent relapses. In comparison, much lower levels were found in stable RRMS patients, which in most studies were not significantly different from levels in healthy controls. Two longitudinal studies on cICAM-1 have been published. Rieckmann et al.[93] found a significant association of cICAM-1 and relapses. Giovannoni et al.[94] could not confirm this finding and described highly variable individual cICAM-1 levels throughout the study.

Disease activity in MS is thought to be associated with Gd-enhancing lesions, and disease outcome may be influenced by the total lesion load. Therefore, cICAM-1 levels and MRI findings were compared. Hartung et al.[95] first described elevated cICAM-1 serum levels in MS patients with Gd-enhancing lesions compared to MS patients without Gd+ lesions. These findings were confirmed and extended by several other groups[93,94,96–100] (Table 12.3). In contrast, one group reports higher cICAM levels in clinically active RRMS without active lesions in MRI.[99] Increased CSF levels and serum/CSF ratios for ICAM-1 have been described in association with an impaired blood–CSF barrier and with disease activity in MRI.[101] Treatment with methylprednisolone either reduced[87] or had no effect[85] on serum cICAM-1; IFN-β1b[102] therapy did not significantly modify cICAM-1 levels.

Less data have been published about cICAM-1 in serum in chronic progressive MS (CPMS). Dore Duffy et al.[103] found higher concentrations of serum cICAM-1 in CPMS than in active RRMS. Similarly, increased levels were noted in primary progressive MS.[104] Hartung et al.[95] describe statistically significantly increased levels of cICAM-1 in CPMS, but these were much lower than in active RRMS.

Circulating VCAM-1 (cVCAM-1)

Circulating VCAM-1 has a molecular mass of approximately 85 kDa and is shed from endothelial cells and macrophages upon activation. In humans, serum levels are comparable to cICAM-1.[90] Serum and CSF cVCAM-1 have been described to be elevated in active RRMA and in CPMS.[93,97,105,106] Others have not found such a correlation.[102,103,107] Elevated serum cVCAM-1 concentrations have been reported to be positively correlated to the presence of Gd-enhancing lesions in MRI.[93,97,105,107] Others could not confirm this association.[94,102] The only longitudinal study published found no significant correlation between relapses and cVCAM-1 levels.[94]

Treatment of MS patients with IFN-β1b resulted in elevated cVCAM-1 serum levels which were correlated with a decreased number of Gd+ lesions in MRI.[102] By contrast, pulse treatment with methylprednisolone had no effect on serum cVCAM.[85]

Circulating E-selectin (cE-selectin)

E-selectin is present only on activated endothelial cells and hence, all cE-selectin is endothelium derived. In humans, serum concentrations of cE-selectin are considerably lower (factor 10) than cICAM-1 or cVCAM-1 levels, and cE-selectin is barely detectable in CSF.[90]

All groups[85,93,102–105,107,108] but one[109] found no significant differences of serum cE-selectin levels between active RRMS and controls (Table 12.3). Serum concentrations did not correlate with clinical disease activity nor with Gd enhancement on MRI. In contrast, patients with CPMS seem to have elevated cE-selectin levels in serum.[103,104,109] These were correlated to clinical disease progression. A possible relationship with MRI findings have not been addressed in these studies (Table 12.3).

Circulating L-selectin (cL-selectin)

cL-Selectin circulates in two isoforms which have a different molecular mass (62 kDa and

Table 12.3 Circulating adhesion molecules in multiple sclerosis

Reference	RRMS Serum	RRMS CSF	CPMS Serum	CPMS CSF	Correlated with CDA	Correlated with EDSS	Correlated with MRI
A. Circulating ICAM-1:							
95	↑ $n = 97$	ND	↑ to ± $n = 50$	ND	+	+	+
181	± $n = 18$	± $n = 18$	± $n = 5$	± $n = 5$	ND	ND	ND
101	± $n = 9$	↑ $n = 9$	ND	ND	ND	ND	ND
98	↑ $n = 38$	↑ $n = 38$	ND	ND	+	ND	ND
182	ND	↑ $n = 25$	ND	↑ $n = 25$	+	ND	ND
100	↑ $n = 25$	ND	± $n = 6$	ND	+	ND	ND
93	↑ $n = 29$	ND	ND	ND	+	ND	+
103	± $n = 44$	± $n = 44$	↑ $n = 14$	± $n = 14$	no	ND	ND
108	↓ $n = 56$	↑ $n = 56$	ND	ND	ND	ND	ND
99	↑ $n = 35$	↑ $n = 35$	ND	ND	+	ND	–
102	± $n = 11$	± $n = 4$	ND	ND	ND	ND	ND
96	↑ $n = 8$	↑ $n = 8$	↑ $n = 8$	↑ $n = 8$	+	+	ND
94	↑ $n = 22$	ND	↑ $n = 25$	ND	no	no	+
97	↑ $n = 46$	↑ $n = 46$	ND	ND	ND	ND	+

Reference	RRMS Serum	RRMS CSF	CPMS Serum	CPMS CSF	Correlated with CDA	Correlated with EDSS	Correlated with MRI
B. Circulating VCAM-1:							
93	↑ $n = 29$	ND	ND	ND	+	ND	+
103	± $n = 44$	± $n = 44$	± $n = 14$	↑ $n = 14$	+ (Trend)	ND	ND
105	↑ $n = 97$	ND	↑ to ± $n = 50$	ND	+	no	+
103	± $n = 56$	↑ $n = 56$	ND	ND	ND	ND	ND
103	↑ $n = 29$	↑ $n = 29$	↑ $n = 10$	↑ $n = 11$	+	ND	ND
107	± $n = 21$	± $n = 21$	ND	ND	ND	ND	+ (Trend)
102	± $n = 11$	± $n = 4$	ND	ND	no	no	no
94	↑(Trend) $n = 22$	ND	↑(Trend) $n = 25$	ND	no	no	no
97	↑ $n = 46$	↑ $n = 46$	ND	ND	ND	ND	+
C. Circulating E-selectin:							
93	± $n = 29$	ND	ND	ND	no	ND	no
103	± $n = 44$	± $n = 44$	↑ $n = 14$	↑ $n = 14$	+	ND	ND
105	± $n = 97$	ND	± $n = 50$	ND	no	no	no
109	↑ $n = 32$	↑ (Trend) $n = 32$	↑ $n = 12$	↑ (Trend) $n = 12$	+	ND	ND

continued

Table 12.3 Continued

Reference	RRMS Serum	RRMS CSF	CPMS Serum	CPMS CSF	Correlated with CDA	Correlated with EDSS	Correlated with MRI
108	± $n = 56$	± $n = 56$	ND	ND	ND	ND	ND
107	± $n = 21$	± $n = 21$	ND	ND	no	ND	no
104	± $n = 9$	ND	↑ $n = 10$	ND	+ (Trend)	+ (Trend)	no
102	± $n = 11$	± $n = 4$	ND	ND	ND	ND	ND
D. Circulating L-selectin:							
93	↑ $n = 29$	ND	ND	ND	no	ND	no
105	↑ $n = 97$	ND	↑ to ± $n = 50$	ND	+	+	+
111	± $n = 20$	± $n = 20$	ND	ND	+ (Trend)	ND	+
102	± $n = 11$	± $n = 4$	ND	ND	ND	ND	ND

Summary of studies published on measurements of circulating adhesion molecule (cAM) in serum and cerebrospinal fluid (CSF) in patients with relapsing–remitting (RR) and chronic progressive (CP) multiple sclerosis (MS). The number of MS patients studied is given as *n*. cAM levels were significantly elevated (↑), decreased (↓) or statistically not significantly different from controls (±). In some studies cAM levels were correlated with clinical disease activity (CDA), to the expanded disability status scale (EDSS) or to cranial magnetic resonance imaging (MRI) findings. + significant positive correlation; – significant negative correlation; no: indicates an absent correlation; + (Trend), positive correlation but failed to reach statistical significance; ND: not done.

75–100 kDa), are differentially glycosylated and are derived from different cell types, namely lymphocytes and neutrophils.[90,110] L-selectin is shed from the leukocyte surface upon activation.

cL-Selectin has been reported to be elevated,[93,105] normal[102,111] or lowered[85] in active RRMS. Two groups found a significant correlation between serum cL-selectin levels and the presence of Gd-enhancing MRI lesions[105,111] (Table 12.3). No longitudinal studies are available. Serum concentrations are not altered by treatment with IFN-β1b.[102] Intravenous high-dose methylprednisolone reduced cL-selectin levels in the first week after treatment.[85]

Circulating adhesion molecules—future prospects

cICAM-1 is the best characterized cAM in MS. Serum levels are consistently elevated in active RRMS and correlate with the presence of Gd-enhancing lesions in MRI. cVCAM-1 has a similar profile, though less data are available and—compared to cICAM-1—MRI findings are less consistent. cE-selectin data are less convincing for RRMS but it could be useful marker to monitor CPMS. Of course, more studies are needed. The few studies published on cL-selectin indicate an elevation in RRMS which is correlated with the presence of Gd+ lesions in MRI. Current available assays measure both forms of L-selectin, neutrophil- and lymphocyte-derived. It would be interesting to quantitate only cL selectin shed from lymphocytes by use of specific assays. This may considerably improve the utility of this marker in MS.

Research on cAM needs to be intensified. More longitudinal studies are warranted to evaluate their usefulness as an easy-to-measure disease activity marker in MS.

cAM in CSF, although of pathophysiological relevance, will most likely not become a routine marker of disease activity.

cAM should not only be studied as indicators of disease, but their pathobiological function in MS requires to be elucidated. Most soluble AM circulate in an active form as monomers, cICAM-1 also as homodimer, and are committed to bind to their ligands either at the site of their release or systemically. Some cAM have been shown to compete with membrane-anchored AM for their ligands. Ligand bound cAM are not detected in serum or CSF measurements but may be responsible for their relevant biological function. Illumination of the pathophysiological role of cAM in MS may also have future therapeutic implications (see below).

Unfortunately, elevated levels of cAM are not specific to MS, being detectable in other acute and chronic inflammatory diseases of the CNS. This poses some problems when targeting AM with putative experimental therapies, as will be discussed below.

POTENTIAL OF AM-DERIVED THERAPIES IN MS

Monoclonal antibodies: tolerance induction

Most of the studies on the effect of antibodies of AM in EAE relied on the acute binding of the antibody to AM and blockade of the corresponding step in the immune response.

Some lymphocyte-directed antibodies when administered to mice in vivo induced tolerance.[110] Physiologically, foreign antigens or grafted allo-derived tissues elicit a rejecting immune response in the recipient mice. However, if the foreign tissue or antigens were grafted under the 'umbrella' of tolerogenic mAbs to AM, such as CD4, CD8, LFA-1, ICAM-1, CD28 and B7, the host-derived rejection response (host versus graft reaction) was attenuated or abolished. This effect lasted several months, and in some instances an indefinite acceptance of a transplanted organ under the 'protection' of CD4 antibodies was achieved.[112–114]

Tolerance induction consists of the 'reprogramming' of the immune system to allow acceptance of antigenic material that would otherwise be rejected; it is a complex, still incompletely understood process.

Transient antigen-independent T-cell hyporesponsiveness

Some of the available antibodies against CD2, ICAM-1 or the B7:CD28/CTLA-4 costimulatory pathway, among others, can induce temporary antigen-independent T-cell hyporesponsiveness. Recent studies in murine EAE demonstrated a long-term inhibition of clinical and histological signs after treatment with the immunoadhesin CTLA-4-Fc[115] (see next section). The potential for antibodies to induce specific tolerance and general T-cell hyporesponsiveness are qualities that add tremendous power to the better-understood, short-term blocking effects of anti-AM-therapy.

Antibody derivatives to AM

In oncology, genetically engineered tumor-specific antibodies are coupled to cytokines, AM or toxins. The basic idea is to deliver the desired therapeutic agent specifically to the tumor. Successful targeting of carcino-embryonic antigen-producing cancers has been achieved in humans.[116] These immunoconjugates could also be promising therapeutics for EAE and in the future for MS.[117] These constructs should consist of a mAb (for example directed to a CNS-specific antigen such as MOG, see below) coupled by genetic engineering to various inflammation-modulating agents such as soluble AM, immunosuppressive cytokines such as interleukin-10 (IL-10), transforming growth factor β (TGF-β), apoptosis-inducing agents such as Fas-ligand, or transcription-regulating factors (Fig. 12.5a) (see below). This field is only emerging and data on chronic inflammatory disease of the CNS are not yet available.[118]

CLINICAL TRIALS WITH ANTIBODIES AGAINST ADHESION MOLECULES

Rheumatoid arthritis

Promising phase II clinical trials with tolerogenic antibody to ICAM-1 are already underway for rheumatoid arthritis, a chronic inflammatory disease of the joints resembling MS in some immunopathological features. Administration of an unmodified murine antibody against ICAM-1 to 13 patients with refractory disease produced clinical improvement in some patients. This was paralleled by: a T-cell hyporesponsiveness lasting up to 5 months after cessation of antibody treatment; reduced IL-6 messenger RNA in patients' lymphocytes; and reduced levels of cICAM-1.[119] Thus, antigen-independent anti-AM-antibody treatment could result in 'reprogramming' of the immune system.

Multiple sclerosis

Monoclonal antibody treatment for MS

There have been some pilot studies of mAb treatment of MS using murine antibodies directed to transmembrane T-cell antigens[11] such as CD2,[120] CD3,[121] CD4,[122–125] and CD6.[126] These elicited anti-idiotypic immune responses and caused acute side-effects such as transient worsening of symptoms, fever, myalgia and hypotension, limiting the usefulness of this approach. Although some improvement was reported in these studies, the clinical benefit was difficult to assess, because no placebo-treated control patients were included.

More recently, in another pilot study, CAMPATH-1H (a humanized mAb to CDw25, a T-cell antigen) was administered to 13 patients with secondary CPMS.[127] The aim was to elaborate possible side-effects and changes in immune parameters. Clinical efficacy was not addressed by this study and will require a future placebo-controlled, double-blind study design.

In an open phase 1 trial, a chimeric 'humanized' mAb to CD4 (cM-T412) was administered as a single dose intravenously to 26 patients with CPMS.[122] Treatment induced a long-lasting depletion of CD4-positive T cells. Side-effects included headache, nausea, myalgia and fever. The single-dose treatment reduced Gd-enhancing lesions as detected on MRI in the first week after injection, and the disability was stable after 6 months.

In a second randomized, double-blind, phase II trial van Oosten and colleagues[124] treated 71 patients suffering from RRMS and CPMS with monthly cM-T412 antibody infusions over 6 months. Besides the expected depletion of CD4-positive T cells they observed a statistically

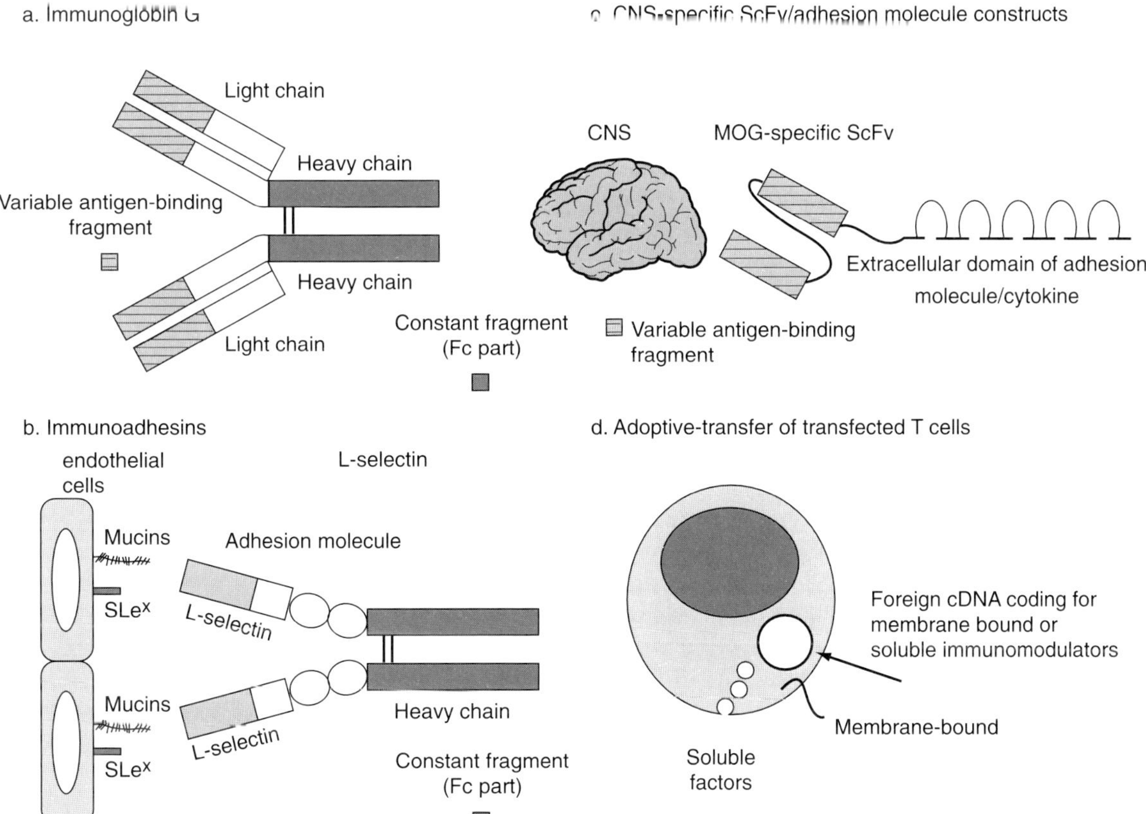

Figure 12.5 Experimental tools to target specifically adhesion molecules involved in experimental autoimmune encephalomyelitis. (a) Immunoglobulins (Igs) are composed of two identical heavy chains, linked together by disulphide bonds, and two identical light chains. They are bifunctional molecules with an antigen-binding region formed by the variable parts of the heavy and light chain. The constant part of both heavy chains confers effector function to the Ig molecule. (b) Immunoadhesins are genetically engineered bifunctional molecules combining the constant region of an immunoglobulin (Fc-fragment) and an adhesion molecule (AM). The AM part directs the action of the construct to a specific AM and can be used to block the corresponding function of the immune response. The added Fc-part increases plasma half-life of the therapeutic and adds, if desired, effector function to the immunoadhesins, allowing the elimination of a determined T-cell subpopulation. In addition the Fc part facilitates purification of immunoadhesins. (c) A single chain construct of the variable antibody fragment (ScFv) reacting with myelin/oligodendrocyte glycoprotein (MOG) selectively expressed in the central nervous system (CNS) could serve as a carrier of immunomodulators such as ICAM-1. These CNS-specific ScFv constructs could exert their activity predominantly in the inflammatory lesion of the CNS where the blood brain barrier is disrupted. Such constructs open the possibility of organ-specific modulation of the immune response—an aim not yet achieved by established treatments in experimental autoimmune encephalomyelitis or multiple sclerosis. (d) T cells offer another possibility of CNS-specific treatment. T cells can be transduced with genes encoding beneficial membrane-bound or secreted immunomodulators to downregulate the adhesion molecules (for details see Fig. 12.6).

significant reduction of 41% in the number of clinical relapses. However, the number of Gd-enhancing lesions was not significantly reduced by cM-T412.

ADHESION MOLECULES AS THERAPEUTIC TARGETS IN EAE AND MS

Therapy of MS with antibodies to AM

Which AM should be targeted in future clinical trials in MS? Until one or more autoantigens are proven to cause MS, antigen-specific intervention during the induction phase of MS is not feasible. Antibody targeting of transendothelial migration of T cells (governed by the selectins, VCAM-1/α4 and LFA-1/ICAM-1) and of monocytes (additionally regulated by PECAM-1) and the use of tolerogenic antibodies provide realistic potential therapeutic options to be evaluated in MS. Major efforts need to be invested to further elucidate the mechanisms underlying the migration of these cells into the CNS with the aim of inhibiting this process. One scenario in which to use blocking antibodies to AM might be acute intervention in severe disease, or for the treatment of lesions affecting crucial structures such as the lower brainstem.

A phase II/III clinical trial with a 'humanized' antibody[128] to the α_4-chain of VLA-4 has been initiated in the UK; 80 MS patients will be enrolled and clinical benefit, drug safety, side-effects and disease activity in MRI will be monitored.

Regulating adhesion molecule expression

Cytokines are the most important soluble mediators of inflammation released by immune cells; they strongly regulate AM expression on both endothelial cells and lymphocytes. There is already a wealth of information on this topic[129–131] and only a few examples will be discussed here. 'Pro-inflammatory' cytokines such as IL-1, tumor necrosis factor-α (TNF-α), and IFN-γ increase the expression of ICAM-1 and IL-1, and TNF-α upregulates VCAM-1 on human and murine endothelial cells.[12] In contrast, TGF-β_2—a cytokine involved in tissue repair among other properties—has been shown to reduce AM expression of murine T cells in vitro;[132] it also diminishes the migration of murine T cells in vitro and their homing into the CNS in EAE in the SJL/J mouse.[132] Thus, treatment strategies aimed at modulating the immune response by interfering with the cytokine network could also indirectly impact on the levels of AM on cell surfaces and hence regulate lymphocyte trafficking.

Surprisingly, transcription of the genes encoding VCAM-1, ICAM-1, PECAM-1 and E-selectin is regulated by the cytokine-inducible nuclear transcription factor kappa-B (NF-κB). The 'pro-inflammatory' cytokines IL-1, IL-2 and TNF-α all activate this shared, regulating pathway and induce upregulation of endothelial AM via NF-κB.[133,134] Curiously, the expression of these cytokines is also regulated by the same factor. In MBP-induced EAE in the Lewis rat, a strong upregulation of transcription factor NF-κB in endothelium, lesion-infiltrating immune cells and CNS-resident microglia correlated with the presence of inflammatory lesions and disease activity.[135] The identification of the NF-κB system as a dominant regulator of endothelial cell AM and proinflammatory cytokine genes suggests that pharmacological inhibition of NF-κB activation could represent an attractive, novel approach to the development of anti-inflammatory therapies.[136] Inhibition of NF-κB activation by immunoconjugates (chimera containing an organ-specific antibody part) and an NF-κB downregulating agent such as small peptidergic or synthetic nonpeptidergic antagonists, represents a single molecular target to suppress simultaneously the expression of multiple genes involved in lymphocyte transmigration and inflammation.[134] The initial in vitro studies using serine protease inhibitors of the NF-κB pathway have yielded promising results; stimulation-induced expression of VCAM-1, ICAM-1 and E-selectin could be blocked in a human endothelial cell line[137] and in vivo.[138] First promising in vivo results showed that antisense oligonucleotides inhibiting NF-κB abrogated experimental colitis in mice.[139] Strategies to target this transcription factor in vivo in rodent EAE animal models are required before this approach could be considered for clinical use.

Soluble natural ligands of AM

Soluble, or circulating, forms of AM are shed from the surface of the endothelium and T cells upon activation by cytokines; they retain their functional and ligand binding capacity, however. In vitro studies revealed that these soluble forms of AM can interfere with the cell surface bound forms thus opening an avenue for potential therapeutic intervention.[140,141] Exogenously applied soluble AM, or stable derivatives of AM in the form of immunoadhesins, provide the opportunity to modulate the immune response at several levels.

Recently, long-term inhibition of murine chronic EAE was achieved with an immunoadhesin[117] combining the immunoglobulin-like extracellular domain of CTLA-4 with the Fc part of an immunoglobulin (CTLA-4-Fc fusion protein).[115] Intraperitoneal injection of CTLA-4-Fc profoundly suppressed clinical and histological manifestations of EAE. More information regarding the long-term effects and side-effects of treatment with natural ligands of AM or with immunoadhesins is now required in EAE before these treatments can enter clinical trials.

Blocking peptides and synthetic antagonists

Synthetic peptides ranging from cyclic 3 to linear 50 amino acids with antagonistic effects on AM binding are ideal targeted drugs. However, pharmacokinetic studies show that such peptides, which are usually water soluble, do not readily cross mucosal surfaces and have a rapid whole-body clearance due to renal excretion and degradation. Chemical modifications of the peptide backbone, such as the use of cycled peptides, may partly overcome these problems. Of primary interest in targeting the AM with blocking peptides is the identification of the three-dimensional structure of the most relevant binding sites on AM. The rational design of the peptides requires an exact fitting of the relative small peptide into the binding epitope. In contrast, blockade of AM by mAbs does not require such exact information about the binding domain; first, because mAbs in their production are tailored to the AM by the immune system of the animals used for fusion, and second because the large immunoglobulin exerts a steric hindrance even if the antibody binds not exactly but in close proximity to the functional epitope.

Inhibition of AM function can be achieved by the use of short peptide sequences based on the structure of VLA-4[142–144] or ICAM-1 in vitro.[145] However, in most applications complex binding regions are prevalent. Recently an innovative approach to peptide-drug development was reported by Wang and colleagues[146] who mapped by three-dimensional crystallography the binding epitopes of VCAM-1. In doing so they highlighted the structural participation of distant epitopes, and most intriguingly designed a short peptide that mimicked the complex binding loop of VCAM-1 and acted as a potent antagonist blocking VCAM-1/α_4-integrin interactions in vitro. It is likely that once a specific peptide blocking an AM–ligand-receptor interaction has been identified a corresponding synthetic compound offering better pharmacokinetic properties (oral bioavailability, longer in vivo half-lives, higher affinities, chemical stability) will be developed.[146]

Targeting the selectins with antagonists

Integrins or AM of the immunoglobulin superfamily mediate multiple functions in the immune response (antigen presentation, transendothelial migration and tolerance); by contrast, the selectins have a much more restricted role directing lymphocyte–endothelial migration into the target organ or within lymph nodes. This makes them particular attractive targets for therapeutic intervention.[147,148] In addition, binding of the lectin domain of selectins is often confined to short carbohydrate structures on a variety of ligands (see Table 12.1)[149] Oligosaccharides with potent antagonistic effect on the sialylLewis^x epitope (ligand of E- and L-selectin) for example, have been developed and tested successfully in vivo in several acute inflammatory disease animal models.[150] The greatest appeal of such agents derives from their particularly safe pharmacotoxicology and pharmacodynamics profile in humans and animals.[148] In contrast to the other therapeutics discussed, oligosaccharides are highly water soluble, easy to sterilize for intravenous application, are identical to natural, endogenous oligosaccharides, and therefore well tolerated. They exhibit a relative lack of immune reactivity with no significant side-effects in vivo and could even be applied orally. Problems arise from the low specificity of the carbohydrates to block single selectins. Another disadvantage is the particular interaction of selectins via carbohydrates with their ligands.[149] The high avidity binding of selectins in contrast to the high affinity binding of integrins make it necessary to create antagonists with a high avidity and not necessarily a high affinity as for peptide analogues. However, synthesis of proteins carrying carbohydrates at high density able to disrupt or antagonize high avidity interactions is a complex task and suitable synthetic substances are beginning to be available.[151] Selectin antagonists are a promising alternative to therapeutic mAbs directed to selectins. Because of the lack of knowledge about long-term beneficial effects such as tolerance induction, the application of these molecules would be restricted primarily to acute intervention in MS. Studies on the long-term effects of continuous application of carbohydrate-based antagonists in chronic and acute EAE are now needed.

Antisense oligonucleotide technology

Oligonucleotides are short antisense DNA sequences binding complementary to a defined messenger RNA (sense) to prevent corresponding protein synthesis.[152] Antisense oligonucleotides display high selectivity and affinity for, as well as reversibility of effects for their nucleic acid targets.[153] Indeed, expression of the endothelial AM crucial for lymphocyte transmigration such as ICAM-1, VCAM-1, L- and E-selectin has been inhibited in vitro by the use of corresponding antisense oligonucleotides.[154] High-affinity oligonucleotide antagonists specific for L-selectin have been developed for future in vivo use.[155,156]

In rat EAE disease severity was ameliorated by intracerebroventricular application of an antisense oligonucleotide directed to murine IFNγ-inducible protein (IP-10), a chemokine attracting mononuclear cells to the CNS lesion.[157] Other data on EAE and AM oligonucleotides have not been published.

Unfortunately, current phase I and II human clinical trials evaluating the pharmacokinetics, effects and side-effects of intravenously infused oligonucleotides show that oligonucleotides administered intravenously have a short plasma half-life and induce side-effects such as prolonged coagulation time, elevation of liver enzymes, splenomegaly, complement activation and cytokine release.[153]

The problem of specificity

As discussed above, AM play a pivotal role in the immune response in EAE and possibly in MS. However, these molecules are also critically important for several physiological functions of the immune system. Thus, therapeutic interventions targeted to AM in MS or other diseases could engender a state of generalized immunosuppression[68]—or even tolerance induction—but perhaps could compromise essential functions of the immune system such as those that control infection. Short-term use of AM-modulating agents might circumvent those unwanted effects. MS is a chronic disease, and little is known about the long-term impact of even transiently stabilizing or resolving individual lesions. It is possible that temporary downregulation of AM expression would allow the disordered immune system to be 'reset' thereby allowing long-term remission.

Can MS therapy be targeted to the CNS?

CNS-specific antibody fragments as potential carriers

Recombinant technologies make it feasible to engineer single recombinant fragments of immunoglobulins. DNA coding for single chain fragments of immunoglobulins. DNA coding for single chain fragments containing the variable part of an immunoglobulin (ScFv) can be isolated and cloned to a DNA of an AM or cytokine to produce a bifunctional molecule. These constructs are expressed in a suitable prokaryotic or eukaryotic expression system and exhibit a dual function. The antibody fragment specific for a given antigen carries the chimera to the desired target and the AM or cytokine coupled to it could exert an immunomodulatory function (Fig. 12.5b). With this approach constructs with IL-2 and IL-8 coupled to a tumor-specific ScFv have been created. ScFv have been shown to target selectively tumor tissue in patients suffering from cancer.[116] Applied to MS one could couple AM—such as the extracellular domain of ICAM-1 or of coaccessory molecule B7-1, or immunosuppressive cytokines such as TGF-β or IL-10—to a ScFv of MOG (a myelin protein expressed exclusively in the CNS). These constructs would enter the CNS only at sites where the BBB is open, corresponding to active Gd-enhanced lesions, and the delivered AM would compete with the natural ligands for AM and possibly locally modulate the immune response (Fig. 12.5).

T cells as 'Trojan horses'?

An 'ideal' immunotherapy would target AM, or their regulators, exclusively in the CNS without interfering with the systemic immune system. Promising strategies based on gene therapy are in sight.[158]

Transduced CNS-specific T cells

A very elegant approach was recently published by two groups.[159,160] Active EAE was induced in mice and autoreactive mouse T cells that were specific for PLP and MBP, respectively, were transfected with a construct containing either the gene of IL-10 or IL-4—two strong immunosuppressive cytokines. After injection of these transfected autoreactive T cells into mice, EAE was ameliorated by the locally-released cytokine.

Future approaches in EAE could use such CNS-specific transfected T cells that retain the capacity to respond specifically to the appropriate antigen and are able to release immunomodulators in the inflamed lesions in the CNS. Thus, these 'therapeutic' T cells could serve as 'Trojan horses', engineered for short-term local delivery of immunomodulating agents to target AM (Fig. 12.5 and Fig. 12.6). In humans, myelin-protein specific T cells form part of the normal T-cell repertoire; this could circumvent any problems of histocompatibility because T cells would be autologous.

Transduced nonspecific T cells

As mentioned above, in murine AT-EAE induced by the transfer of MBP-specific T cells, only 5% of the T cells present in the lesion are myelin reactive. Almost all T cells are nonspecific. If activated nonspecific T cells are injected into rats together with the MBP-specific T cells the animals develop EAE, and a considerable proportion of the co-injected nonspecific T cells accumulates in the lesion, a factor × 20 more than if the nonspecific T cells are injected alone.[161] This confirms that regardless of their antigenic specificity, activated T cells are attracted to the lesion by chemokines and cytokines in EAE. Therefore, as a second experimental treatment approach, T cells taken from the peripheral blood could be activated and transfected with immunosuppressive agents or soluble AM or apoptosis-inducing agents in vitro and then injected back to the donor (Fig. 12.6). These nonspecific transfected T cells could then accumulate in the lesions and secrete their AM or immunosuppressive cytokines. Although adoptive T-cell transfer is already under clinical evaluation in patients with viral diseases,[162] more extensive research in EAE is required before these future CNS-targeted treatments may be subjected to a clinical trial.

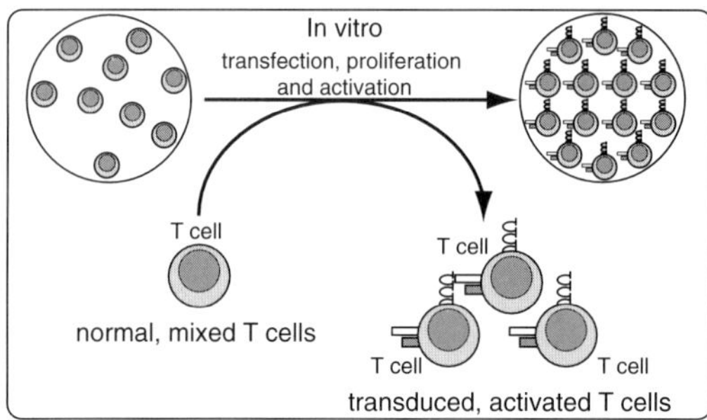

1. Venous blood is taken from a MS patient.
2. T cells are isolated *in vitro.*

3a. Myelin-specific T cells are generated and transduced

3b Nonspecific T cells are transduced and activated.

3. 'Therapeutic' T cells are reinjected into the patients vein.
4. Injected T cells modulate immune response in the MS lesion.

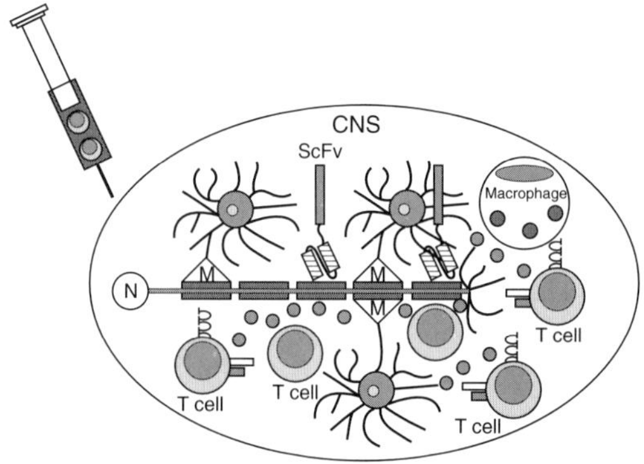

Figure 12.6 Adoptive transfer of T cells as a future treatment of experimental autoimmune encephalomyelitis and multiple sclerosis. T cells can be isolated from blood, transfected with the desired immunomodulator, expanded by mitogenic substances and activated to express adhesion molecules—a prerequisite to migrate through the blood–brain barrier (BBB). With this approach nonspecific 'harmless' T cells can be expanded. To generate CNS-specific T cells in vitro antigen presentation by monocytes of the same patient's blood can be used. These 'therapeutic' T cells are then reinjected into the donor. Problems of histocompatibility should therefore not arise. The activated T cells will enter the CNS across the BBB and stimulated by the 'proinflammatory' cytokines present in the chronic inflamed tissue will release the immunomodulator (dark small circles) in the lesion. Abbreviations: O: oligodendrocytes; N: neurons; M: myelin.

FUTURE PROSPECTS

It is reasonable to presume that AM are of central importance in the pathogenesis of EAE and could be important and useful targets for therapeutic agents in MS. The functional consequences of targeting these molecules with antibodies (monoclonal or chimeric forms), conjugated antibodies, peptides, synthetic compounds or carbohydrates are currently being evaluated in animal models and in human diseases. The apparent widespread involvement of AM in immune-mediated disorders in general diseases, has attracted the attention of all major biotechnology companies. Use of such novel agents either alone, or in combination with established anti-inflammatory therapies, might improve the prognosis and quality of life of patients suffering from multiple sclerosis.

REFERENCES

1. Hohlfeld R. Biotechnological agents for the immunotherapy of multiple sclerosis. *Brain* 1997; **120**: 865–916.
2. Cook SD, ed. *Handbook of Multiple Sclerosis*, 2nd edn. New York: Marcel Dekker, 1996.
3. Raine CS, McFarland HF, Tourtellotte WW, eds. *Multiple Sclerosis: Clinical and Pathogenetic Basis.* London: Chapman & Hall, 1997.
4. Steinman L. Multiple sclerosis: a coordinated immunological attack against myelin in the central nervous system. *Cell* 1996; **85**: 299–302.
5. Raine CS. Multiple sclerosis: a pivotal role for the T cell in lesion development. *Neuropath Appl Neurobiol* 1991; **17**: 265–274.
6. Swanborg RH. Experimental autoimmune encephalomyelitis in rodents as a model for human demyelinating disease. *Clin Immol Immunopathol* 1995; **77**: 4–13.
7. Genain CP, Nguyen MH, Letvin NL et al. Antibody facilitation of multiple sclerosis-like lesions in a nonhuman primate. *J Clin Invest* 1995; **96**: 2966–2974.
8. Massacesi L, Genain CP, Lee-Parritz D et al. Active and passively induced experimental autoimmune encephalomyelitis in common marmosets: a new model for multiple sclerosis. *Ann Neurol* 1995; **37**: 519–530.
9. Raine CS. The lesion in multiple sclerosis and chronic relapsing experimental allergic

encephalomyelitis: a structural comparison. In: Raine CS, McFarland HF, Tourtellotte, eds. *Multiple Sclerosis: Clinical and Pathogenetic Basis*. London: Chapman and Hall, 1997: 243–286.

10. Abbas AK, Murphy KM, Sher A. Functional diversity of helper T lymphocytes. *Nature* 1996; **383**: 787–793.
11. Panitch HS. Investigational drug therapies for treatment of multiple sclerosis. *Multiple Sclerosis* 1996; **2**: 66–77.
12. Bevilacqua MP, Nelson RM, Mannori G et al. Endothelial–leukocyte adhesion molecules in human disease. *Ann Rev Med* 1994; **45**: 361–378.
13. Butcher E, Picker LJ. Lymphocyte homing and homeostasis. *Science* 1996; **272**: 60–66.
14. Oppenheimer-Marks N, Lipsky PE. Adhesion molecules as targets for the treatment of autoimmune diseases. *Clin Immunol Immunopathol* 1996; **79**: 203–210.
15. Springer TA. Traffic signals for lymphocyte recirculation and leukocyte emigration: the multistep paradigm. *Cell* 1994; **76**: 301–314.
16. Lassmann H, Rössler K, Zimprich F et al. Expression of adhesion molecules and histocompatibility antigens at the blood–brain barrier. *Brain Pathol* 1991; **115**: 115–123.
17. Sligh JE Jr, Ballantyne CM, Rich SS et al. Inflammatory and immune responses are impaired in mice deficient in intercellular adhesion molecule 1. *Proc Natl Acad Sci USA* 1993; **90**: 8529–8533.
18. Arabonés ML, Ord DC, Ley K et al. Lymphocyte homing and leukocyte rolling and migration are impaired in L-selectin-deficient mice. *Immunity* 1994; **1**: 147–260.
19. Labow AA, Norton CR, Rumberger JM et al. Characterization of E-selectin-deficient mice: demonstration of overlapping function of the endothelial selectins. *Immunity* 1994; **1**: 709–720.
20. Steeber DA, Green NE, Sato S et al. Lymphocyte migration in L-selectin-deficient mice. Altered subset migration and aging of the immune system. *J Immunol* 1996, **157**: 1096–1106.
21. Tedder TF, Steeber DA, Pizcueta P. L-selectin-deficient mice have impaired leukocyte recruitment into inflammatory sites. *J Exp Med* 1995; **181**: 2259–2264.
22. Tivol EA, Borriello F, Schweitzer AN et al. Loss of CTLA-4 leads to massive lymphoproliferation and fatal multiorgan tissue destruction, revealing a critical negative regulatory role of CTLA-4. *Immunity* 1995; **3**: 541–547.
23. Grewal IS, Foellmer HG, Grewal KD et al. Requirement for CD40 ligand in costimulation induction, T cell activation, and experimental allergic encephalomyelitis. *Science* 1996; **273**: 1864–1867.
24. Karandikar NJ, Vanderlugt CL, Walunas TL et al. CTLA-4: a negative regulator of autoimmune disease. *J Exp Med* 1996; **184**: 783–788.
25. Kuchroo VK, Das MP, Brown JA et al. B7-1 and B7-2 costimulatory molecules activate differentially the Th1/Th2 developmental pathways: application to autoimmune disease therapy. *Cell* 1995; **80**: 707–718.
26. Reiser H, Stadecker MJ. Costimulatory B7 molecules in the pathogenesis of infectious and autoimmune diseases. *New Engl J Med* 1996; **335**: 1369–1377.
27. Johnston B, Walter UM, Issekutz AC et al. Differential roles of selectins and the α_4-integrin in acute, subacute, and chronic leukocyte recruitment in vivo. *J Immunol* 1997; **159**: 4514–4523.
28. Pryce G, Male D, Campbell I et al. Factors controlling T-cell migration across rat cerebral endothelium in vitro. *J Neuroimmunol* 1997; **75**: 84–94.
29. DeGrendele HC, Estess P, Siegelman MH. Requirement for CD44 in activated T cell extravasation into an inflammatory site. *Science* 1997; **278**: 672–675.
30. Cross AH, Cannella B, Brosnan CF et al. Homing to central nervous system vasculature by antigen-specific lymphocytes. I. Localization of 14C-labeled cells during acute, chronic, and relapsing experimental allergic encephalomyelitis. *Lab Invest* 1990; **63**: 162–170.
31. Cross AH, O'Mara T, Raine CS. Chronologic localization of myelin-reactive cells in the lesion of relapsing EAE: implications for the study of multiple sclerosis. *Neurology* 1993; **43**: 1028–1033.
32. Steinman L. A few autoreactive cells in an autoimmune infiltrate control a vast population of nonspecific cells: a tale of smart bombs and the infantry. *Proc Natl Acad Sci USA* 1996; **93**: 2253–2256.
33. Lehmann PV, Forsthuber T, Miller A et al. Spreading of T-cell autoimmunity to cryptic determinants of an autoantigen. *Nature* 1992; **358**: 155–157.
34. Vanderlugt CT, Miller SD. Epitope spreading. *Curr Opin Immunol* 1996; **8**: 831–836.

35. Jansson L, Diener P, Engstrom A et al. Spreading of the immune response to different myelin basic protein peptides in chronic experimental autoimmune encephalomyelitis in B10.RIII mice. *Eur J Immunol* 1995; **25**: 2195–21200.
36. McRae BL, Vanderlugt CL, Dal Canto MC et al. Functional evidence for spreading in the relapsing pathology of experimental autoimmune encephalomyelitis. *J Exp Med* 1995; **182**: 75–85.
37. Miller SD, Vanderlugt CL, Lenschow DJ et al. Blockade of CD28/B7-1-interaction prevents epitope spreading and clinical relapses of murine EAE. *Immunity* 1995; **3**: 739–745.
38. Miller SD, Vanderlugt, Smith Begolka W et al. Persistent infection with Theiler's virus leads to CNS autoimmunity via epitope spreading. *Nat Med* 1997; **3**: 1133–1136.
39. Vanderlugt CT, Karandikar NJ, Lenschow DJ et al. Treatment with intact anti-B7-1 mAB during disease remission enhances epitope spreading and exacerbates relapses in R-EAE. *J Neuroimmunol* 1997; **79**: 113–118.
40. Voskuhl RR, Farris II RW, Nagasato K et al. Epitope spreading occurs in active but not passive EAE induced by myelin basic protein. *J Neuroimmunol* 1996; **70**: 103–111.
41. Yu M, Johnson JM, Tuohy VK. A predictable sequential determinant spreading cascade invariably accompanies progression of experimental autoimmune encephalomyelitis: a basis for peptide-specific therapy after onset of clinical disease. *J Exp Med* 1996; **183**: 1777–1788.
42. O'Neill JK, Butter C, Baker D et al. Expression of vascular addressins and ICAM-1 by endothelial cells in the spinal cord during chronic relapsing experimental allergic encephalomyelitis in the Biozzi AB/H mouse. *Immunology* 1991; **72**: 520–525.
43. Raine CS. Multiple sclerosis: immune system molecule expression in the central nervous system. *J Neuropathol Exp Neurol* 1994; **53**: 328–337.
44. Wilcox CE, Ward AMV, Evans A et al. Endothelial cell expression of the intercellular adhesion molecule-1 (ICAM-1) in the central nervous system of guinea pigs during acute and chronic relapsing experimental allergic encephalomyelitis. *J Neuroimmunol* 1990; **30**: 43–51.
45. Dopp JM, Brenemann SM, Olschowska JA. Expression of ICAM-1, VCAM-1, L-selectin, and leukosialin in the mouse central nervous system during the induction and remission stages of experimental allergic encephalomyelitis. *J Neuroimmunol* 1994; **54**: 129–144.
46. Engelhardt B, Vestweber D, Hallmann R et al. E- and P-selectin are not involved in the recruitment of inflammatory cells across the blood–brain barrier in experimental autoimmune encephalomyelitis. *Blood* 1997; **90**: 4459–4472.
47. Lindsey JW, Steinman L. Competitive PCR quantification CD4, CD8, ICAM-1, VCAM-1, and MHC class II mRNA in the central nervous system during development and resolution of experimental allergic encephalomyelitis. *J Neuroimmunol* 1993; **48**: 227–234.
48. Williams KC, Zhao RW, Ueno K. PECAM-1 (CD31) expression in the central nervous system and its role in experimental allergic encephalomyelitis in the rat. *J Neurosci Res* 1996; **45**: 747–757.
49. Cannella B, Cross AH, Raine CS. Upregulation and coexpression of adhesion molecules correlate with relapsing autoimmune demyelination in the central nervous system. *J Exp Med* 1990; **172**: 1521–1524.
50. Cannella B, Cross AH, Raine CS. Adhesion-related molecules in the central nervous system. Upregulation correlates with inflammatory cell influx during experimental autoimmune encephalomyelitis. *Lab Invest* 1991; **6**: 23–31.
51. Raine CS, Cannella B, Duijvestijn AM et al. Homing to central nervous system vasculature by antigen-specific lymphocytes. II. Lymphocyte/endothelial cell adhesion during the initial stages of autoimmune demyelination. *Lab Invest* 1990; **63**: 476–489.
52. Allen SJ, Baker D, O'Neill JK et al. Isolation and characterization of cells infiltrating the spinal cord during the course of chronic relapsing experimental allergic encephalomyelitis in the Biozzi AB/H mouse. *Cell Immunol* 1993; **146**: 335–350.
53. Engelhardt B, Conley FC, Kilshaw PJ et al. Lymphocytes infiltrating the CNS during inflammation display a distinctive phenotype and bind to VCAM-1 but not to MAdCAm-1. *Int Immunol* 1995; **7**: 481–491.
54. Kalman B, Alder H, Lublin FD. Characteristics of the T lymphocytes involved in experimental allergic encephalomyelitis. *J Neuroimmunol* 1995; **61**: 107–116.
55. Mix E, Fiszer U, Olsson T et al. V delta 1 gene usage, interleukin-2 receptors and adhesion

molecules on gamma delta+ T cells in inflammatory diseases of the nervous system. *J Neuroimmunol* 1994; **49**: 59–66.

56. Karpus WJ, Lukacs NW, McRae BL et al. An important role for the chemokine macrophage inflammatory protein-1α in the pathogenesis of the T cell-mediated autoimmune disease, experimental autoimmune encephalomyelitis. *J Immunol* 1995; **155**: 5003–5010.
57. Cannella B, Cross AH, Raine CS. Anti-adhesion molecule therapy in experimental autoimmune encephalomyelitis. *J Neuroimmunol* 1993; **46**: 43–56.
58. Welsh CT, Rose JW, Hill KE et al. Augmentation of adoptively transferred experimental allergic encephalomyelitis by administration of a monoclonal antibody specific for LFA-1α. *J Neuroimmunol* 1993; **43**: 161–168.
59. Staunton DE, Merluzzi VJ, Rothlein R et al. A cell adhesion molecule, ICAM-1, is the major surface receptor for rhinoviruses. *Cell* 1989; **56**: 849–853.
60. Bergelson JM, Chan BM, Finberg RW et al. The integrin VLA-2 binds echovirus 1 and extracellular matrix ligands by different mechanisms. *J Clin Invest* 1993; **92**: 232–239.
61. Falkow S, Isberg RR, Portnoy DA. The interaction of bacteria with mammalian cells. *Ann Rev Cell Biol* 1992; **8**: 333–363.
62. Hogg N, Berlin C. Structure and function of adhesion receptors in leukocyte trafficking. *Immunol Today* 1995; **16**: 327–330.
63. Petruzzelli L, Maduzia L, Springer L et al. Activation of lymphocyte function-associated molecule-1 (CD11a/CD18) and MAC-1 (CD11b/CD18) mimicked by an antibody directed against CD18. *J Immunol* 1995; **155**: 854–866.
64. Berman ME, Xie Y, Muller WA. Roles of platelet/endothelial cell adhesion molecule-1 (PECAM-1, CD31) in natural killer cell transendothelial migration and β_2 integrin activation. *J Immunol* 1996; **156**: 1515–1524.
65. Liao F, Huynh HK, Eiroa A et al. Migration of monocytes across endothelium and passage through extracellular matrix involve separate molecular domains of PECAM 1. *J Exp Med* 1995; **182**: 1337–1343.
66. Newman PJ. The biology of PECAM-1. *J Clin Invest* 1997; **99**: 3–8.
67. Zocchi MR, Ferrero E, Leone BE et al. CD31/PECAM-1-driven chemokine independent transmigration of human T lymphocytes. *Eur J Immunol* 1996; **26**: 759–767.
68. Archelos JJ, Jung S, Mäurer M et al. Inhibition of experimental autoimmune encephalomyelitis by an antibody to the intercellular adhesion molecule ICAM-1. *Ann Neurol* 1993; **34**: 145–154.
69. Soilu-Hänninen M, Roytta M, Salmi A et al. Therapy with antibody against leukocyte integrin VLA-4 (CD49d) is effective and safe in virus-facilitated experimental allergic encephalomyelitis. *J Neuroimmunol* 1997; **72**: 95–105.
70. Morrissey SP, Deichmann R, Syha J et al. Partial inhibition of AT-EAE by an antibody to ICAM-1: clinico-histological and MRI studies. *J Neuroimmunol* 1996; **69**: 85–93.
71. Namer IJ, Steibel J, Piddlesden SJ et al. Magnetic resonance imaging of antibody-mediated demyelinating experimental allergic encephalomyelitis. *J Neuroimmunol* 1994; **54**: 41–50.
72. Seeldrayers PA, Syha J, Morrissey SP et al. Magnetic resonance imaging investigation of blood–brain barrier damage in adoptive transfer experimental autoimmune encephalomyelitis. *J Neuroimmunol* 1993; **46**: 199–206.
73. Hawkins CP, Munroe PMG, MacKenzie F et al. Duration and selectivity of blood–brain barrier breakdown in chronic relapsing experimental allergic encephalomyelitis studied by gadolinium-DTPA and protein markers. *Brain* 1990; **113**: 365–367.
74. Kent SJ, Karlik SJ, Rice GPA et al. A monoclonal antibody to α_4 integrin reverses the MRI-detectable signs of experimental allergic encephalomyelitis in the guinea pig. *J Mag Res Imaging* 1995; **5**: 535–540.
75. Morrissey SP, Stodal H, Zettl U. In vivo MRI and its histological correlates in acute adoptive transfer experimental allergic encephalomyelitis. Quantification of inflammation and oedema. *Brain* 1996; **119**: 239–248.
76. Namer IJ, Steibel J, Poulet P et al. Blood–brain barrier breakdown in MBP-specific T cell induced experimental allergic encephalomyelitis. A quantitative in vivo MRI study. *Brain* 1993; **116**: 147–159.
77. Bö L, Peterson JW, Mork S et al. Distribution of immunoglobulin superfamily members ICAM-1, -2, -3, and the β_2 integrin LFA-1 in multiple sclerosis. *J Neuropathol Exp Neurol* 1996; **55**: 1060–1072.
78. Brosnan C, Cannella B, Battistini L et al. Cytokine localization in multiple sclerosis lesions: correlation with adhesion molecule expression and reactive nitrogen species. *Neurology* 1995; **45 (suppl 6)**: S16–S21.

79. Cannella B, Raine CS. The adhesion molecule and cytokine profile of multiple sclerosis lesions. *Ann Neurol* 1995; **37**: 424–435.
80. DeSimone R, Giampaola A, Giometto B et al. The costimulatory molecule B7 is expressed on human microglia in culture and in multiple sclerosis lesions. *J Neuropathol Exp Neurol* 1995; **54**: 175–187.
81. Girgrah N, Letarte M, Becker LE et al. Localization of the CD44 glycoprotein to fibrous astrocytes in normal white matter and to reactive astrocytes in active lesions in multiple sclerosis. *J Neuropathol Exp Neurol* 1991; **50**: 779–792.
82. Sobel RA, Mitchell M, Fondren G. Intercellular adhesion molecule-1 (ICAM-1) in cellular immune reactions in the human central nervous system. *Am J Pathol* 1990; **136**: 1309–1316.
83. Windhagen A, Newcombe J, Dangond F et al. Expression of costimulatory molecules B7-1 (CD80), B7-2 (CD86), and interleukin 12 cytokine in multiple sclerosis. *J Exp Med* 1995; **182**: 1985–1996.
84. Stüber A, Martin R, Stone LA et al. Expression pattern of activation and adhesion molecules on peripheral blood CD4+ T-lymphocytes in relapsing–remitting multiple sclerosis patients: a serial analysis. *J Neuroimmunol* 1996; **66**: 147–151.
85. Droogan AG, Crockard AD, McMillan SA et al. Effects of intravenous methylprednisolone therapy on leukocyte and soluble adhesion molecule expression in MS. *Neurology* 1998; **50**: 224–229.
86. Soilu-Hänninen M, Salmi A, Salonen R. Interferon-beta downregulates expression of VLA-4 antigen and antagonizes interferon-gamma-induced expression of HLA-DQ on peripheral blood monocytes. *J Neuroimmunol* 1996; **60**: 99–106.
87. Pitzalis C, Sharrack B, Gray IA et al. Comparison of the effects of oral versus intravenous methylprednisolone regimens on peripheral blood T lymphocyte adhesion molecule expression, T cell subsets distribution and TNF alpha concentrations in multiple sclerosis. *J Neuroimmunol* 1997; **74**: 62–68.
88. Svenningsson A, Hansson GK, Andersen O et al. Adhesion molecule expression on cerebrospinal fluid T lymphocytes: evidence for common recruitment mechanisms in multiple sclerosis, aseptic meningitis, and normal controls. *Ann Neurol* 1993; **34**: 155–161.
89. Svenningsson A, Dotevall L, Stemme S et al. Increased expression of B2-7 costimulatory molecule on cerebrospinal fluid cells of patients with multiple sclerosis and infectious central nervous system disease. *J Neuroimmunol* 1997; **75**: 59–68.
90. Gearing AJH, Newman W. Circulating adhesion molecules in disease. *Immunol Today* 1993; **14**: 506–512.
91. Hartung HP, Archelos JJ, Zielasek J et al. Circulating adhesion molecules and inflammatory mediators in demyelination. *Neurology* 1995; **45 (suppl 6)**: S22–S32.
92. Martin S, Rieckmann P, Melchers I et al. Circulating forms of ICAM-3 (cICAM-3). Elevated levels in autoimmune diseases and lack of association with cICAM-1. *J Immunol* 1995; **154**: 1951–1955.
93. Rieckmann P, Martin S, Weichselbraun I et al. Serial analysis of circulating adhesion molecules and TNF receptor in serum from patients with multiple sclerosis: cICAM-1 receptor in serum from patients with multiple sclerosis: cICAM-1 is an indicator for relapse. *Neurology* 1994; **44**: 2367–2372.
94. Giovannoni G, Lai M, Thorpe J et al. Longitudinal study of soluble adhesion molecules in multiple sclerosis: correlation with gadolinium enhanced magnetic resonance imaging. *Neurology* 1997; **48**: 1557–1565.
95. Hartung HP, Michels M, Reiners RH et al. Soluble ICAM-1 serum levels in multiple sclerosis and viral encephalitis. *Neurology* 1993 **43**: 2331–2335.
96. Franciotta D, Piccolo G, Zardine E et al. Soluble CD8 and ICAM-1 in serum and CSF of MS patients treated with 6-methylprednisolone. *Acta Neurol Scand* 1997; **95**: 275–279.
97. Rieckmann P, Altenhofer B, Riegel A et al. Soluble adhesion molecules (sVCAM-1 and sICAM-1) in cerebrospinal fluid and serum correlate with MRI activity in multiple sclerosis. *Ann Neurol* 1997; **41**: 326–333.
98. Sharief MK, Noori MA, Ciardi M et al. Increased levels of circulating ICAM-1 in serum and cerebrospinal fluid of patients with active multiple sclerosis. Correlation with TNF-alpha and blood–brain barrier damage. *J Neuroimmunol* 1993; **43**: 15–21.
99. Trojano M, Avolio C, Simone IL. Soluble intercellular adhesion molecule-1 in serum and cerebrospinal fluid of clinically active relapsing–remitting multiple sclerosis. *Neurology* 1996; **47**: 1535–1541.

100. Tsukada N, Miyagi K, Matsuda M et al. Increased levels of circulating intercellular adhesion molecule-1 in multiple sclerosis and human T-lymphotropic virus type-1-associated myelopathy. *Ann Neurol* 1993; **33**: 646–649.
101. Rieckmann P, Nunke K, Burchhardt M et al. Soluble intercellular adhesion molecule-1 in cerebrospinal fluid: an indicator for the inflammatory impairment of the blood–cerebrospinal fluid barrier. *J Neuroimmunol* 1993; **47**: 133–140.
102. Calabresi PA, Tranquill LR, Dambrosia JM et al. Increases in soluble VCAM-1 correlate with a decrease in MRI lesions in multiple sclerosis treated with interferon β-1b. *Ann Neurol* 1997; **41**: 669–674.
103. Dore-Duffy P, Newman W, Balabanov R et al. Circulating, soluble adhesion proteins in cerebrospinal fluid and serum of patients with multiple sclerosis: correlation with clinical activity. *Ann Neurol* 1995; **37**: 55–62.
104. Giovannoni G, Thorpe J, Kidd D et al. Soluble E-selectin in multiple sclerosis: raised concentrations in patients with primary progressive disease. *J Neurol Neurosurg Psychiatry* 1996; **60**: 20–26.
105. Hartung HP, Reiners KH, Archelos JJ et al. Circulating adhesion molecules and TNF receptor (60 kDa) in multiple sclerosis: correlation with MRI and comparison with viral encephalitis. *Ann Neurol* 1995; **38**: 186–193.
106. Matsuda M, Tsukada N, Miyagi K et al. Increased levels of soluble vascular cell adhesion molecule-1 (VCAM-1) in the cerebrospinal fluid and sera of patients with multiple sclerosis and human T lymphotropic virus type-1-associated myelopathy. *J Neuroimmunol* 1995; **59**: 35–40.
107. Mössner R, Fassbender K, Kühnen J et al. Vascular cell adhesion molecule – a new approach to detect endothelial cell activation in MS and encephalitis in vivo. *Acta Neurol Scand* 1996; **93**: 118–122.
108. Droogan AG, McMillan SA, Douglas JP et al. Serum and cerebrospinal fluid levels of soluble adhesion molecules in multiple sclerosis: predominant intrathecal release of vascular cell adhesion molecule-1. *J Neuroimmunol* 1996; **64**: 185–191.
109. Tsukada N, Miyagi K, Matsuda M et al. Soluble E-selectin in the serum and cerebrospinal fluid of patients with multiple sclerosis and human T-lymphotropic virus type 1-associated myelopathy. *Neurology* 1995; **45**: 1914–1918.
110. Schleiffenbaum B, Spertini O, Tedder TF. Soluble L-selectin is present in human plasma at high levels and retains functional activity. *J Cell Biol* 1992; **119**: 229–238.
111. Mössner R, Fassbender K, Kühnen J et al. Circulating L-selectin in multiple sclerosis patients with active, gadolinium-enhancing brain plaques. *J Neuroimmunol* 1996; **65**: 61–65.
112. Waldmann H, Cobbold S. The use of monoclonal antibodies to achieve immunological tolerance. *Immunol Today* 1993; **14**: 247–251.
113. Biasi G, Facchinetti A, Monastra G et al. Protection from experimental autoimmune encephalomyelitis (EAE): non-depleting anti-CD4 mAb treatment induces peripheral T-cell tolerance to MBP in PL/J mice. *J Neuroimmunol* 1997; **73**: 117–123.
114. Isobe M, Yagita H, Okumura K et al. Specific acceptance of cardiac allograft after treatment with antibodies to ICAM-1 to LFA-1. *Science* 1992; **255**: 1125–1158.
115. Cross AH, Girard TJ, Giacoletto KS et al. Long-term inhibition of murine experimental autoimmune encephalomyelitis using CTLA-4-Fc supports a key role for CD28 costimulation. *J Clin Invest* 1995; **95**: 2783–2789.
116. Begent RH, Verhaar MJ, Chester KA et al. Clinical evidence of efficient tumor targeting based on single-chain Fv antibody selected from a combination library. *Nat Med* 1996; **2**: 979–984.
117. Chamow SM, Ashkenazi A. Immunoadhesins: principles and applications. *Trends Biotechnol* 1996; **14**: 52–60.
118. Chester KA, Hawkins RE. Clinical issues in antibody design. *Trends Biotechnol* 1995; **13**: 294–300.
119. Davis LS, Kavanaugh AF, Nichols LA et al. Induction of persistent T cell hyporesponsiveness in vivo by monoclonal antibody to ICAM-1 in patients with rheumatoid arthritis. *J Immunol* 1995; **154**: 3525–3537.
120. Hafler DA, Weiner HL. Immunosuppression with monoclonal antibodies in multiple sclerosis. *Neurology* 1988; **38 (suppl 2)**: 42–47.
121. Weinshenker BG, Bass B, Karlik S et al. An open trial of OKT3 in patients with multiple sclerosis. *Neurology* 1991; **41**: 1047–1052.
122. Lindsey JW, Hodgkinson S, Mehta R et al. Phase 1 clinical trial of chimeric monoclonal anti-CD4 antibody in multiple sclerosis. *Neurology* 1994; **44**: 413–419.
123. Llewellyn-Smith N, Lai M, Miller DH et al. Effects of anti-CD4 antibody treatment on lymphocyte subsets and stimulated tumor

necrosis factor alpha production: a study of 29 multiple sclerosis patients entered into a clinical trial of cM-T412. *Neurology* 1997; **48**: 810–816.

124. van Oosten BW, Lai M, Hodgkinson S et al. Treatment of multiple sclerosis with the monoclonal anti-CD4 antibody cM-T412. Results of a randomized, double-blind, placebo-controlled, MR-monitored phase II trial. *Neurology* 1997; **49**: 351–357.
125. Racadot E, Rumbach L, Bataillard M et al. Treatment of multiple sclerosis with anti-CD4 monoclonal antibody. *J Autoimmun* 1993; **6**: 771–786.
126. Hafler DA, Fallis RJ, Dawson DM et al. Immunologic responses of progressive multiple sclerosis patients treated with an anti-T-cell monoclonal antibody, anti-T12. *Neurology* 1986; **36**: 777–784.
127. Moreau T, Coles A, Wing M et al. Transient increase in symptoms associated with cytokine release in patients with multiple sclerosis. *Brain* 1996; **119**: 225–237.
128. Leger OJ, Yednock TA, Tanner L et al. Humanization of a mouse antibody against human alpha-4 integrin: a potential therapeutic for the treatment of multiple sclerosis. *Human Antibodies* 1997; **8**: 3–16.
129. Benveniste EN. Cytokines in the central nervous system. In: DG Remick, JS Friedland, eds. *Cytokines in Health and Disease*, 2nd edn. New York: Marcel Dekker; 1997, 531–536.
130. Merrill JE, Benveniste EN. Cytokines in inflammatory brain lesions: helpful and harmful. *Trends Neurosci* 1996; **19**: 331–338.
131. Navikas V, Link H. Review: cytokines and the pathogenesis of multiple sclerosis. *J Neurosci Res* 1996; **45**: 322–333.
132. Fabry Z, Topham DJ, Fee D et al. TGF-β_2 decreases migration of lymphocytes in vitro and homing of cells into the central nervous system. *J Immunol* 1995; **155**: 325–332.
133. Baeuerle PA, Henkel T. Function and activation of NF-κB in the immune system. *Ann Rev Immunol* 1994; **12**: 141–179.
134. Baldwin AS. The NF-κB proteins: new discoveries and insights. *Ann Rev Immunol* 1996; **14**: 649–681.
135. Kaltschmidt C, Kaltschmidt B, Lannes-Vieira J et al. Transcription factor NF-κB is activated in microglia during experimental autoimmune encephalomyelitis. *J Neuroimmunol* 1994; **55**: 99–106.
136. Van der Burg B, Liden J, Okret S et al. Nuclear factor-κB repression in antiinflammation and immunosuppression by glucocorticoids. *Trends Endocrinol Metab* 1997; **8**: 152–157.
137. Chen C, Rosenbloom CL, Anderson DC et al. Selective inhibition of E-selectin, vascular cell adhesion molecule-1, and intercellular adhesion molecule-1 expression by inhibitors of IκB-α phosphorylation. *J Immunol* 1995; **155**: 3538–3545.
138. Pierce JW, Schoenleber R, Jesmok G et al. Novel inhibitors of cytokine-induced Iκ-Ba phosphorylation and endothelial cell adhesion molecule expression show anti-inflammatory effects in vivo. *J Biol Chem* 1997; **272**: 21096–21103.
139. Neurath MF, Pettersson S, Büschenfelde KH et al. Local administration of antisense phosphorothioate oligonucleotides to the p65 subunit of NF-κB abrogates established experimental colitis in mice. *Nat Med* 1996; **2**: 998–1004.
140. Meyer DM, Dustin ML, Carron CP. Characterization of intercellular adhesion molecule-1 ectodomain (sICAM-1) as an inhibitor of lymphocyte function-associated molecule-1 interaction with ICAM-1. *J Immunol* 1995; **155**: 3578–3584.
141. Rieckmann P, Michel U, Albrecht M et al. Soluble forms of intercellular adhesion molecule-1 (ICAM-1) block lymphocyte attachment to cerebral endothelial cells. *J Neuroimmunol* 1995; **60**: 9–15.
142. McIntyre BW, Woodside DG, Caruso DA et al. Regulation of human T lymphocyte coactivation with an α_4 integrin antagonist peptide. *J Immunol* 1997; **158**: 4180–4186.
143. Newham P, Craig SE, Seddon GN et al. α_4 Integrin binding interface on VCAM-1 and MAdCAM-1. *J Biol Chem* 1997; **272**: 19429–19440.
144. Vanderslice P, Ren K, Revelle JK et al. A cyclic hexapeptide is a potent antagonist of α_4 integrin. *J Immunol* 1997; **158**: 1710.
145. Fecondo JV, Kent SBH, Boyd AW. Inhibition of intercellular adhesion molecule-1 dependent biological activities by a synthetic peptide analog. *Proc Natl Acad Sci USA* 1991; **88**: 2879–2882.
146. Wang JH, Pepinsky RB, Stehle T et al. The crystal structure of an N-terminal two-domain fragment of vascular cell adhesion molecule 1 (VCAM-1): a cyclic peptide based on the domain 1 C–D loop can inhibit VCAM-1–α_4 integrin interaction. *Proc Natl Acad Sci USA* 1995; **92**: 5714–5718.
147. Lowe JB, Ward PA. Therapeutic inhibition of carbohydrate–protein interactions in vivo *J Clin Invest* 1997; **99**: 822–826.

148. Zopf D, Roth S. Oligosaccharide anti-infective agents. *Lancet* 1996; **347**: 1017–1021.
149. Varki A. Selectin ligands: will the real ones please stand up? *J Clin Invest* 1997; **99**: 158–162.
150. Rosen SD, Bertozzi CR. The selectins and their ligands. *Curr Opin Cell Biol* 1994; **6**: 663–673.
151. Todderud G, Nair X, Lee D et al. BMS-190394, a selectin inhibitor, prevents rat cutaneous inflammatory reactions. *J Pharmacol Exp Ther* 1997; **282**: 1298–1304.
152. Wagner RW. Gene inhibition using antisense oligodeoxynucleotides. *Nature* 1994; **372**: 333–335.
153. Agrawal S. Antisense oligonucleotides: towards clinical trials. *Trends Biotechnol* 1996; **14**: 376–387.
154. Bennett CF, Condon TP, Grimm S et al. Inhibition of endothelial cell adhesion molecule expression with antisense oligonucleotides. *J Immunol* 1994; **152**: 3530–3540.
155. Hicke B, Watson SR, Koenig A et al. DNA aptamers block L-selectin function in vivo. Inhibition of human lymphocyte trafficking in SCID mice. *J Clin Invest* 1996; **98**: 2688–2692.
156. O'Connell D, Koenig A, Jennings S et al. Calcium-dependent oligonucleotide antagonists specific for L-selectin. *Proc Natl Acad Sci USA* 1996; **93**: 5883–5887.
157. Wojcik WJ, Swoveland P, Zhang X et al. Chronic intrathecal infusion of phosphorothioate or phosphodiester antisense oligonucleotides against cytokine response gene-2/IP-10 in experimental allergic encephalomyelitis of Lewis rat. *J Pharmacol Exp Ther* 1996; **278**: 404–410.
158. Ridet JL, Privat A. Gene therapy in the central nervous system: direct versus indirect gene delivery. *J Neurosci Res* 1995; **42**: 289–293.
159. Mathisen PM, Yu M, Johnson JM et al. Treatment of experimental autoimmune encephalomyelitis with genetically modified memory T cells. *J Exp Med* 1997; **186**: 159–164.
160. Shaw MK, Lorens JB, Dhawan A et al. Local delivery of interleukin 4 by retrovirus transduced T lymphocytes ameliorates experimental autoimmune encephalomyelitis. *J Exp Med* 1997; **185**: 1711–1714.
161. Ludowyk PA, Willenborg DO, Parish CR. Selective localization of neuro-specific T lymphocytes in the central nervous system. *J Neuroimmunol* 1992; **37**: 237–250.
162. Riddell SR, Greenberg PD. Principles for adoptive T cell therapy of human viral diseases. *Annu Rev Immunol* 1995; **13**: 545–586.
163. Adams DH, Lloyd AR. Chemokines: leucocyte recruitment and activation cytokines. *Lancet* 1997; **349**: 490–495.
164. Howard OMZ, Ben-Baruch A, Oppenheim JJ. Chemokines: progress toward identifying molecular targets for therapeutic agents. *Trends Biotechnol* 1996; **14**: 46–51.
165. Yednock TA, Cannon C, Fritz LC et al. Prevention of experimental autoimmune encephalomyelitis by antibodies against $\alpha_4\beta_1$ integrin. *Nature* 1992; **356**: 63–66.
166. Couraud PO. Interactions between lymphocytes, macrophages, and central nervous system cells. *J Leukocyte Biol* 1994; **56**: 407–415.
167. Baron JL, Madri JA, Ruddle NH et al. Surface expression of α_4 integrin by CD4 T cells is required for their entry into brain parenchyma. *J Exp Med* 1993; **177**: 57–68.
168. Kent SJ, Karlik SJ, Cannon C et al. A monoclonal antibody to α_4 integrin suppresses and reverses active experimental allergic encephalomyelitis. *J Neuroimmunol* 1995; **58**: 1–10.
169. Keszthelyi E, Karlik S, Hyduk S et al. Evidence for a prolonged role of α_4 integrin throughout active experimental allergic encephalomyelitis. *Neurology* 1996; **47**: 1053–1059.
170. Willenborg DO, Simmons RD, Tamatani T. ICAM-1-dependent pathway is not critically involved in the inflammatory process of autoimmune encephalomyelitis or in cytokine-induced inflammation of the central nervous system. *J Neuroimmunol* 1993; **45**: 147–154.
171. Gordon EJ, Myers KJ, Dougherty JP et al. Both anti-CD11a (LFA-1), and anti-CD11b (MAC-1) therapy delay the onset and diminish the severity of experimental autoimmune encephalomyelitis. *J Neuroimmunol* 1995; **62**: 153–160.
172. Willenborg DO, Staykova MA, Miyasaka M. Short term treatment with soluble neuroantigen and anti-CD11a (LFA-1) protects rats against autoimmune encephalomyelitis: treatment abrogates autoimmune disease but not autoimmunity. *J Immunol* 1996; **157**: 1973–1980.
173. Kawai K, Kobayashi Y, Shiratori M et al. Intrathecal administration of antibodies against LFA-1 and against ICAM-1 suppresses experimental allergic encephalomyelitis in rats. *Cell Immunol* 1996; **171**: 262–268.
174. Huitinga I, Damoiseaux JGMC, Dopp EA et al. Treatment with anti-CR3 antibodies ED7 and ED8 suppresses experimental allergic encephalomyelitis in Lewis rats. *Eur J Immunol* 1993; **23**: 709–715.

175. Archelos JJ, Jung S, Rinner W et al. Role of leukocyte adhesion molecule L-selectin in experimental autoimmune encephalomyelitis. *J Neurol Sci* 1998 (in press).
176. Racke MK, Scott DE, Quigley L et al. Distinct roles for B7-1 (CD80) and B7-2 (CD86) in the initiation of experimental allergic encephalomyelitis. *J Clin Invest* 1995; **96**: 2195–2203.
177. Perrin PJ, Scott D, Davis TA et al. Opposing effects of CTLA-Ig and anti-CD80 (B7-1) plus anti-CD86 (B7-2) on experimental allergic encephalomyelitis. *J Neuroimmunol* 1996; **65**: 31–39.
178. Hurwitz AA, Sullivan TJ, Krummel MF et al. Specific blockade of CTLA/B7 interactions results in exacerbated clinical and histologic disease in an actively-induced model of experimental allergic encephalomyelitis. *J Neuroimmunol* 1997; **73**: 57–62.
179. Jung S, Toyka KV, Hartung HP. Suppression of experimental autoimmune encephalomyelitis in Lewis rats by antibodies against CD2. *Eur J Immunol* 1995; **25**: 1391–1398.
180. Gerritse K, Laman JD, Noelle RJ et al. CD40–CD40 ligand interaction in experimental allergic encephalomyelitis and multiple sclerosis. *Proc Natl Acad Sci USA* 1996; **93**: 2499–2504.
181. Jander S, Heidenreich F, Stoll G. Serum and CSF levels of soluble intercellular adhesion molecule-1 (ICAM-1) in inflammatory neurologic diseases. *Neurology* 1993; **43**: 1809–1813.
182. Tsakuda N, Matsuda M, Miyagi K. Increased levels of intercellular adhesion molecule-1 (ICAM-1) and tumor necrosis factor receptor in the cerebrospinal fluid in patients with multiple sclerosis. *Neurology* 1993; **43**: 2679–2682.

13

Immunological parameters and magnetic resonance imaging activity

Peter Rieckmann and Boris Kallmann

INTRODUCTION

Magnetic resonance imaging (MRI) is currently used as an important paraclinical surrogate marker for disease activity in patients with multiple sclerosis (MS).[1,2] Of particular interest is the temporal variation of gadolinium-enhancing lesions, as they reflect ongoing inflammation, disturbance of the blood–brain barrier and represent an early stage of new lesion development.[3–5] Histopathological studies have demonstrated that transmigration of lymphocytes across the endothelial cell monolayer occurs at sites of gadolinium (Gd) enhancement.[3,6,7] This process involves the coordinated release of cytokines, upregulation of cellular adhesion molecules, contact and signalling between lymphocytes and cerebral endothelial cells—the major constituents of the blood–brain barrier—as well as proteolytic disruption of the extracellular matrix by proteinases (for review see Hohlfeld[8]). Until recently the avenues of MRI research and immunopathogenetic aspects of MS have run in parallel. With the advent of new immunomodulating drugs, which demonstrated an impressive effect on disease activity as measured by cranial MRI, we are now in the position to directly compare changes in the immune system—relevant to MS pathology—and the temporospatial variations of MRI lesions during the initiation and continuation of immunomodulatory treatment. Therefore, a major goal of current research is to establish a quantitative correlation between the number and volume of Gd-enhancing lesions and the immunological parameters which are involved in the transmigration process of lymphocytes across the blood–brain barrier.

THEORETICAL CONSIDERATIONS

An immunological marker which reflects disease activity in patients with MS should fulfil the following criteria:

(a) association with known pathophysiological events during the disease process
(b) cellular expression during different stages of MS plaque development
(c) easily accessible (soluble or cell-associated) in blood, urine or cerebrospinal fluid (CSF)
(d) standardized techniques for quantification and minor fluctuations during stable phases of the diseases and in healthy controls
(e) cellular expression or levels in body fluids influenced by immunomodulation.

In practice, none of the known immunological parameters currently under scrutiny will fit all the above-mentioned criteria. Therefore, a rational approach should focus on factors which can be closely monitored to evident disease activity as visualized by active Gd enhancing lesions on cranial MRI. In addition, MRI as an accepted paraclinical surrogate marker is clearly influenced by immunomodulatory treatment modalities, like interferon beta (IFN-β) or corticosteroids.[9,10] Another advantage is the fact that Gd enhancement which can be visualized in vivo clearly indicates blood–brain barrier dysfunction, an important prerequisite for immune cell invasion of the central nervous system (CNS). The important steps of transmigration have been clearly described in vitro and in animal models of the disease.[8,11–13]

CASCADE OF EVENTS DURING IMMUNE CELL TRANSMIGRATION

In MS, antigen-induced activation of lymphocytes most likely occurs initially outside the CNS in compartmentalized lymphoid organs, probably via molecular mimicry.[12,14–16] These activated cells are in general capable of crossing the blood–brain barrier and entering the CNS.[17] The initial contact between lymphocytes and cerebral endothelial cells is mediated by a random interaction between constitutively expressed endothelial selectins (E-selectin) and exposed sugar residues (Lewis^x) on the lymphocytes. Firm attachment of these cells is mediated by the contact between the integrins lymphocyte function-associated molecule-1 (LFA-1) and very late antigen-4 (VLA-4) on the surface of the lymphocyte and the immunoglobulin-like molecules intercellular adhesion molecule-1 (ICAM-1) and vascular cell adhesion molecule-1 (VCAM-1) on the endothelial cells.[18,19] Increased expression and higher avidity of these molecules are induced by the release of pro-inflammatory cytokines, like tumor necrosis factor-alpha (TNF-α), interferon-gamma (IFN-γ) or interleukin-1 (IL-1), which are produced locally by activated lymphocytes.[20,21] This adhesion molecule-mediated contact between lymphocytes and endothelial cells enables further communication and release of matrix-degrading metalloproteinases, which leads to transmigration of lymphocytes across the endothelial cell barrier.[22,23] During this process, soluble adhesion molecules are released from the surface of the participating cells (Fig. 13.1) and can be detected in the blood circulation as well as in the CSF.[24–29]

MS PATHOLOGY AND MRI

Although MRI is an important marker of subclinical disease activity in MS, standard techniques do not allow discrimination between inflammatory changes, demyelination and axonal loss. Recent advances, like magnetization transfer imaging (MTI) or MR spectroscopy (MRS) have provided important clues for the detection of macromolecular associated alterations in MS lesions.[30,31] These techniques will help us to delineate further the pathological process during the evolution of new lesions and the progress of demyelination in vivo, but this technology is not yet available for routine examination. Therefore, established MRI monitoring of MS focuses on the detection of inflammatory disease activity as evidenced by enlarging T2-weighted lesions or Gd enhancement.[1] It has been clearly demonstrated from autopsy and diagnostic brain biopsy studies that increased cellular infiltrates and alterations of the blood–brain barrier are the characteristic features of Gd-enhancing lesions.[3,6,32] From serial MRI studies it is well known that Gd-enhancing lesions occur on average 5–10 times more often than clinical relapses.[4,33] Therefore, this paraclinical surrogate marker of disease activity in MS is currently used in prospective studies to evaluate the significance of various immunological parameters.

COMPLEX KINETICS AND TOPOLOGICAL ASPECTS OF MS IMMUNOPATHOLOGY

Unlike experimental autoimmune encephalomyelitis, an animal model of MS, the exact disease onset in an individual MS patient cannot be identified by any means available

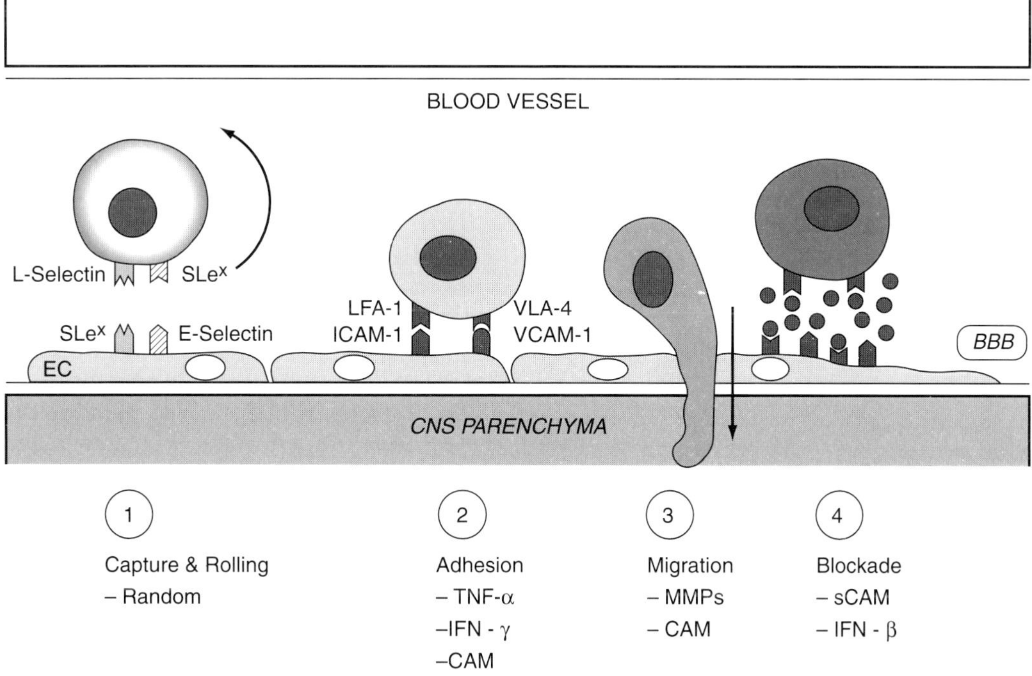

Figure 13.1 Modulation of lymphocyte adhesion to the blood–brain barrier. 1. Blood lymphocyte flow within the microvessel is reduced and cells are tethered to the endothelium by a random contact between selectins and sLewis^x antigen. 2. In the presence of ongoing inflammation the cellular adhesion molecules (CAM) ICAM-1 and VCAM-1 are upregulated and the avidity of their counter-ligands LFA-1 and VLA-4 is increased. 3. This enables firm adhesion of both cell types and the initiation of transmigration by release of matrix-degrading proteases (MMPs). 4. At later time points an increased release of soluble cellular adhesion molecules (sCAM) may block the interaction of lymphocytes and cerebral cells and therefore reduce cellular transmigration. This immunomodulatory event is probably enhanced by interferon-beta (IFN-β).[4] Adapted with permission.[11]

today. In many patients with a clinical presentation suggestive of disseminated encephalomyelitis, signal abnormalities on MRI are already present and intrathecal immunoglobulin G (IgG) production indicates an ongoing CNS-confined humoral immune process.[34] Serial MRI studies revealed that in patients with very active disease there is an overlap of evolving, full-blown and remitting Gd-enhancing lesions; therefore it was suggested that the underlying immunopathological disease process may be constitutively active and the transmigration of activated immune cells occurs only at random locations within the brain or spinal cord.[35,36] However, prospective longitudinal studies have shown that there is an activity associated variation of certain immunological parameters with an increase of pro-inflammatory cytokines, like TNF-α and IFN-γ, as early as 4 weeks before a clinical relapse,[37,38] and immunomodulatory cytokines (e.g. IL-10 and transforming growth factor-β) (TGF-β) expressed at higher levels during stable phases of the relapsing–remitting disease.[38–40]

To detect these complex changes during the disease process it is essential to perform timely correlated longitudinal analyses of frequent

MRI scans, clinical examinations and body fluid sampling for the determination of immunological markers.[41,42] We know from animal studies that the relative changes in cytokine pattern (e.g. Th1/Th2 shift) associated with disease fluctuation are more important than purely absolute levels of a single cytokine.[40,43] It is therefore of paramount importance to analyse synergistic as well as opposing/antagonistic factors in parallel.

The initial immune activation in MS most likely occurs outside the CNS in the peripheral lymphatic tissue.[14] There are indications that this process involves mechanisms, like molecular mimicry or superantigen activation of autoreactive T cells[12,15,16] followed by complex immunoregulatory events which are mediated by various cytokines.[38,44] It is not clear how long these events last before individual cells will enter the CNS and induce new lesion formation, but during this time immune cells involved in this process may be detectable in the circulating blood. Initial cellular migration may cause an early local upregulation of proinflammatory molecules at the blood–brain barrier and thereby recruit further activated autoantigen specific, as well as unspecific, immune cells to orchestrate the evolving new lesion.[19] Within several days to weeks these events may lead to a new Gd-enhancing lesion and possibly create clinical symptoms either via inflammatory mediators, local oedema or incipient demyelination.[8,21]

The initial steps of autoantigen recognition and immune cell activation which occur outside the CNS in lymphoid tissue and which are part of the complex immunoregulatory events in MS are probably not detectable on cranial MRI (Fig. 13.2). The subsequent steps of transmigration and blood–brain barrier disturbance are best seen on Gd-enhancing lesions, whereas tissue destruction and possibly early reconstitution can be detected on T2- or T1-weighted lesions.[35,45] Newly developed MTI, as well as MRS are able to detect demyelinating areas as well as neuronal damage, and will in the future supplement the in vivo demonstration of ongoing pathophysiological events during the course of the disease.[46]

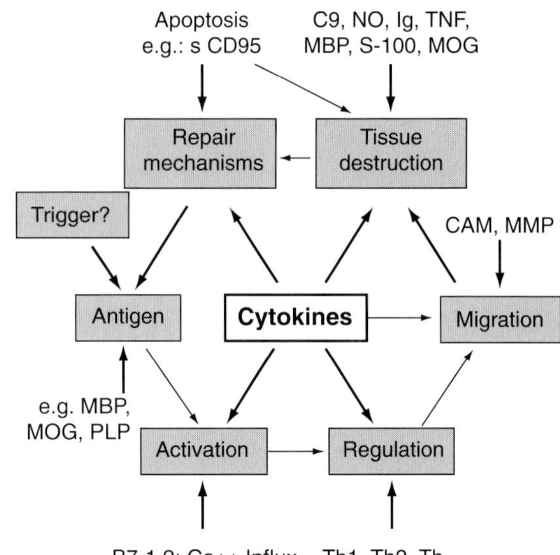

Figure 13.2 Important steps of the immunopathogenesis in MS and their relation to biological activity markers. The initial autoantigen presentation is most likely induced by an environmental trigger and leads to the activation of autoreactive immune cells. This process is dependent on the availability of costimulatory molecules (e.g. B7) on the cellular surface and is regulated by various cytokines. Once the immune cell is fully activated, firm adhesion to the cerebral endothelial cells mediated via adhesion molecules occurs and transmigration is initiated by matrix-degrading proteases (MMP). Once the cells have entered the target organ, cytotoxic substances (TNF-α, nitric oxide, complement) may be released and tissue destruction occurs. Subsequent repair mechanisms, like the induction of apoptotic cell death of the invading immune cells will initiate a remyelination process. Examples are given for biological activity markers which are involved in certain steps of this pathogenetic cascade. For details see text. (MBP, myelin basic protein; MOG, myelin oligodendrocyte glycoprotein; PLP, proteolipid protein.)

VARIATION OF BIOLOGICAL MARKERS RELATED TO MS PATHOLOGY AND MRI

To compare MR pathology with the molecular events associated with these changes, it is important to define activity and, preferentially, cell type specific markers that are stable and easily accessible in body fluids and can therefore be analysed in parallel to serial MRI scans. Initial studies have been performed recently that describe associations between MRI activity and the corresponding biological markers to a varying extent.

For example, myelin basic protein-like material in the urine may indicate ongoing demyelination and correlated with chronic progression disease course and with the number and total area of lesions on subsequent cranial MRI scans.[47] Peak levels of urinary neopterin secretion, a marker of IFN-γ-induced macrophage activity were detected more often in patients during an acute relapse and were associated with contrast-enhancing lesions on MRI.[48] Another (IFN-γ) induced activation marker of T lymphocytes, a specific transplasmalemma Ca^{2+} influx, was demonstrated to precede clinical attacks and coincide with MRI evidence of inflammation.[49]

A serial analysis of activation molecules on CD4+ peripheral blood lymphocytes in relapsing–remitting MS patients revealed no coincidence of relevant changes in the surface expression of these molecules with signs of increased disease activity on MRI.[50] Rosenberg et al. reported increased matrix metalloproteinase-9 (MMP-9; gelatinase B) levels in the CSF of MS patients.[51] This enzyme is involved in the proteolytic disruption of extracellular matrix and damage to the blood–brain barrier.[23] Interestingly, in patients with Gd-enhancing lesions, gelatinase B activity significantly decreased after high-dose methylprednisolone treatment, accompanied by a reduction in contrast-enhancing lesions.[51]

Two studies reported soluble cytokine levels in CSF and serum of MS patients in comparison to active MRI scans and did not detect a significant correlation between number of active lesions and levels of interleukin-1 beta (IL-1β), interleukin-6 (IL-6) and TNF-α in either compartment,[52,53] but patients who were prospectively monitored with monthly MRI demonstrated measurable TNF levels in the CSF associated with Gd-enhancing lesions on MRI.[53] As it is known that cytokines act mainly at paracrine distances and have a short biological half-life in body fluids, it may be difficult to detect subtle changes within the finely tuned cytokine network in compartments with a high turnover rate, such as the peripheral blood or the CSF.[54] There have been no reported studies on cell-associated cytokine expression in comparison to MRI activity that may help to clarify this issue.

CELLULAR ADHESION MOLECULES AND BLOOD–BRAIN BARRIER DYSFUNCTION

As mentioned above, levels of soluble adhesion molecules may be likely candidates for correlative analysis with Gd enhancing MRIs, as both are associated with inflammatory mediated blood–brain barrier dysfunction. Therefore, several studies have focused on either cross-sectional or longitudinal analysis of soluble adhesion molecules in blood or CSF and correlated their results to MRI activity.

In an early cross-sectional study higher serum levels for sICAM-1 were detected in MS patients with Gd-enhancing lesions when compared to those without MRI activity.[55] A clear positive correlation was observed between the total area and number of Gd-enhancing lesions per scan and the intrathecal production as well a serum levels for sVCAM-1 and to a lesser extent sICAM-1 in patients with newly diagnosed MS.[26] This correlation (for ICAM-1) was not apparent in an investigation which included patients with longer disease duration.[28]

Another study reported higher serum levels of sVCAM-1 and L-selectin in patients with Gd-enhancing lesions in comparison to those without MRI disease activity.[25] A longitudinal analysis by Giovannoni et al. found high serum levels for sICAM-1 together with a greater number of contrast-enhancing lesions.[24] These findings tended to be associated with short-term clinical disease progression. In this study, no such association was found for sVCAM-1.[24] The reported studies are not directly comparable as they all allowed different time frames for the interval between MRI and blood/CSF sampling which may impact on the different results (see later for discussion).

The first reports on soluble adhesion molecules in patients which were started on immunomodulatory treatment with interferon beta-1b (IFN–β1b) revealed interesting results. Determination of sVCAM-1 during the initiation of IFN-β1b indicated increasing serum levels (Fig. 13.3) which were associated with a decrease in the number of contrast-enhancing lesions on cranial MR images.[41,42] These changes were accompanied by a significant decrease of very late antigen-4 (VLA-4) expression on peripheral blood lymphocytes which is the ligand for VCAM-1 during the adhesion process.[56]

Furthermore, we also observed a relation between sVCAM-1 increase and response to treatment after 1 year as measured by MRI T2 lesion load. Patients with new T2 lesions had no or a much smaller increase in sVCAM-1 serum levels than patients who demonstrated a stable or even lower T2 lesion load after 1 year of treatment with subcutaneous IFN-β1b.[41]

In addition to the role of sVCAM-1 as an early indicator of blood–brain barrier disturbance, this adhesion molecule may also serve as a marker of treatment response in MS-patients. This aspect of sVCAM-1 in MS may be related to its function as an active immunomodulator.

Initially, upregulation of proinflammatory cytokine production (TNF-α and IFN-γ) by peripheral blood mononuclear cells may initiate an immunopathological cascade, which will lead to the upregulation of adhesion molecules (sVCAM-1 and sICAM-1) on cerebral endothelial cells and transmigration of activated T cells across the blood brain barrier. This scenario will lead to new lesions, which can be visualized on Gd-enhancing MRI, and eventually produce new clinical symptoms (relapse). As a consequence, soluble adhesion molecules, which are functionally active and can block cellular interactions,[57,58] may be released from the cytokine-activated endothelial cells. This immunoregulatory event to reduce further immune cell invasion of the CNS is reflected by increased levels of soluble adhesion molecules in the circulation, which can be detected at the time of a clinical relapse or a new lesion on cranial MRI. IFN-β may exert part of its beneficial activity in MS via an enhanced release of sVCAM-1 from pre-activated endothelial cells and therefore leads to a further and stable increase in sVCAM-1 serum levels, which in turn may block cellular traffic across the blood–brain barrier and reduce the development of new inflammatory lesions (Fig. 13.1).

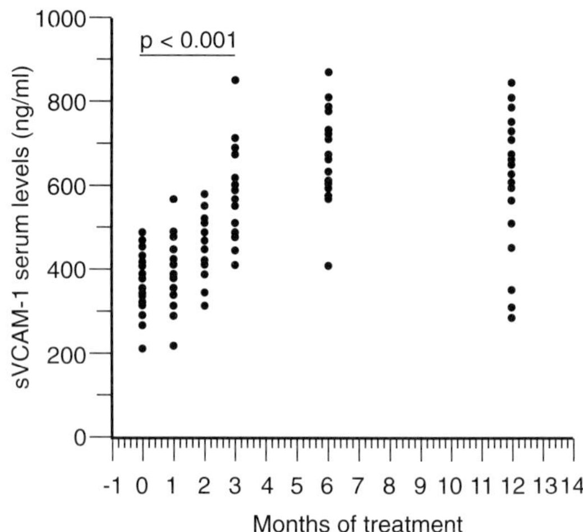

Figure 13.3 Longitudinal analysis of serum levels of serum levels for soluble VCAM-1 during the treatment with subcutaneous interferon beta-1b in 19 patients with relapsing–remitting MS. A significant increase in sVCAM-1 levels was detected between month 0 and 3 ($p < 0.001$).

As it is known from histopathological studies of brain lesions from MS patients that adhesion molecules are upregulated in areas of ongoing blood–brain barrier dysfunction—as indicated by Gd enhancement—cerebral endothelial cells which are a major constituent of this selective tissue interface appear to be a good model to study further molecular events in vitro.[59]

Current research will focus on the in vitro modulation of adhesion molecule expression as well as cellular adhesion events and transmigration of lymphocytes to elucidate the pathophysiological events during immune cell traffic into the CNS, which is a major step during the evolution of new lesions, can be visualized by contrast-enhancing MRI and may be an important target for the development of new drugs to modify positively the disease course in patients with MS.

ACKNOWLEDGEMENT

Part of the work presented in this manuscript was supported by grants from Gemeinnützige Hertie-Stiftung and the Deutsche Multiple Sklerose Gesellschaft (DMSG).

REFERENCES

1. Miller DH, Albert PS, Barkhof F et al. Guidelines for the use of magnetic resonance techniques in monitoring the treatment of multiple sclerosis. *Ann Neurol* 1996; **39**: 6–16.
2. Barkhof F, Filippi M, Miller DH et al. Strategies for optimizing MRI techniques aimed at monitoring disease activity in multiple sclerosis treatment trials. *J Neurol* 1997; **244**: 76–84.
3. Kermode AG, Thompson AJ, Tofts PS. Breakdown of the blood–brain barrier precedes symptoms and other MRI signs of new lesions in multiple sclerosis: pathogenetic and clinical implications. *Brain* 1990; **113**: 1477–1489.
4. Miller DH, Barkhof F, Nauta JP. Gadolinium enhancement increases the sensitivity of MRI in detecting disease activity in multiple sclerosis. *Brain* 1993; **116**: 1077–1094.
5. Koudriavtseva T, Thompson AJ, Fiorelli M et al. Gadolinium enhanced MRI predicts clinical and MRI disease activity in relapsing–remitting sclerosis. *J Neurol Neurosurg Psychiatry* 1997; **62**: 285–287.
6. Katz D, Taubenberger JK, Cannella B et al. Correlation between magnetic resonance imaging findings and lesion development in chronic, active multiple sclerosis. *Ann Neurol* 1993; **34**: 661–669.
7. Newcombe J, Hawkins CP, Henderson CL et al. Histopathology of multiple sclerosis lesions detected by magnetic resonance imaging in unfixed postmortem central nervous system tissue. *Brain* 1991; **114**: 1013–1023.
8. Hohlfeld R. Biotechnological agents for the immunotherapy of multiple sclerosis. *Brain* 1997; **120**: 865–916.
9. Barkhof F, Tas MW, Frequin ST et al. Limited duration of the effect of methylprednisolone on changes on MRI in multiple sclerosis. *Neuroradiology* 1994; **36**: 382–387.
10. Stone LA, Frank JA, Albert PS et al. The effect of interferon-beta on blood–brain barrier disruptions demonstrated by contrast-enhanced magnetic resonance imaging in relapsing–remitting multiple sclerosis. *Ann Neurol* 1995; **37**: 611–619.
11. Hartung HP. Pathogenesis of inflammatory demyelination: implications for therapy. *Curr Opin Neurol* 1995; **8**: 191–199.
12. Steinman L. Multiple sclerosis: a coordinated immunological attack against myelin in the central nervous system. *Cell* 1996; **85**: 299–302.
13. Lucchinetti C, Rodriguez M. The controversy surrounding the pathogenesis of the multiple sclerosis lesion. *Mayo Clin Proc* 1997; **72**: 665–678.
14. Hafler DA, Weiner HL. MS: a CNS and systemic autoimmune disease. *Immunol Today* 1989; **10**: 104–108.
15. Wucherpfennig KW, Strominger JL. Molecular mimicry in T cell-mediated autoimmunity: viral peptides activate human T cell clones specific for myelin basic protein. *Cell* 1995; **80**: 695–705.
16. Hemmer B, Fleckenstein BT, Vergelli M et al. Identification of high potency microbial and self ligands for a human autoreactive class II-restricted T cell clone. *J Exp Med* 1997; **185**: 1651–1659.
17. Wekerle H, Linington C, Lassman H et al. Cellular immune reactivity within the CNS. *Trends Neurosci* 1986; **6**: 271–277.
18. Springer T. Traffic signals for lymphocyte recirculation and leukocyte emigration: the multistep paradigm. *Cell* 1994; **76**: 301–314.
19. Archelos JJ, Hartung HP. The role of adhesion molecules in multiple sclerosis: biology, pathogenesis and therapeutic implications. *Mol Med Today* 1997; **3**: 310–321.
20. de Vries HE, Kuiper J, Boer AG de et al. The blood–brain barrier in neuroinflammatory disease. *Pharmacol Rev* 1997, **49**: 143–155.
21. Storch M, Lassmann H. Pathology and pathogenesis of demyelinating diseases. *Curr Opin Neurol* 1997; **10**: 186–192.
22. Cuzner ML, Gveric D, Strand C et al. The expression of tissue-type plasminogen activator, matrix metalloproteinases and endogenous inhibitors in the central nervous system in multiple sclerosis: comparison of stages in lesion

evolution. *J Neurolpathol Exp Neurol* 1996; **55**: 1194–1204.

23. Leppert D, Waubant E, Burk MR et al. Interferon beta-1b inhibits gelatinase secretion and in vitro migration of human T cells: a possible mechanism for treatment efficacy in multiple sclerosis. *Ann Neurol* 1996; **40**: 846–852.
24. Giovannoni G, Lai M, Thorpe J et al. Longitudinal study of soluble adhesion molecules in multiple sclerosis: correlation with gadolinium enhanced magnetic resonance imaging. *Neurology* 1997; **48**: 1557–1565.
25. Hartung HP, Reiners K, Archelos JJ et al. Circulating adhesion molecules and tumor necrosis factor receptor in multiple sclerosis: correlation with magnetic resonance imaging. *Ann Neurol* 1995; **38**: 186–193.
26. Rieckmann P, Altenhofen B, Riegel A et al. Soluble adhesion molecules (sVCAM-1 and sICAM-1) in cerebrospinal fluid and serum correlate with MRI activity in multiple sclerosis. *Ann Neurol* 1997; **41**: 326–333.
27. Rieckman P, Martin S, Albrecht M et al. Serial analysis of circulating adhesion molecules and TNF receptor in serum from patients with multiple sclerosis: cICAM-1 is an indicator for relapse. *Neurology* 1994; **44**: 2367–2372.
28. Trojano M, Avolio C, Simone IL et al. Soluble intercellular adhesion molecule-1 in serum and cerebrospinal fluid of clinically active relapsing–remitting multiple sclerosis: correlation with Gd-DTPA magnetic resonance imaging-enhancement and cerebrospinal fluid findings. *Neurology* 1996; **47**: 1535–1541.
29. Tsukada N, Matsuda M, Miyagi K et al. Adhesion of cerebral endothelial cells to lymphocytes from patients with multiple sclerosis. *Autoimmunity* 1993; **14**: 329–333.
30. Kimura H, Grossman RI, Lenkinski RE et al. Proton MR spectroscopy and magnetization transfer ratio in multiple sclerosis: correlative findings of active versus irreversible plaque disease. *AJNR* 1997; **17**: 1539–1547.
31. van Waesberghe JH, Castelijns JA, Scheltens P et al. Comparison of four potential MR parameters for severe tissue destruction in multiple sclerosis lesions. *Magn Res Imaging* 1997; **15**: 155–162.
32. Brück W, Porada P, Poser S et al. Monocyte/macrophage differentiation in early multiple sclerosis lesions. *Ann Neurol* 1995; **38**: 788–796.
33. Bastianello S, Pozzilli C, Bernardi S et al. Serial study of gadolinium-DTPA MRI enhancement in multiple sclerosis. *Neurology* 1990; **40**: 591–595.
34. Optic Neuritis Study Group. The 5-year risk of MS after optic neuritis. Experience of the optic neuritis treatment trial. *Neurology* 1997; **49**: 1404–1413.
35. Paty DW. Magnetic resonance in multiple sclerosis. *Curr Opin Neurol Neurosurg* 1993; **6**: 202–208.
36. Calabresi PA, Stone LA, Bash CN et al. Interferon beta results in immediate reduction of contrast-enhanced MRI lesions in multiple sclerosis patients followed by weekly MRI. *Neurology* 1997; **48**: 1446–1448.
37. Beck J, Rondot P, Catinot L et al. Increased production of interferon gamma and tumor necrosis factor precedes clinical manifestation in multiple sclerosis: do cytokines trigger off exacerbations? *Acta Neurol Scand* 1988; **78**: 318–323.
38. Rieckmann P, Albrecht M, Kitze B et al. Tumor necrosis factor-α messenger RNA expression in patients with relapsing–remitting multiple sclerosis is associated with disease activity. *Ann Neurol* 1995; **37**: 82–88.
39. Rieckmann P, Albrecht M, Kitze B et al. Cytokine mRNA levels in mononuclear blood cells from patients with multiple sclerosis. *Neurology* 1994; **44**: 1523–1526.
40. Olsson T. Role of cytokines in multiple sclerosis and experimental autoimmune encephalomyelitis. *Eur J Neurol* 1994; **1**: 7–19.
41. Rieckmann P, Kallmann B, Altenhofen B et al. Correlation of soluble adhesion molecules in blood and cerebrospinal fluids with magnetic resonance imaging activity in patients with multiple sclerosis. *Multiple Sclerosis* 1998 (in press).
42. Calabresi PA, Tranquill LR, Dambrosia JM et al. Increases in soluble VCAM-1 correlate with a decrease in MRI lesions in multiple sclerosis treated with interferon beta-1b. *Ann Neurol* 1997; **41**: 669–674.
43. Kennedy MK, Torrance DS, Picha KS et al. Analysis of cytokine mRNA expression in the central nervous system of mice with experimental autoimmune encephalomyelitis reveals that IL-10 mRNA expression correlates with recovery. *J Immunol* 1992; **149**: 2496–2505.
44. Arnason BGW, Reder AT. Interferons and multiple sclerosis. *Clin Neuropharmacol* 1994; **17**: 495–547.

45. Miller DA. Magnetic resonance in monitoring the treatment of multiple sclerosis. *Ann Neurol* 1994; **36**: S91–S94.
46. Erickson BJ, Noseworthy JH. Value of magnetic resonance imaging in assessing efficacy in clinical trials of multiple sclerosis. *Mayo Clin Proc* 1997; **71**: 1080–1089.
47. Whitaker JN, Kachelhofer RD, Bradley EL et al. Urinary myelin basic protein-like material as a correlate of the progression of multiple sclerosis. *Ann Neurol* 1995; **38**: 625–632.
48. Giovannoni G, Lai M, Kidd D et al. Daily urinary neopterin excretion as an immunological marker of disease activity in multiple sclerosis. *Brain* 1997; **120**: 1–13.
49. Martino G, Filippi M, Martinelli V et al. Interferon-gamma induced increases in intracellular calcium in T lymphocytes from patients with multiple sclerosis precede clinical exacerbations and detection of active lesions on MRI. *J Neurol Neurosurg Psychiatry* 1997; **63**: 339–345.
50. Stuber A, Martin R, Stone LA et al. Expression pattern of activation and adhesion molecules on peripheral blood CD4+ T-lumphocytes in relapsing–remitting multiple sclerosis patients: a serial analysis. *J Neuroimmunol* 1996; **66**: 147–151.
51. Rosenberg GA, Dencoff JE, Correa N et al. Effect of steroids on CSF matrix metalloproteinases in multiple sclerosis: relation to blood–brain barrier injury. *Neurology* 1996; **46**: 1626–1632.
52. Rovaris M, Barnes D, Woodrofe N et al. Patterns of disease activity in multiple sclerosis patients: a study with quantitative gadolinium-enhanced brain MRI and cytokine measurement in different clinical subgroups. *J Neurol* 1996; **243**: 536–542.
53. Spuler S, Yousry T, Scheller A et al. Multiple sclerosis: prospective analysis of TNF-alpha and 55 kDa TNF receptor in CSF and serum in correlation with clinical and MRI activity. *J Neuroimmunol* 1996; **66**: 57–64.
54. Hartung HP. Immune-mediated demyelination. *Ann Neurol* 1993; **33**: 563–567.
55. Hartung HP, Michels M, Reiners K et al. Soluble ICAM-1 serum levels in multiple sclerosis and viral encephalitis. *Neurology* 1993; **43**: 2331–2335.
56. Calabresi PA, Pelfrey CM, Tranquill LR et al. VLA-4 expression on peripheral blood lymphocytes is downregulated after treatment of multiple sclerosis with interferon beta. *Neurology* 1997; **49**: 1111–1116.
57. Chuluyan HE, Osborn L, Lobb R et al. Domains 1 and 4 of vascular cell adhesion molecule-1 (CD 106) both support very late activation antigen-4 (CD49d/CD29)-dependent messocyte transendothelial migration. *J Immunol* 1995; **155**: 3135–3143.
58. Rieckmann P, Michel U, Albrecht M et al. Cerebral endothelial cells are a major source for soluble intercellular adhesion molecule-1 in the human central nervous system. *Neurosci Lett* 1995; **186**: 61–64.
59. Cannella B, Raine CS. The adhesion molecule and cytokine profile of multiple sclerosis lesions. *Ann Neurol* 1995; **37**: 424–435.

14

Immunomodulation in multiple sclerosis and cytokine response

Ariel Miller, Sarah Shapiro and Nitza Lahat

INTRODUCTION

Multiple sclerosis (MS) is presumed to be a $CD4^+$ T-cell-mediated central nervous system (CNS) autoimmune disease. It is characterized by elevated levels of the pro-inflammatory cytokines such as interferon-γ (IFN-γ), tumor necrosis factor α/β (TNF-α/β), interleukin (IL)-1, IL-2 and IL-12, in the peripheral blood, cerebrospinal fluid (CSF) and brain lesions. The association of these inflammatory cytokines with disease activity implies that $CD4^+$ T cells of the T helper type 1 (Th1) phenotype and macrophages play a pivotal role in the immunopathogenesis of the CNS demyelinating disease.[1] A major contribution to the understanding of the role of Th1/Th2 paradigm in the immunopathogenesis of MS results from the extensive studies in experimental autoimmune encephalomyelitis (EAE), a $CD4^+$ Th1-cell-mediated demyelinating disease of the CNS that is used as a model for the human disease MS.[2] The established theory of functional dichotomy among $CD4^+$ T cells sets the stage for studies directed at the mechanisms of Th1 to Th2 shift and immune deviation as a therapeutic strategy in the treatment of MS.

THE TH1/TH2 DICHOTOMY

Studies of the dual requirement T lymphocytes for cell-mediated and humoral immunities have clarified that there are two distinct subsets of $CD4^+$ T cells, each associated with a different arm of the immune system. The work of Mosmann and Coffman[3] has demonstrated that the so-called T helper 1 (Th1) subset of cloned lines makes predominantly IL-2 and IFN-γ. These cytokines are known to be involved in classic cell-mediated functions such as clonal expansion of cytotoxic T lymphocytes (CTLs), macrophage activation and class-switch to immunoglobulin G (IgG) isotypes that mediate complement lysis of sensitized cells. By contrast, another subset of cells (called Th2) make the functionally opposite cytokines IL-4, IL-5 and IL-10, which are known to activate B cells to switch to neutralizing antibodies (IgG1 in the mouse) and IgE, the initiator of immediate hypersensitivity. These findings were followed by extensive research demonstrating the role of Th1 and Th2 $CD4^+$ T cells in the pathogenesis of organ-specific autoimmune diseases.[1–6]

Thus, cytokines produced by Th1 cells (IFN-γ, TNF-α/β, IL-2 and IL-12) are inflammatory mediators of various autoimmune processes, including autoimmune demyelinating diseases where oligodendrocytes are a target for immune attack. Cytokines produced by Th2 cells (IL-4, IL-5 and IL-10) or by Th3 cells (transforming growth factor β (TGF-β) mediate antibody production, anti-inflammatory cascade, and resolution of inflammatory and autoimmune processes.

MS AS A TH1-MEDIATED DISEASE OF THE CNS

MS is an inflammatory disease of the CNS of suspected autoimmune origin. Studies in MS and its animal model EAE, suggest that MS results from immune dysregulation and aberrant activation, whereby CNS myelin proteins serve as autoantigens leading to a T-cell-driven inflammatory and demyelinating process.[7–9] The immune dysregulation in MS involves both cellular and humoral arms of the immune response and can be identified in the peripheral blood, CSF and CNS. These include: defective immune-suppressor response[10]; elevated T-cell reactivity against various myelin antigens, such as myelin basic protein (MBP), proteolipid protein (PLP) or myelin oligodendrocyte glycoprotein (MOG)[10]; increased expression of major histocompatibility complex (MHC) class II molecules on antigen presenting cells (APCs), monocytes, endothelial as well as glial cells; elevated levels of circulating memory T cells ($CD4^+$/IL–2R+/$CD45RO^+$)[7–9]; raised levels of cell surface adhesion molecules on T cells and macrophages.[1–14] The elevated levels of adhesion molecules correlate with the degree of blood–brain barrier (BBB) eruption.[15,16] MS is also characterized by elevated levels of pro-inflammatory cytokines such as TNF-α, IL-1, IL-2 and IFN-γ in the peripheral blood,[17–19] CSF[20,21] and in brain lesions.[22] The association of these inflammatory cytokines with disease activity,[19–21] implies that $CD4^+$ T cells of Th1[23,24] and macrophages,[25,26] play a pivotal role in the immunopathogenesis of the CNS demyelinating disease. Moreover, the relative low levels and defective production of IL-10, IL-4 and TGF-β in patients with active multiple sclerosis[27] and their protective role in EAE,[28–34] suggest that T cells of the Th2 and Th3 phenotypes and their characteristic cytokine products may be involved in induction of remission and in suppression of the disease process (Figure 14.1a,b).

IMMUNOTHERAPIES AND CYTOKINE SHIFT IN MS

Increased understanding of the EAE model and the human demyelinating disease MS has recently led to the implementation of a number of immunomodulatory strategies, some already approved as effective in the treatment of the human disease, while others are still in clinical trials or are examined in the animal disease model. These immune interventions include: regulatory cytokines, cytokine antagonists, antigen-driven therapeutic strategies as well as other immunomodulatory agents (Table 14.1)

Table 14.1. Therapeutic strategies associated with cytokine shift and immune deviation
Cytokine-mediated immune deviation:
Downregulatory cytokines
IFN-β (1b/1a)
IL-4, IL-10
TGF-β
Cytokine antagonists:
Anti-TNF-α antibodies
Soluble TNF-α receptors (sTNFα-R)
TNFα knock-out
Antigen-driven immune deviation:
Oral tolerance (oral myelin)
Glatiramer acetate (copolymer-1; Copaxone®)
Altered peptide ligands
Vaccination with T-cell receptor peptides
DNA immunization
Others:
Linomide
Pentoxifylline (PTX)
Rolipram
Retinoids
Cyclophosphamide
Corticosteroids

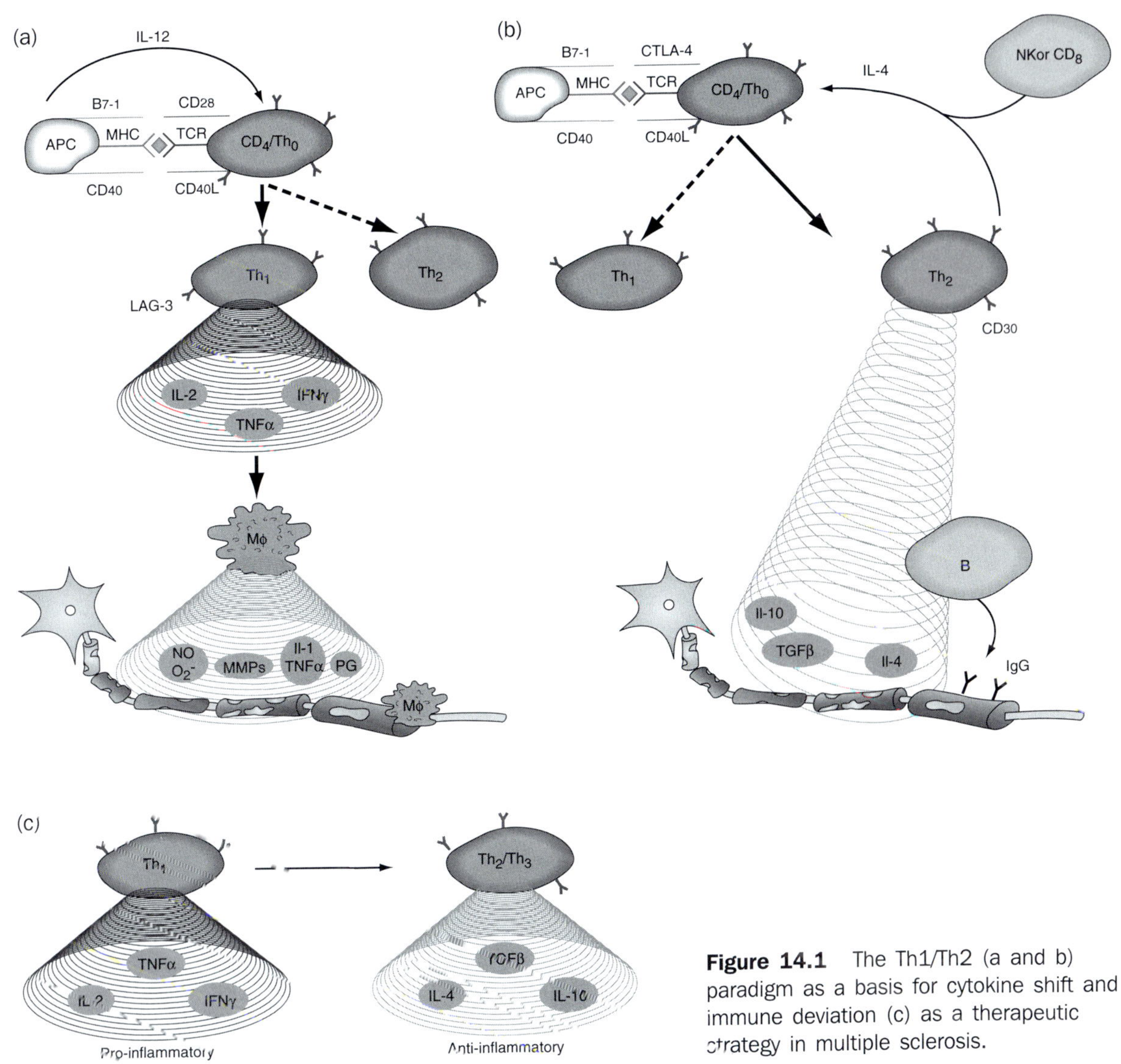

Figure 14.1 The Th1/Th2 (a and b) paradigm as a basis for cytokine shift and immune deviation (c) as a therapeutic strategy in multiple sclerosis.

that share cytokine-shift and immune deviation as common mechanisms of immunoregulation (Figure 14.1C).

Cytokine-mediated immune deviation

The complex pro-inflammatory cytokine cascade in the pathogenesis of MS has become the target of a number of suppressor cytokines as anti-inflammatory drugs (SCAIDs) and specific antagonists of pro-inflammatory cytokines for the treatment of experimental as well as human inflammatory and autoimmune diseases.[35]

Interferon-β (IFN-β)

IFN-β, the first treatment approved as effective in reduction of disease activity in MS patients,[36–39] has demonstrated unique downregulatory effects on Th1 cytokines. Preliminary studies by Arnason suggested that IFN-β seems to induce immune cells capable of mediating suppressor activity.[40] Recent studies, however, have clarified that the activities of both Th1 cytokines (TNFα and IFN-γ) are antagonized by IFN-β.[41,42] Additionally, IFN-β has demonstrated direct suppressor effects mediated by the induction of the Th2 cytokines IL-4 and IL-10, both in vitro,[43,44] as well as in vivo in MS patients treated with IFN-β.[45] Induction of the Th2 cytokines following IFN-β treatment was correlated with a beneficial clinical effect in the MS patients as well as with a reduced encephalitogenicity in the animal disease model.[45]

Although some of the effects of IFN-β are antagonistic to Th1 cytokines, others are clearly agonistic to Th1 activities. For example, although IFN-β antagonizes the upregulatory effects of IFN-γ on MHC class II molecules expressed on antigen presenting cells, both cytokines synergize for the induction of cell surface MHC class I molecules.[41] This synergistic effect of the interferons for the induction of class I molecules may be part of the induction of suppressor T cells restricted to MHC I. Nevertheless, clear pro-inflammatory effects of IFN-β are the well known 'flu-like symptoms' associated with IFN-β treatment in MS patients. These clinical symptoms may result because TNF suppression is accompanied by induction of IL-6.[42] Thus, although IFN-β has clear and predominant downregulatory effects in MS, some pro-inflammatory activities may be demonstrated at least as part of its initial effect.

IL-4, IL-10, TGF-β and Th1 cytokine antagonists

Modulation of an immune response from one dominated by excessive Th1 activity to one dominated by the protective cytokines produced by Th2/Th3 cells, has been demonstrated as an effective immunomodulatory and therapeutic strategy in certain experimental autoimmune diseases. For example, IL-4 treatment in EAE resulted in amelioration of clinical disease, inhibition of the synthesis of inflammatory cytokines, the induction of MBP-specific TGF-β-producing Th2/Th3 cells, and diminished CNS demyelination.[28] Similarly, induction of IL-10 mRNA expression was reported to correlate with recovery in EAE.[30] Some reports have indicated that IL-10 failed to suppress EAE,[46] but others have demonstrated that Th2 cells producing IL-10 inhibit encephalitogenic Th1 cells and suppress EAE.[24,28]

TGF-βs are a family of multipotent regulatory proteins, known to modulate proliferation and differentiation of many cell types. The available data suggest that TGF-βs are involved in a multitude of processes in autoimmune diseases such as rheumatoid arthritis and MS. Studies that demonstrate the downregulatory effects of TGF-β on T-cell responses in vitro,[47] accompanied by experiments in the EAE model that emphasize its prominent involvement as part of the endogenous mechanisms of natural recovery, as well as its suppressive effects on autoimmune processes when administered exogenously,[48,49] support the view of TGF-β as a promising candidate for the treatment of MS patients. The protective role played by TGF-β in suppressing EAE is attributed in part to the direct anti-inflammatory effects of TGF-β as well as to the antagonism between TGF-β and TNF-α.[47] However, the complex activities and multi-effects of TGF-β may explain the difficulties and side-effects associated with its systemic administration and the obligation to abandon its use in a clinical trial in MS patients (personal data).

Immunotherapies using Th1 cytokine antagonists such as antitumor necrosis factor antibodies and soluble tumor necrosis factor receptors (sTNF-r) were also demonstrated to suppress effectively experimental models of both chronic and relapsing inflammatory CNS disease.[50–52] However, these strategies were not found to be successful when implemented in MS patients,[53] and probably require further evaluation before being used as treatments of the human disease.

Antigen-driven immune deviation

A promising approach toward the prevention and treatment of autoimmune diseases involves identifying the mediating antigen and then tolerizing the autoreactive T cells with the corresponding antigen. Antigen-driven immune-intervention using analogues of autoantigens been known to protect animals from the induction of autoimmune disease and has been implemented recently as a therapeutic strategy in MS. This immune intervention in MS includes: copolymer-1 (Cop-1), oral tolerance, altered peptide ligands (APL), and vaccination with T-cell receptor (TCR) peptides. In all these approaches there is evidence for the involvement of immune deviation and bystander suppression mechanisms.

Copolymer-1/glatiramer acetate

The synthetic polypeptide copolymer-1 (Cop-1; Copaxone®, glatiramer acetate), a synthetic amino acid copolymer of alanine, glutamic acid, lysine and tyrosine, was originally synthesized with the aim of mimicking the myelin antigen MBP. In vitro, Cop-1 inhibits the proliferative response to MBP of T-cell lines and clones of various MHC restrictions of both mouse as well as human origin. Cop-1 treatment suppresses EAE induced in a variety of species,[54] and has been demonstrated to reduce clinical disease activity in humans with relapsing–remitting disease.[55–57] It has been proposed that the predominant mechanism underlying the immunomodulatory activities of Cop-1 resides in the immunological cross-reactivity of Cop-1 with MBP and its competition with MBP for MHC class II presentation. This may result in the inhibition of MBP-specific T-cell activation.[55,58–60] Nevertheless, molecular mimicry to MBP and blocking of MBP-specific autoimmune T cells does not explain recent observations suggesting that the effect of Cop-1 in EAE is not restricted to a particular encephalitogen, but rather suppresses disease induced by various myelin antigens such as PLP[61] and MOG.[62] The suppressive activity of Cop-1 has, however, been shown to be organ-specific and limited to inflammatory and autoimmune diseases involving CNS myelin, such as EAE, although no effect was demonstrated in SLE or other autoimmune diseases.[63] Studies using experimental animals have indeed suggested that the effectiveness of Cop-1 in preventing EAE results also from the induction of antigen-specific suppressor T cells that cross-react with MBP.[54] Cop-1-specific suppressor T cells isolated from rodents showed polarized secretion of Th2 type cytokines.[64] However, active suppression as a possible mechanism for the beneficial effect of Cop-1 in humans with MS has been described only recently. To further evaluate Cop-1 immunomodulatory activities, we have conducted a clinical and immunological study in relapsing-remitting MS patients treated with Copaxone® for 12 months in an open trial. Clinical improvement in Cop-1-treated patients was accompanied by a reduction in IL-2 soluble receptor but elevation of serum IL-10 levels, suppression of the pro-inflammatory cytokine TNF-α mRNA, but elevation of the anti-inflammatory cytokines TGF-β and IL-4 mRNA. Thus, the Th1 to Th2/Th3 immune deviation demonstrated in our study, implicating mechanisms of bystander suppression,[65] may explain the effects of Cop-1 on PLP- and MOG-induced experimental diseases.[61,62] Immune reactivity to these myelin antigens, as well as spreading autoimmunity to other putative neuro-antigens, may be downregulated by the anti-inflammatory mediators released at the microenvironment of the target organ.

Oral tolerance

The first demonstration of the clinical potential of immune deviation as a therapeutic strategy in inflammatory and autoimmune diseases came from studies of the basic mechanisms of oral tolerance and the characterization of the phenomenon entitled 'bystander suppression' and its beneficial effects in suppressing inflammatory diseases of the CNS such as EAE. Oral tolerance is a well-known method to induce peripheral immune tolerance and to downregulate the immune response (reviewed in Weiner[66]). Orally administered antigen induces tolerance primarily by the generation of active suppression. The regulatory cells that mediate active suppression act via the secretion of suppressive cytokines such as TGF-β and IL-4 after being triggered by the oral tolerogen.[67] Furthermore, Th2-like clones derived from mucosa and induced by oral antigen and secrete TGF-β can actively regulate immune responses in vivo and may represent a different subset of T cells—the Th3 type regulatory cells.[68]

Orally administered autoantigens suppress several experimental autoimmune models in a disease- and antigen-specific fashion; the diseases include EAE, uveitis, myasthenia, collagen- and adjuvant-induced arthritis, and diabetes in the NOD mouse.[66] Feeding mice with MBP was shown to suppress PLP-induced EAE,[69] emphasizing the potential therapeutic role of bystander suppression in autoimmune disease. Initial clinical trials of oral tolerance in MS, rheumatoid arthritis, and uveitis have demonstrated positive clinical effects with no apparent toxicity and decreases in T-cell autoreactivity.[70] The mechanism of immune deviation following oral tolerance in humans with autoimmune disease has been confirmed by Fukaura et al[71] who have demonstrated a marked increase in the relative frequencies of both MBP and PLP specific TGF-β-secreting T-cell lines in the MS patients treated with myelin as compared with untreated MS patients. Because the regulatory cells generated following oral tolerization are triggered in an antigen-specific fashion but suppress in an antigen-nonspecific fashion, they mediate bystander suppression when they encounter the fed antigen.[72]

Altered peptide ligands

Using a soluble peptide variant of an MBP epitope, altered peptide ligands (APLs), several investigators[73–75] have reported a reversal of EAE and the modulation of human autoreactive cells. In addition to TCR antagonism, the use of APL was shown to implicate modulation of the cytokine patterns of human autoreactive cells. Following a single amino acid substitution of their encephalitogenic peptide ligand, MBP peptide 85–99-reactive Th0 T-cell clones, for example, demonstrated a shift from Th1 to Th2 (IFN-γ to TGF-β) cytokine secretion pattern and bystander suppression.[76,77]

T-cell receptor (TCR) peptide vaccination and DNA immunization

A recent study by Vandenbark et al[77] shows that TCR peptide vaccination may also involve a mechanism of bystander suppression. TCR vaccination of patients with progressive resulted in stabilization of the disease clinically and was associated with the generation of peptide-specific Th-2 cells that directly inhibited MBP-specific Th-1 cells in vitro through the release of IL-10, thereby implicating mechanisms of bystander suppression. Similarly, DNA immunization by vaccination with naked DNA encoding TCR V β 8.2, protected mice from EAE and was associated with a reduction in the Th1 cytokines IL-2 and INF-γ but an elevation in the production of IL-4.[78]

Antigen-driven bystander suppression

The extensive studies on oral tolerance followed by other antigen-driven immune intervention using analogues or autoantigens, have clarified that it may not be necessary to identify the target autoantigen to suppress an organ-specific autoimmune disease via antigen-driven tolerance; it is necessary only to administer a protein capable of inducing regulatory cells that secrete suppressive cytokines when the autoantigen is encountered at the target organ.[66] This characteristic phenomenon of suppressor cytokines, which may shut-down the Th1-mediated inflammatory process independently of the primary autoantigen or of the antigen-specificity of the autoimmune cells, has been defined as antigen-driven bystander suppression.[66,72] Antigen-driven bystander suppression seems to be an important mechanism for the mediation of antigen-driven peripheral tolerance after administration of antigen, and presumably occurs in the microenvironment accounting for the antigen specificity of suppression generated by tolerization to antigens.[72] Therapeutic strategies based on antigen-driven bystander suppression carry two major advantages. Firstly, these strategies provide a unique delivery system of downregulatory/suppressor factors that are released at the target organ. This specific targeting of regulatory agents prevents the risks and side-effects associated with systemic administration of those agents. Secondly, these strategies solve the problem of the elusive autoantigen responsible for the elicitation of the CNS-inflammatory and autoimmune process in MS. The primary autoantigen, which may be MBP, PLP, MOG or an as yet unidentified myelin antigen, may differ between individuals. Moreover, the myelin autoantigen may vary not only among different individuals but also in the same individual during the course of the disease as part of the phenomenon of 'spreading autoimmunity'.[79]

Other immune-suppressor drugs associated with immune deviation

Successful treatment of Th1-mediated diseases like MS by reversal of the autoimmune response from a Th1 to a Th2 cytokine pattern has been documented as a common denominator of several additional immunotherapeutic strategies, in both EAE and MS. The treatment of EAE with retinoid revealed that an improved disease course was correlated with IL-4 production.[80] Pentoxifylline (PTX), a phosphodiesterase inhibitor that is known to suppress TNF-α and IFN-γ, used for the treatment of relapsing–remitting MS patients was associated with a marked reduction in intercellular adhesion molecule 1 (ICAM-1) and IL-2R expression as well as a decrease of TNF-α, IFN-γ and IL-12, whereas production of IL-4 and IL-10 increased.[81] Suppression of Th1 cytokine production and prevention of autoimmune encephalomyelitis was demonstrated also following treatment with the antidepressant rolipram.[82,83] The results of the phase-II clinical trial of linomide in progressive MS patients have shown that effective treatment is correlated with a significant reduction of memory T cells ($CD45RO^+$), an increase in the natural killer (NK) cell ($CD56^+$) and induction of Th2 cytokines.[84] Similarly, cyclophosphamide/methylprednisolone treatment of MS was recently found to be associated with increased IL-4 production.[85]

It is of interest that some of the beneficial effects of glucocorticosteroids in the treatment of acute exacerbation appear to involve inhibition of TNF-α and lymphocyte adhesion as well as the induction of anti-inflammatory Th2/Th3 cytokines such as TGF-β. Thus, glucocorticosteroids seem to shift the balance of the cytokine profile to favour the 'counterinflammatory' Th2 response. $CD4^+$ T cells activated in the presence of corticosteroids express higher levels of IL-4, IL-10 and IL-13, whereas synthesis of IFN-γ and TNF-α was diminished in comparison with cells activated in the absence of corticosteroids.[86–88]

POTENTIAL RISKS OF IMMUNE DEVIATION IN MS

It should be noted, however, that a shift from a Th1 to a Th2 cytokine production phenotype may carry the risk of elicitation of the humoral arm of the immune response in a dysregulated manner, with potential aggravation of the autoimmune process. Lafaille et al[89] recently reported that MBP-specific Th2 cells cause EAE in immune-deficient hosts rather than protect them from the disease. Similarly, Genain et al[90] have demonstrated that enhanced titers of autoantibodies to MOG may mediate the late complications of immune-deviation therapy in EAE. These findings should be evaluted carefully together with evidence of increased MRI activity and immune activation in two MS patients treated with the monoclonal antitumor necrosis factor antibody cA2.[53] Hence, careful follow-up of both clinical and immunological parameters may be required in patients treated with therapeutic strategies implicating immune deviation, in order to identify such possible delayed complications, particularly since a Th1 to Th2 shift may carry the risk of elicitation of the humoral arm of the immune response in a dysregulated manner.

CONCLUSIONS

Several immunomodulatory strategies that suppress MS or its experimental animal model (EAE), such as IFN-β, Cop-1, oral tolerance and T-cell vaccination, have demonstrated a common mechanism of action: promotion of immune deviation, i.e. the Th1 to Th2 shift and bystander suppression. Thus, Th1 to Th2 immune deviation seems to represent a common denominator for the successful immunotherapy of MS. Although the Th1 to Th2 shift seems to be an essential mechanism, it is not sufficient by itself. Combined Th1 to Th2 shift with modulation of T-cell subsets, adhesion molecules and NK cell activity seems to be required for effective treatment.[91]

ACKNOWLEDGEMENTS

The authors are grateful to the Technion Israel Institute of Technology, the Rappapot Family Institute for Research in the Medical Sciences and the Israeli Ministry of Health, for supporting their research studies.

REFERENCES

1. Olsson T. Critical influences of the cytokine orchestration on the outcome of myelin antigen-specific T-cell autoimmunity in experimental autoimmune encephalomyelitis and multiple sclerosis. *Immunol Rev* 1995; **144**: 245–268.
2. Cohen IR, Miller A (eds). *Autoimmune Disease Models—A Guidebook*. San Diego: Academic Press, 1994.
3. Mosmann TR, Coffman RL. Th1 and Th2 cells different patterns of lymphokine secretion lead to different functional properties. *Ann Rev Immunol* 1989; **7**: 145–173.
4. Liblau RS, Singer SM, McDevitt HO. Th1 and Th2 CD4+ T cells in the pathogenesis of organ-specific autoimmune diseases. *Immunol Today* 1995; **16**: 34–38.
5. Rocken M, Shevach EM. Immune deviation—the third dimension of nondeletional T cell tolerance. *Immunol Rev* 1996 **149**: 175–194.
6. Romagnani S. The Th1/Th2 paradigm. *Immunol Today* 1997; **18**: 263–266.
7. Martin R, McFarland HF, McFarlin DE. Immunological aspects of demyelinating diseases. *Ann Rev Immunol* 1992; **10**: 153–187.
8. Steinman L, Miller A, Bernard CCA et al. The epigenetics of multiple sclerosis: clues to etiology and a rationale for immune therapy. *Annu Rev Neurosci* 1994; **17**: 247–265.
9. Hafler DA, Weiner HL. Immunologic mechanisms and therapy in multiple sclerosis. *Immunol Rev* 1995; **144**: 75–107.
10. Antel JP, Owens T. The attraction of adhesion molecules [editorial]. *Ann Neurol* 1993; **34**: 123–124.
11. Steinman L, Waisman A, Altmann D. Major T-cell responses in multiple sclerosis. *Mol Med Today* 1995; **1**: 79–83.
12. Cannella B, Raine CS. The adhesion molecule and cytokine profile of multiple sclerosis lesions. *Ann Neurol* 1995; **37**: 424–435.
13. Navikas V, Link H. Cytokines and the pathogenesis of multiple sclerosis. *J Neurosci Res* 1996; **45**: 322–333.
14. Weller RO, Engelhardt B, Philips MJ. Lymphocyte targeting of the central nervous system: a review of afferent and efferent CNS-immune pathways. *Brain Pathol* 1996; **6**: 275–288.
15. Sharief MK, Noori MA, Ciardi M et al. Increased levels of circulating ICAM-1 in serum and cerebrospinal fluid of patients with active multiple sclerosis: correlation with TNF-α and blood–brain barrier damage. *J Neuroimmunol* 1993; **43**: 15–22.
16. Rieckmann P, Martin S, Weichselbraun I et al. Serial analysis of circulating adhesion molecules and TNF receptor in serum from patients with multiple sclerosis: sICAM-1 is an indicator for relapse. *Neurology* 1994; **44**: 2367–2372.
17. Trotter JL, Collins KG, van der Veen RC. Serum cytokine levels in chronic progressive multiple sclerosis: interleukin-2 levels parallel tumor necrosis factor-alpha levels. *J Neuroimmunol* 1991; **33**: 29–36.
18. Sharief MK, Hentges R. Association between tumor necrosis factor-α and disease progression in patients with multiple sclerosis. *N Engl J Med* 1991; **325**: 467–472.
19. Hartung HP, Reiners K, Archelos JJ et al. Circulating adhesion molecules and tumor necrosis factor receptor in multiple sclerosis: correlation with magnetic resonance imaging. *Ann Neurol* 1995; **38**: 186–193.
20. Hauser SL, Doolittle TH, Lincoln R et al. Cytokine accumulation in CSF of multiple sclerosis patients: frequent detection of interleukin-1 and tumor necrosis factor but not interleukin-6. *Neurology* 1990; **40**: 1735–1739.
21. Rudick RA, Ransohoff RM. Cytokine secretion by multiple sclerosis monocytes. Relationship to disease activity. *Arch Neurol* 1992; **49**: 265–270.

22. Hofmann FM, Hinton DR, Johnson K et al. Tumor necrosis factor identified in multiple sclerosis. *J Exp Med* 1980; **170**: 607–612.
23. Voshuhl RR, Martin R, Bergman C et al. T helper (Th1) functional phenotype of human myelin basic protein-specific T lymphocytes. *Autoimmunity* 1993; **15**: 137–143.
24. Windhagen A, Nicholson LB, Weiner HL et al. Role of Th1 and Th2 cells in neurologic disorders. *Chem Immunol* 1996; **63**: 171–186.
25. Cua DJ, Hinton DR, Kirkman L et al. Macrophages regulate induction of delayed-type hypersensitivity and experimental allergic encephalomyelitis in SJL mice. *Eur J Immunol* 1995; **25**: 2318–2324.
26. van der Laan LJ, Ruuls SR, Weber KS et al. Macrophage phagocytosis of myelin in vitro determined by flow cytometry: phagocytosis is mediated by CR3 and induces production of tumor necrosis factor-alpha and nitric oxide. *J Neuroimmunol* 1996; **70**: 145–152.
27. Mokhtarian F, Shi Y, Shirazian D et al. Defective production of anti-inflammatory cytokine TGF-beta by T cell lines from patients with active multiple sclerosis. *J Immunol* 1994; **152**: 6003–6010.
28. Van der Veen RC, Stohlman SA. Encephalitogenic Th_1 cells are inhibited by Th_2 cells with related peptide specificity, relative roles of IL-4 and IL-10. *J Neuroimmunol* 1993; **48**: 213–217.
29. Kennedy JK, Torrance DS, Picka KS et al. Analysis of cytokine mRNA expression in the central nervous system of mice with experimental autoimmune encephalomyelitis reveals that IL-10 mRNA expression correlates with recovery. *J Immunol* 1992; **149**: 2496–2505.
30. Falcone M, Bloom BR. A T helper cell 2 (Th2) immune response against non-self antigens modifies the cytokine profile of autoimmune T cells and protects against experimental allergic encephalomyelitis. *J Exp Med* 1997; **185**: 901–907
31. Johns LD, Flanders KC, Ranges GE et al. Successful treatment of experimental allergic encephalomyelitis with transforming growth factor-beta 1. *J Immunol* 1991; **147**: 1792–1796.
32. Racke MK, Dhib-Jalbut S, Cannella B et al. Prevention and treatment of chronic relapsing experimental allergic encephalomyelitis by transforming growth factor-beta 1. *J Immunol* 1991; **146**: 3012–3017.
33. Kuruvilla AP, Shah R, Hochwald GM et al. Protective effect of transforming growth factor beta 1 on experimental autoimmune diseases in mice. *Proc Natl Acad Sci USA* 1991; **88**: 2918–2921.
34. Fabry Z, Topham DJ, Fee D et al. TGF-β2 decreases migration of lymphocytes in vitro and homing of cells into the central nervous system in vivo. *J Immunol* 1995; **155**: 325–332.
35. Racke MK, Bonomo A, Scott DE et al. Cytokine-induced immune deviation as a therapy for inflammatory autoimmune disease. *J Exp Med* 1994; **180**: 1961–1966.
36. IFNβ Multiple Sclerosis Study Group. Interferon beta-1b is effective in relapsing–remitting multiple sclerosis. Clinical results of multicenter, randomized, double-blind, placebo-controlled trial. *Neurology* 1993; **43**: 655–661.
37. Paty DW. MS/MRI Study Group and the IFNβ Multiple Sclerosis Study Group. Interferon beta-1b is effective in relapsing–remitting multiple sclerosis. II. MRI analysis of multicenter, randomized, double-blind, placebo-controlled trial. *Neurology* 1993; **43**: 662–667.
38. Jacobs L., Cookfair D, Rudick R et al. Results of phase III trial of intramuscular recombinant beta interferon as treatment of multiple sclerosis. *Ann Neurol* 1994; **36**: 256–262.
39. Pozzilli C, Bastianello S, Koudriavtseva T et al. Magnetic resonance imaging changes with recombinant human interferon-beta-1a: a short term study in relapsing–remitting multiple sclerosis. *J Neurol Neurosurg Psychiatry* 1996; **61**: 251–258.
40. Arnason BG. Interferon beta in multiple sclerosis. *Clin Immunol Immunopathol* 1996; **81**: 1–11.
41. Miller A, Lanir N, Shapiro S et al. Immunoregulatory effects of interferon-beta and interacting cytokines on human vascular endothelial cells. Implications for multiple sclerosis and other autoimmune diseases. *J Neuroimmunol* 1996; **64**: 151–161.
42. Brod SA, Marshall GD Jr, Henninger EM et al. Interferon-beta 1b treatment decreases tumor necrosis factor-alpha and increases interleukin-6 production in multiple sclerosis. *Neurology* 1996; **46**: 1633–1638.
43. Rep MH, Hintzen RQ, Polman CH et al. Recombinant interferon beta blocks proliferation but enhances interleukin-10 secretion by activated human T-cells. *J Neuroimmunol* 1996; **67**: 111–118.
44. Porrini AM, Gambi D, Reder AT. Interferon effects on interleukin-10 secretion. Mononuclear cell response to interleukin 10 is normal in multiple sclerosis patients. *J Neuroimmunol* 1995; **61**: 27–34.

45. Rudick RA, Ranshoff RM, Lee JC et al. In vivo effects of interferon beta-1a on immunosuppressive cytokines in multiple sclerosis. *Neurology* 1998; **50**: 1294–1300.
46. Cannella B, Gao YL, Brosman C et al. IL-10 fails to abrogate experimental autoimmune encephalomyelitis. *J Neurosci Res* 1996; **45**; 735–746.
47. Merrill JE. Proinflammatory and antiinflammatory cytokines in multiple sclerosis and central nervous system acquired immunodeficiency syndrome. *J Immunother* 1992; **12**: 167–170.
48. Racke MK, Dhib-Jalbut S, Cannella B et al. Prevention and treatment of chronic relapsing experimental allergic encephalomyelitis by transforming growth factor-beta 1. *J Immunol* 1991; **146**: 3012–3017.
49. Kuruvilla AP, Shah R, Hochwald GM et al. Protective effect of transforming growth factor beta 1 on experimental autoimmune diseases in mice. *Proc Natl Acad Sci USA* 1991; **88**: 2918–2921.
50. Martin D, Near SL, Bendele A et al. Inhibition of tumor necrosis factor is protective against neurologic dysfunction after active immunization of Lewis rats with myelin basic protein. *Exp Neurol* 1995; **131**: 221–228.
51. Selmaj KW, Raine CS. Experimental autoimmune encephalomyelitis: immunotherapy with anti-tumor necrosis factor antibodies and soluble tumor necrosis factor receptors. *Neurology* 1995; **45**: S44–49.
52. Selmaj K, Papierz W, Glabinski A et al. Prevention of chronic relapsing experimental autoimmune encephalomyelitis by soluble tumor necrosis factor receptor I. *J Neuroimmunol* 1995; **56**: 135–141.
53. van Oosten BW, Barkhof F, Truyen L et al. Increased MRI activity and immune activation in two multiple sclerosis patients treated with the monoclonal anti-tumor necrosis factor antibody. *Neurology* 1996; **47**: 1531–1534.
54. Teitlebaum, D, Arnon R, Sela M. Copolymer 1: from basic research to clinical application. *Cell Mo Life Sci* 1997; **53**: 24–28.
55. Abramsky O, Teitelbaum D, Arnon R. Effect of a synthetic polypeptide (copolymer 1) on patients with multiple sclerosis and acute disseminated encephalomyelitis: preliminary report. *J Neurol Sci* 1977; **31**: 433–438.
56. Bornstein MB, Miller A, Slagle S et al. A pilot trial of Cop 1 in exacerbating–remitting multiple sclerosis. *N Engl J Med* 1987; **317**: 408–414.
57. Johnson KP, Brooks BR, Cohen JA et al. Copolymer 1 reduces relapse rate and improves disability in relapsing–remitting multiple sclerosis: results of a phase III multicenter, double-blind placebo-controlled trial. *Neurology* 1995; **45**: 1268–1276.
58. Teitelbaum D, Milo R, Arnon R et al. Synthetic copolymer 1 inhibits human T-cell lines specific factor myelin basic protein. *Proc Natl Acad Sci USA* 1991; **898**: 137–141.
59. Racke MK, Martin R, McFarland H et al. Copolymer 1-induced inhibition of antigen-specific T-cell activation: interference with antigen presentation. *J Neuroimmunol* 1992; **37**: 75–84.
60. Fridkis-Hareli M, Teitelbaum D, Gurevitch E et al. Direct binding of myelin basic protein and synthetic copolymer 1 to class II major histocompatibility complex molecules on living antigen presenting cells – specificity and promiscuity. *Proc Natl Acad Sci USA* 1994; **91**: 4872–4876.
61. Teitelbaum D, Fridkis-Hareli M, Arnon R et al. Copolymer 1 inhibits chronic relapsing experimental allergic encephalomyelitis induced by proteolipid protein (PLP) peptides in mice and interferes with PLP-specific T cell response. *J Neuroimmunol* 1996; **64**: 209–217.
62. Ben-Nun A, Mendel I, Bakimer R et al. The autoimmune reactivity to myelin oligodendrocyte glycoprotein (MOG) in multiple sclerosis is potentially pathogenic: effect of copolymer 1 on MOG induced disease. *J Neurol* 1996; **243**: S14–22.
63. Arnon R, Sela M, Teitelbaum D. New insights into the mechanism of action of copolymer 1 in experimental allergic encephalomyelitis and multiple sclerosis. *J Neurol* 1996; **243**: S8–13.
64. Aharoni R, Teitelbaum D, Sela M et al. Copolymer 1 induces T cells of the T helper type 2 that crossreact with myelin basic protein and suppress experimental autoimmune encephalomyelitis. *Proc Natl Acad Sci USA* 1997; **94**: 10821–10826.
65. Miller A, Shapiro S, Kinarty A et al. Treatment of multiple sclerosis with copolymer-1: implicating mechanisms of Th1 to Th2/Th3 immune-deviation. *J Neuroimmunol* 1998; in press.
66. Weiner HL. Oral tolerance: immune mechanisms and treatment of autoimmune diseases. *Immunol Today* 1997; **18**: 335–343.
67. Miller A, Lider O, Roberts AB et al. Suppressor T cells generated by oral tolerization to myelin

basic protein suppress both in vitro and in vivo immune responses by the release of TGF-β after antigen-specific triggering. *Proc Natl Acad Sci USA* 1992; **89**: 421–425.

68. Chen Y, Kuchroo VK, Inobe J et al. Regulatory T cell clones induced by oral tolerance: suppression of autoimmune encephalomyelitis. *Science* 1994; **265**: 1237–1240.
69. Al-Sabbagh AA, Miller A, Santos LMB et al. Antigen driven tissue-specific suppression following oral tolerance: orally administered myelin basic protein suppresses PLP induced experimental autoimmune encephalomyelitis in the SJL mouse. *Eur J Immunol* 1994; **24**: 2104–2109.
70. Weiner HL, Mackin GA, Matsui M et al. Double-blind pilot trial of oral tolerization with myelin antigens in multiple sclerosis. *Science* 1993; **259**: 1321–1324.
71. Fukaura H, Kent SC, Pietrusewicz MJ et al. Induction of circulating myelin basic protein and proteolipid protein-specific transforming growth factor-beta 1-secreting Th3 T cells by oral administration of myelin in multiple sclerosis patients. *J Clin Invest* 1996; **98**: 70–77.
72. Miller A, Lider O, Weiner LH. Antigen driven bystander suppression after oral administration of antigens. *J Exp Med* 1991; **174**: 791–798.
73. Karin N, Mitchell DJ, Brocke S et al. Reversal of experimental autoimmune encephalomyelitis by a soluble peptide variant of a myelin basic protein epitope: T cell receptor antagonism and reduction of interferon gamma and tumor necrosis factor alpha production. *J Exp M ed* 1994; **180**: 2227–2237.
74. Nicholson LB, Greer JM, Sobel RA et al. An altered peptide ligand mediates immune deviation and prevents autoimmune encephalomyelitis. *Immunity* 1995; **3**: 397–405.
75. Nicholson LB, Murtaza A, Hafler BP et al. A T cell receptor antagonist peptide induces T cells that mediate bystander suppression and prevent autoimmune encephalomyelitis induced with multiple myelin antigens. *Proc Natl Acad Sci USA* 1997; **94**: 9279–9284.
76. Gaur A, Boehme SA, Chalmers D et al. Amelioration of relapsing experimental autoimmune encephalomyelitis with altered myelin basic protein peptides involves different cellular mechanisms. *J Neuroimmunol* 1997; **74**: 149–158.
77. Vandenbark AA, Chou YK, Whitham R et al. Treatment of multiple sclerosis with T-cell receptor peptides: results of a double-blind pilot trial. *Nat Med* 1996; **2**: 1109–1115.
78. Waisman A, Ruiz PJ, Hirschberg DL et al. Suppressive vaccination with DNA encoding a variable region gene of the T-cell receptor prevents autoimmune encephalomyelitis and activates Th2 immunity. *Nat Med* 1996; **8**: 899–905.
79. Lehmann PV, Forsthuber T, Miller A et al. Spreading of T-cell autoimmunity to cryptic determinants of an autoantigen. *Nature* 1992; **358**: 155–157.
80. Racke MK, Burnett D, Pak SH et al. Retinoid treatment of experimental allergic encephalomyelitis. IL-4 production correlates with improved disease course. *J Immunol* 1995; **154**: 450–458.
81. Rieckmann P, Weber F, Gunther A et al. Pentoxifylline, a phosphodiesterase inhibitor, induces immune deviation in patients with multiple sclerosis. *J Neuroimmunol* 1996; **64**: 193–200.
82. Sommer N, Loschmann PA, Northoff GH et al. The antidepressant rolipram suppresses cytokine production and prevents autoimmune encephalomyelitis. *Nat Med* 1995; **3**: 244–248.
83. Jung S, Zielasek J, Kollner G et al. Preventive but not therapeutic application of rolipram ameliorates experimental autoimmune encephalomyelitis in Lewis rats. *J Neuroimmunol* 1996; **68**: 1–11.
84. Karussis DM, Meiner Z, Lehmann D et al. Immunomodulation of experimental autoimmune encephalomyelitis (EAE and CR-EAE) and of multiple sclerosis with quinoline-3-carboxamide. *J Neuroimmunol* 1995; **suppl 1**: 15.
85. Smith DR, Balashov K, Hafler DA et al. Immune deviation following pulse cyclophosphamide/methylprednisolone treatment of multiple sclerosis: increased IL-4 production and associated eosinophilia. *Ann Neurol* 1997; **42**: 313–318.
86. Pitzalis C, Sharrack B, Gray IA et al. Comparison of the effcts of oral versus intravenous methylprednisolone regimens on peripheral blood T lymphocyte adhesion molecule expression, T cell subsets distribution and TNF alpha concentrations in multiple sclerosis. *J Neuroimmunol* 1997; **74**: 62–68.
87. Zabiaga AM, Munoz E, Huber BT. IL-4 and IL-2 selectively rescue Th cell subsets from glucosteroid-induced apoptosis. *J Immunol* 1992; **70**: 1–5.
88. Ramierz F, Fowell DJ, Puclavec M et al. Glucocorticoids promote a Th2 cytokine response by $CD4^+$ T cells in vitro. *J Immunol* 1996; **156**: 2406–2412.

89. Lafaille JJ, Van de Keere F, Hsa AL et al. Myelin basic protein-specific T helper 2 (Th2) cells cause experimental encephalomyelitis in immunodeficient hosts rather than protect them from the disease. *J Exp Med* 1997; **186**: 307–312.

90. Genain CP, Abel K, Belmar N et al. Late complications of immune-deviation therapy in a nonhuman primate. *Science* 1996; **274**: 2054–2057.

91. Zhang J, Hohlfeld R, Hafler D et al. (eds). *Immunotherapy in Neuroimmunologic Diseases*. London: Martin Dunitz, 1998.

15

Future prospects of cytokines in the pathogenesis and management of multiple sclerosis

Tomas Olsson

INTRODUCTION

In multiple sclerosis (MS) and its model, experimental autoimmune encephalomyelitis (EAE), activated immunocompetent cells in the systemic circulation enter the central nervous system (CNS) where they provoke a further recruitment of inflammatory cells. Immune-medicated mechanisms then lead to damage to myelin sheaths and neurons/axons. Cytokines are by definition important for the outcome of MS and EAE, since they are peptides responsible both for effector functions of immunocompetent cells and their intercellular communication.[1] Thus studies of cytokines are very important for the understanding of the natural course of MS, the effects of therapy and genetic factors. The cytokine production by lymphoid cells can be polarized into T1 and T2-cells.[2,3] T1-cells are involved in delayed-type hypersensitivity reactions and produce lymphotoxin (LT) or tumor necrosis factor-beta (TNF-β) and interferon-gamma (TNF-γ), while T2-cells produce cytokines involved in B-cell proliferation and differentiation, such as interleukins (IL)-4, 5, 6, 10 and 13. Often the T1 and T2 subsets interact and may counteract each other. Pioneering studies have demonstrated that infections, genetic and environmental influences determine T1–T2 bias and host defence. A successful host defence against intracellular micro-organisms depend on a T1-biased immunity as shown in *Leishmania*,[4] as in leprosy.[5] Defence against extracellular micro-organisms such as *Trypanosoma brucei* depends on the humoral immune response, in part dependent on a genetic, strain-dependent ability to produce T2 cytokines.[6] Similar published and future studies in putatively autoimmune diseases such as MS will be important, and this review deals with selected aspects of these matters.

CYTOKINE CHARACTER—METHODOLOGICAL PRECAUTIONS

The character of cytokines necessitates caution both in studies of their expression and their experimental manipulations. First, cytokines are redundant in a sense that multiple cytokines signalling through the same or different receptors can induce similar cell responses. With the technical invention of genomic deletions in mice, this has been applied to cytokine genes. In view of the redundancy of cytokine function, studies on deleted cytokine genes may not be so informative.

Secondly most cytokines act autocrinely or paracrinely. Assays of free levels in body fluids therefore poorly reflect their local actions. It is therefore preferable to study cellular production of cytokines, in tissues or cell suspensions. This may be done by measuring mRNA for the produced cytokine by the polymerase chain reaction (PCR) or in situ hybridization,[7,8] secreted cytokines either in supernatants with enzyme-linked immunosorbent assay (ELISA) or single cells secreting the cytokines enumerated in enzyme-linked immunosorbent spot (ELISPOT) assays[9–12] or immunostaining of cytokines.

A third complication in studies of cytokines is their mutual interactions. This type of regulation should be kept in mind during in vitro culture. The addition of cytokines to cultures such as interleukin (IL)-2 and IL-4[13] or substances such as glutathione[14] will strongly direct the differentiation into certain cytokine profiles.

Fourthly, the effect of cytokines are time, dose and site dependent. Furthermore, cytokines given systemically may disturb a variety of feedback regulations with a paradoxical outcome. Accordingly, a cytokine given to an animal may induce production of antibodies against a cytokine, and thereby neutralize its effect. Similar paradoxical effects may appear with anticytokine antibodies or soluble receptors as has been observed for IL-6[15] and TNF.[16]

Thus, cytokines are difficult to study and cytokines or anticytokine reagents may be difficult to apply as therapeutic agents themselves, especially in view of difficulties and predicting outcomes from in vitro studies and experimental studies.

EXPRESSION AND MANIPULATIONS OF CYTOKINES IN EAE AND MS

Much of our understanding of cytokines in neuroinflammatory disease stems from various models of EAE, including studies on their tissue expression and role in T-cell transferred EAE, effects of immunomodulatory treatments, and in context with selective in vivo cytokine manipulations.

The prevalent opinion that T1-biased autoreactive T cells are important for inducing autoimmune neuroinflammation in EAE and MS largely stems from T-cell transfer experiments. Thus, myelin antigen specific T1-cells transfer acute monophasic EAE[17–20] while T2-cells transferred into an immunocompetent host failed to mediate disease.[19,20] Standard T2-biased cells do not protect against EAE while IL-4 treatment does.[21] However, encephalitogenic T cells transduced with a retroviral gene constructed to express IL-4 reduce severity of EAE[22] as well as transgenically IL-10 expressing autoreactive T cells.[23] Thus, under certain conditions, T2-cytokines, may protect. A form of allergic EAE was recently demonstrated after transfer of myelin basic protein (MBP)-specific T2-cells into immunocompromised hosts,[24] suggesting that T2-cytokines may be disease promoting under other conditions.

The clearly defined disease phases in an acute monophasic disease as in actively induced EAE in the Lewis rat enables correlative studies of putative disease up- and downregulatory cytokines in the target tissue. Using mRNA for in situ hybridization[25–27] we have demonstrated the appearance of cells in the CNS expressing LT and IL-12 shortly before clinical onset of disease. Roughly paralleling clinical signs, TNF-α and IFN-γ are abundantly expressed both at the mRNA level[25,26] and at the protein level.[28,29] In the interphase between maximum disease and recovery, transforming growth factor-β (TGF-β) appears and in the recovery period there is increased expression of IL-10.[25,26,30] In dark agouti (DA) rats immunized with the same protocol protracted relapsing disease course ensues. The CNS expression of IL-10 and TGF-β is deficient in these rats suggesting a causal relationship between strain-dependent efficient expression of these downregulatory cytokines and chronicity.[27]

Thus, data from transfer experiments and tissue expression of particular cytokines in most cases makes sense in autoimmune neuroinflammation when comparing to functions of particular cytokines analysed in vitro.

Apart from infiltrating lymphoid cells, CNS residents such as microglia, astrocytes and even neurons may also produce cytokines. There is evidence to suggest that such target production of immunoregulatory molecules may effect the outcome of CNS-directed autoimmune response or other insults to the CNS. This is exemplified by the observation that a distal peripheral nerve trauma was accompanied by induction of immunological recognition and effect of molecules in neurons and surrounding glia such as major histocompatibility complex (MHC) class I and class II molecules and an IFN-γ immunoreactive molecule.[31–34] Combination of this procedure with active EAE induction resulted in a stronger infiltration of lymphoid cells in the vicinity of the reacting nerve cell bodies.[34,35] IFN-γ like material has detected that sensory neurons regulate endogenous MHC class I.[36–38] Axotomized neurons also produce IL-6 and GMCSF[39,40] as well as TGF-β.[41] Taken together these studies suggest that neurons regulate the degree of intra-CNS immune reactivity and that target immune reactivity is important for the outcome of CNS inflammation. It will be important to take into account such findings in the context of human disease.

Cytokine expression and polarization is also affected by immunomodulatory treatments. Certain low molecular immunosuppressive drugs convert monophasic EAE to chronic EAE paralleled by increased production of IFN-γ in the CNS.[42,43] Rolipram inhibiting production of pro-inflammatory cytokines, also ameliorates EAE.[44,45] More or less immune specific treatments also affect cytokine expression. A T2-biased immune response ensues upon neonatal or peroral tolerance with MBP.[46,47] Accordingly, altered peptide ligand treatment of mouse EAE generates T2-biased antigen-specific T cells[48,49] as does DNA-vaccination T-cell receptor (TCR) construct for encephalitogenic T cells.[50] These studies have employed probably quite pure T1-mediated disease. Their applicability for human disease is complicated by the probably more complex immune pathogenesis in MS. Autoantibody-mediated attack is an additional noxious mechanism. A T2-biased immune response with stimulation of such autoantibody production is apparent in myelin oligodendrocyte glycoprotein (MOG)-induced EAE in the marmoset where a tolerogenic protocol promoting T2-cytokines occurred in parallel with exacerbated disease.[51] In any case the observations encourage studies of cytokine production during a variety of therapeutic studies both in animals and humans, to understand their mode of action.

More selective experimental manipulations using cytokine anticytokine reagents have been less easy to interpret straightforwardly. IFN-γ is hereby of particular interest. This cytokine activates macrophages; microglial cells;[52,53] induces MHC expression on glial, endothelial cells and neurons;[32,37,38,54–56] induces IL-1 and TNF-α production;[57] induces T-cell homing;[58] promotes B-cell differentiation;[59] activates astrocytes;[60] and kills oligodendrocytes.[61] These effects would suggest a disease-promoting role of IFN-γ. Counterintuitively, IFN-γ treatment protected against EAE while anti-IFN-γ worsened disease and in accordance, EAE is inducible in both IFN-γ receptor and IFN-γ knock-out mice.[62–66] Thus, IFN-γ is not the only cytokine that can promote neuroinflammatory disease. Furthermore the findings may be explained if considering the redundancy in the cytokine system as well as time-, dose- and site-dependent effects. Transgenic expression of IFN-γ induces hypomyelination reactive gliosis upregulation of MHC molecules and lymphocytes infiltration,[67,68] findings keeping IFN-γ on the list of putative disease-promoting cytokines in MS and EAE. Consistent with this, IL-12—a potent inducer of IFN-γ production—has an important role in EAE. In vivo blocking with antibodies ameliorates EAE[69] while cytokine administration promotes disease.[70] In a similar way it has been difficult to categorize TNF or LT in EAE and MS. TNF and LT damage oligodendrocytes[71,72] and they are expressed in the CNS during acute EAE.[25,26,73–75] In vivo blocking ameliorates EAE[76–78] and injection of TNF cause EAE-relapse,[79,80] and transgenic CNS expression of TNF leads to demyelinating inflammatory disease.[81] However, mice deleted both of LT and TNF can develop EAE.[82,83] Two MS patients treated with anti-TNF deteriorated.[84]

Potential disease downregulatory cytokines have been analysed in similar ways. Treatment with IL-4 simultaneously with the transfer of encephalitogenic T cells and MBP ameliorates EAE.[21] The closely related IL-13 acting on the same receptor abrogates EAE.[85] Standard T2 IL-4 producing myelin specific T cells do not protect against EAE,[86] while genetically modified IL-4 expressing cells do.[22] IL-4 knockout mice develop EAE[87] while transfer of T2-cells to immunocompromised mice induce a form of allergic EAE.[24] The potent immunosuppressive abilities of IL-10 makes data from this cytokine intriguing. For example, IL-10 is more potent than IL-4 in inhibiting encephalitogenic T1-cells.[88] Also here, data are not coherent. IL-10 treatment prevents EAE in rats,[89] while it worsens disease in mice.[90] TGF-β is also very interesting with regard to immunosuppression. Its genomic deletion results in widespread inflammatory disease[91] and TGF-β treatment or blocking results in suppression or enhancement of EAE, respectively.[92–94]

Note that additional complications arise when studying cytokines in human diseases of the CNS. First MS is chronic and important cytokine deviations may well be indiscernible at the time points for access of samples. A chaotic dysregulation may prevail where clear-cut correlations to cytokines may be difficult to detect even if they indeed perform their function as suspected from in vitro and in vivo experimental systems. Secondly, the target tissue is relatively inaccessible and the local character of cytokines prompt investigations of local productions. Biopsies or autopsy specimens are seldom accessible. Most observations are therefore restricted to peripheral blood specimens. Samples from cerebrospinal fluid (CSF) may better reflect events ongoing in the CNS. When assessing data in MS, it is important to distinguish between analyses of nonmanipulated fresh samples and data obtained after various periods of in vitro culture. The last mentioned assays are subject to possible in vitro distortion of patterns that may be have occurred in vivo.

In MS, putative disease-promoting cytokines such as TNF-α, LT and IFN-γ have been localized to MS lesions.[95–97] IFN-γ producing cells are detected at increased levels in the CSF of MS patients as compared to controls.[11] There are increased levels of TNF in the CSF correlating to active disease[98] and mRNA for TNF appear before clinical relapses.[99] With in situ hybridization using synthetic oligonucleotide probes we have demonstrated that MS patients display increased numbers of cells in their peripheral blood expressing mRNA for proinflammatory cytokines, strongly enriched to the CSF,[100–102] Combined with surface phenotype staining we recently demonstrated that approximately 30% of the IFN-γ mRNA expressing cells belong to the CD8+ phenotype suggesting that MHC class I restricted cells may be active during MS (Wallström, Khademi, Andersson, Olsson, unpublished). This is interesting in view of recent descriptions of an increased risk for MS is having certain class I alleles.[103] As to putative immunodownmodulatory cytokines, we have observed increased numbers of cells expressing mRNA, IL-4, IL-10 and IL-13.[104,105] Numbers of cells expressing TGF-β were higher in patients with mild MS than severe MS.[101] With all other cytokines we have found no clear-cut correlation to clinical variables. This, however, does not exclude important disease regulatory effects of these cytokines.

Cytokine production as a consequence of antigen-induced activation can be regarded as a measure of T cells with certain specificities. This has traditionally been measured with assays of proliferation or T-cell cloning frequencies. Bulk culture proliferation and T-cell cloning procedures have mainly failed to reveal any differences in myelin antigen autoreactive T-cells between MS-patients and controls.[106–109] With cytokine production as assay for myelin antigen responses, there are increased numbers of cells in MS-patients compared to controls that recognize series of myelin antigens such as MBP, PLP and MOG.[11,104,110–113] Recently we examined responses to MOG peptides in DR 2 MS patients as compared to healthy DR 2 controls. One peptide was immunodominant (MOG 63–87; Wallström, Khademi, Andersson, Weissert, Linington, Olsson, unpublished). Thus, there are prospects for definition of limited sets of myelin antigen epitopes that could be approached with specific immunotherapy. Since MOG-induced IFN-γ production, but not MOG-induced proliferation, discriminated between disease susceptibility and resistance in EAE (see below), this may be a valid way to measure autoimmune responses that are relevant for disease in humans.

INF-β has a proven effect on the natural course of MS making it attractive to analyse how this treatment affects cytokine expression systemically and in the CNS. Dyal et al.[114] reported an increased number of cells in peripheral blood producing IFN-γ in response to concanavalin A (Con A). In contrast, Rudick et al.[115] reported an induced IL-10 production. Two to six months after initiating therapy, and when therapeutic effects are evident, we observed decreased numbers of IL-10 expressing cells.[116] It is still unclear if these cytokine deviations have causal relationships to therapeutic effects or if they represent disease-promoting phenomena, while the therapeutic effects target other mechanisms or represent inert epiphenomena.

GENETICS OF CYTOKINE EXPRESSION IN EAE AND MS

There is a strong genetic influence on both MS and EAE.[117,118] The exact definition of the genetic influences may disclose targets for therapy. Cytokines are key regulators of pathogenic immune responses and it is likely that polymorphic genes which determine disease outcome may act by influencing cytokine production or their action on target cells. This may come about by polymorphisms in cytokine or receptor genes themselves or in any step-regulating cytokine interactions. Thus, assay of cytokines may give important clues on how genetic influences are mediated and helpful in phenotypic evaluations in context with positional cloning events. There are influences both from genes in the MHC complex and non-MHC background genes on MS and EAE,[118–122] which are discussed separately in the following.

Polymorphisms of genes within the MHC-complex affects cytokine expression, correlating to disease course in EAE. This has been demonstrated in experiments with MHC-congenic rats with either a monophasic or relapsing disease course. DA rats develop chronic EAE.[27,123,124] We showed that a relapsing disease correlated with the RT1AV1 MHC-haplotype, and strains with this MHC-complex lacked expression of putatively immunodownmodulatory cytokines, TGF-β and IL-10 in the CNS. Strains with other MHC-haplotypes displaying only monophasic disease had a conspicuous expression of these cytokines.[124] The particular genes within the MHC-complex responsible for this regulatory influence have not yet been positioned. The MHC class I and class II genes, however, are strong candidates for a variety of influences on cytokine differentiation. Experiments using MHC-congenic rats on the Lewis background, subjected to immunizations with encephalitogenic peptides (MBP 63-88 or 89-101[125–127]) revealed three forms of MHC-haplotype influences. First, certain MHC-haplotypes are disease permissive and in these, the T-cell responses are T1 biased. Secondly, disease-resistant MHC-haplotypes can lack T-cell responses to the peptide owing to the absence of MHC class II molecule peptide binding or thymic deletion of autoreactive T-cells. The third category of MHC-haplotypes are disease resistant but display autoreactive responses to the peptide characterized by additional T2 cytokine and TGF-β production. These responses are peptide specific suggesting that the MHC class I or class II molecules themselves are responsible rather than neighbouring genes.[127] Allele-specific protection has been mapped to the class I region[126] and can be abrogated by CD8+ cell depletion in vivo, suggesting the existence of 'class I restricted suppressor cells'.[126]

It is not clear if parts of the MHC influences on human MS can be explained by similar regulations of cytokine spectrum. One recent study demonstrated that T-cell lines obtained from DR2+ donors secreted significantly more TNF-α and LT than T cell lines from DR2-donors.[128] No influences by polymorphisms of TNF and LT, located in the MHC-complex, independent from class II gene influence has been substantiated.[129,130]

Studies on gene influences on cytokine expression in MS is so far only in its infancy, while in EAE such data have started to emerge. A possible role of such a genetic influence in MS is suggested by a study in which immunoglobulin (IgE)-mediated disease, known to be T2 biased, was strongly underrepresented in MS patients.[131] In mouse EAE, a strain-dependent resistance to EAE induction correlated to an inability of T cells to produce IFN-γ in vitro, which was unmasked by IL-12 treatment.[70] Genetically regulated T1-T2 bias correlated to the ability of T-cell lines to transfer EAE, mapping outside the MHC.[132] In rat EAE, the non-MHC genetic resistance correlated to the ability of lymphoid cells to express mRNA for TGF-β.[133] Using MOG-induced EAE in the rat, resulting in a very MS-like disease clinically and histologically, we have observed that non-MHC background genes determine low susceptibility to disease in turn correlating to the inability of lymphoid cells to produce IFN-γ in response to antigen (Weissert, Wallström, Storch, Stefferl, Lorentzen, Lassmann, Linnington, Olsson, unpublished data). These types of influences are accessible for positional cloning using modern mapping techniques. Thus, there are non-MHC background influences on both EAE and cytokine differentiation that will be important to clone positionally and examine for their relevance in MS.

CONCLUSION

In conclusion, by definition cytokine interplay is important for the outcome of autoimmune neuroinflammatory disease. The basic character of cytokines being local hormones, redundant and having time-, site- and level-dependent effects calls for caution when designing and evaluating studies. However, if properly studied, very important information can be obtained with regard to T-cell specificity, genetics and in context with therapeutic trials. Thus, continued intense studies of cytokines are important for our further understanding of the pathogenesis of both EAE and MS.

ACKNOWLEDGEMENTS

The authors' laboratory have received grant support from The Swedish Medical Research Council, The Swedish Society for Neurologically Disabled, Petrus and Augusta Hedlunds' Foundation, Bibbi and Nils Jensens' Foundation and the EC Biomed 2 Program.

REFERENCES

1. Paul WE, Seder RA. Lymphocyte responses and cytokines. *Cell* 1994; **76**: 145–173.
2. Mossman TR, Coffman RL. Th1 and Th2 cells: different patterns of lymphokine secretion leads to different functional properties. *Ann Rev Immunol* 1989; **7**: 145–173.
3. Romagnani S. Human Th1 and Th2 subsets: doubt no more. *Immunol Today* 1991; **12**: 256–257.
4. Heinzel FP, Saidck MD, Holaday BJ. Reciprocal expression of interferon-γ or interleukin 4 during the resolution of progression of murine leishmaniasis. *J Exp Med* 1989; **169**: 59–73.
5. Salgame P, Abrams JS, Clayberger C. Differing lymphokine profiles of functional subsets of human CD4 and CD8 T cell clones. *Science* 1991; **254**: 279–282.
6. Bakhiet M, Jansson L, Büscher P et al. Control of parasitemia and survival during *Trypanosoma brucei brucei* infection is related to strain-dependent ability to produce IL-4. *J Immunol* 1996; **157**: 351. 8–26.
7. Dagerlind Å, Friberg K, Bean AJ et al. Sensitive mRNA detection using unfixed tissues: combined radioactive and non-radioactive in situ hybridization histochemistry. *Histochemistry* 1992; **98**: 39–49.
8. Olsson T, Bakhiet M, Höjeberg B et al. CD8 is critically involved in lymphocyte activation by a *T.b. brucei* released molecule. *Cell* 1993; **72**: 715–727.
9. Czerkinsky C, Andersson B, Ekre HP et al. Reverse ELISPOT assay for clonal analysis of cytokine production. I. Enumeration of gamma-interferon secreting cells. *J Immunol Meth* 1988; **25**: 29–36.
10. Kabilan L, Andersson G, Lolli F et al. Detection of intracellular expression and secretion of IFN-gamma at the single cell level after activation of human T cells with tetanus toxoid *in vitro*. *Eur J Immunol* 1990; **20**: 1085–1089.
11. Olsson T, Zhi W, Höjeberg B et al. Autoreactive T lymphocytes in multiple sclerosis determined

by antigen-induced secretion of interferon-gamma. *J Clin Invest* 1990; **86**: 981–985.

12. El Ghazali GEB, Paulie S, Andersson G et al. Number of IL-4 and IFN-γ secreting human T cells reactive with tetanus toxoid and the mycobacterial antigen (PPD) or phytohemagglutinin (PHA): distinct response profiles depending on the type of antigen used for activation. *Eur J Immunol* 1993; **23**: 2740–2745.
13. O'Garra A, Murphy K. T-cell subsets in autoimmunity. *Curr Opin Immunol* 1993; **5**: 880.
14. Van der Meide PH, de Labie MCDC. Botman CAD et al. Mercuric chloride downregulates T cell interferon-γ production in Brown Norway but not in Lewis rats; role of glutathione. *Eur J Immunol* 1993; **23**: 675–681.
15. Heremans H, Dillen C, Put W et al. Protective effect of anti-interleukin (IL)-6 antibody against endotoxin, associated with paradoxically increased IL-6 levels. *Eur J Immunol* 1992; **22**: 2395–2401.
16. Grau GE, Maenell DN. TNF inhibition and sepsis-sounding a cautionary note. *Nature Medicine* 1997; **3**: 1193.
17. Sedgwick JD, McPhee JHM, Puklawec M. Isolation of encephalitogenic CD4+ T cell clones in the rat. Cloning methodology and IFN-γ secretion. *J Immunol Meth* 1989; **143**: 3492–3497.
18. Ando DG, Clayton J, Kono D et al. Encephalitogenic T cells in the B10. PL model of experimental allergic encephalomyelitis (EAE) are of the Th-1 lymphokine sybtype. *Cell Immunol* 1989; **124**: 132–143.
19. Baron JL, Madri JA, Ruddle NH et al. Surface expression of a VLA-4 integrin by CD4 T cells is required for their entry into brain parenchyma. *J Exp Med* 1993; **177**: 57–68.
20. Van der Veen R, Kapp JA, Trotter JL. Fine-specificity differences in the recognition of an encephalitogenic peptide by T helper 1 and 2 cells. *J Neuroimmunol* 1993; **48**: 221–226.
21. Röcken M, Racke M, Shevach EM. IL-4 induced immune deviation as antigen-specific therapy for inflammatory autoimmune disease. *Immunol Today* 1996; **17**: 225–231.
22. Shaw M, Lorens J, Dhawan A et al. Local delivery of interleukin 4 by retrovirus-transduced T lymphocytes ameliorates experimental autoimmune encephalomyelitis. *J Exp Med* 1997; **185**: 1711–1714.
23. Mathisen P, Yu M, Johnson J et al. Treatment of experimental autoimmune encephalomyelitis with genetically modified T cells. *J Exp Med* 1997; **186**: 159–164.
24. Lafaille JJ, Van de Keere F, Hsu AL et al. Myelin basic protein-specific T helper 2 (Th2) cells cause experimental autoimmune encephalomyelitis in immunodeficient hosts rather than protect them from disease. *J Exp Med* 1986; **186**: 307–312.
25. Issazadeh S, Mustafa M, Ljungdahl Å et al. Interferon-gamma, interleukin 4 and transforming growth factor beta in experimental autoimmune encephalomyelitis in Lewis rats: dynamics of cellular mRNA expression in the central nervous system and lymphoid cells. *J Neurosci Res* 1995; **40**: 579–590.
26. Issazadeh S, Ljungdahl Å, Höjeberg B et al. Cytokine production in the central nervous system of Lewis rats with experimental autoimmune encephalomyelitis: dynamics of mRNA expression for interleukin 10, interleukin 12, cytolysin, tumor necrosis factor-alfa and beta. *J Neuroimmunol* 1995; **61**: 205–212.
27. Issazadeh S, Lorentzen J, Mustafa M et al. Cytokines in relapsing experimental autoimmune encephalomyelitis in DA rats: Persistent mRNA expression of proinflammatory cytokines and absent expression of IL-10 and TGF-beta. *J Neuroimmunol* 1996; **69**: 103–115.
28. Mustafa M, Diener P, Höjeberg B et al. T cells immunity and interferon-γ secretion during experimental allergic encephalomyelitis in Lewis rats. *J Neuroimmunol* 1991; **31**: 19–26.
29. Villarroya H, Violleau K, Younes-Chennoufi AB et al. Myelin-induced experimental allergic encephalomyelitis in Lewis rats: tumor necrosis factor α levels in serum and cerebrospinal fluid. Immunohistochemical expression in glial cells and macrophages of optic nerve and spinal cord. *J Neuroimmunol* 1996; **64**: 55–61.
30. Kennedy MK, Torrance DS, Picha KS et al. Analysis of cytokine mRNA expression in the central nervous system of mice with experimental autoimmune encephalomyelitis reveals that IL-10 mRNA expression correlated with recovery. *J Immunol* 1992; **149**. 2496–2505.
31. Maehlen J, Daa-Schroder H, Klareskog L et al. Axotomy induces MHC class I antigen expression on rat nerve cells. *Neurosci Lett* 1988; **92**: 8–13.
32. Lindå H, Hammarberg H, Cullheim S et al. Expression of MHC class I and β2-microglobulin in rat spinal motorneurons; regulatory influences by IFN-gamma and axotomy. *Exp Neurol* 1998 (in press).

33. Olsson T, Ljungdahl Å, Kristensson K et al. Gamma-interferon-like immunoreactivity in axotomized rat motor neurons. *J Neurosci* 1989; **89**: 3870–3876.
34. Olsson T, Diener P, Ljungdahl Å et al. Facial nerve transection causes expansion of myelin autoreactive T cells in regional lymph nodes and T cell homing to the facial nucleus. *Autoimmunity* 1992; **13**: 117–126.
35. Maehlen J, Olsson T, Zachau A et al. Local enhancement of MHC class I and II expression and cell infiltration in experimental allergic encephalomyelitis around axotomized motor neurons. *J Neuroimmunol* 1989; **23**: 125–132.
36. Olsson T, Kelic S, Edlund C et al. Neuronal interferon-gamma immunoreactive molecule, bioactivities and purification. *Eur J Immunol* 1994; **24**: 308–314.
37. Eneroth A, Bakhiet M, Olsson T et al. Bidirectional signals between *Trypanosoma brucei brucei* and dorsal root ganglia neurons. *J Neurocytol* 1992; **21**: 846–852.
38. Neumann H, Schmidt H, Wilharm E et al. Interferon-gamma gene expression in sensory neurons: evidence for autocrine gene regulation. *J Exp Med* 1997; **186**: 2023–2031.
39. Raivich G, Bluethmann H, Kreutzberg GW. Signaling molecules and neuroglial activation in the injured central nervous system. *Keio J Med* 1996; **45**: 239–247.
40. Kreutzberg GW. Microglia: a sensor for pathological events in the CNS. *Trends Neurosci* 1996; **19**: 312–318.
41. Colosetti P, Olsson T, Miyazono K et al. Axotomy of rat facial nerve induced TGF-β and the latent TGF-β binding protein. *Brain Res Bull* 1995; **37**: 561–567.
42. Correale J, Olsson T, Björk J et al. Sulfasalazine treatment of experimental allergic encephalomyelitis in Lewis rats: disease relapse and increase of autoreactive T cells. *J Neuroimmunol* 1991; **34**: 109–120.
43. Mustafa M, Diener P, Sun JB et al. Immunopharmacological modulation of experimental allergic encephalomyelitis: low-dose cyclosporin A treatment causes disease relapse and increased systemic T and B cell-mediated myelin-directed autoimmunity. *Scand J Immunol* 1993; **38**: 499–507.
44. Sommer N, Löschmann P-A, Northoff GH et al. The antidepressant rolipram suppresses cytokine production and prevents autoimmune encephalomyelitis. *Nature Med* 1995; **1**: 244–248.
45. Genain CP, Roberts T, Davis RL et al. Prevention of autoimmune demyelination in non-human primates by a cAMP-specific phosphodiesterase inhibitor. *Proc Natl Acad Sci USA* 1995; **92**: 3601–3605.
46. Forsthuber T, Yip HC, Lehmann PV. Induction of Th1 and Th2 immunity in neonatal mice. *Science* 1996; **271**: 1728–1730.
47. Khoury SJ, Hancock WW, Weiner HL. Oral tolerance to myelin basic protein and natural recovery from experimental autoimmune encephalomyelitis are associated with downregulation of inflammatory cytokines and differential upregulation of transforming growth factor β, interleukin 4 and prostaglandin E expression in the brain. *J Exp Med* 1992; **176**: 1355–1364.
48. Brocke S, Gijbels K, Allegretta M et al. Treatment of experimental encephalomyelitis with peptide analogue of myelin basic protein. *Nature* 1996; **379**: 343–346.
49. Nicholson LB, Greer JM, Sobel RA et al. An altered peptide ligand mediates immune deviation and prevents autoimmune encephalomyelitis. *Immunity* 1995; **3**: 397–405.
50. Waisman A, Ruiz PJ, Hirschberg DL et al. Suppressive vaccination with DNA encoding a variable region gene of the T-cell receptor prevents autoimmune encephalomyelitis and activates Th2 immunity. *Nature Med* 1996; **2**: 899–905.
51. Genain CP, Abel K, Belmar N et al. Late complications of immune deviation therapy in a nonhuman primate. *Science* 1996; **274**: 2054–2057.
52. Adams DO, Hamilton TA. Molecular trasnductional mechanisms by which IFN-gamma and other signals regulate macrophage development. *Immunol Rev* 1987; **97**: 5–27.
53. Goldberg M, Belkowski LS, Bloom BR. Regulation of macrophage function by interferon-gamma. Somatic cell genetic approaches in murine macrophage cell lines to mechanisms of growth inhibition, the oxidative burst, and expression of the chronic granulomatous disease gene. *J Clin Invest* 1990; **85**: 563–569.
54. Fontana A, Fierz W, Wekerle H. Astrocyte present myelin basic protein to encephalitogenic T cell lines. *Nature* 1984; **307**: 273–276.
55. Steiniger B, van der Meide P. Rat ependyma and microglia cells express class II MHC antigens

after intravenous infusion of recombinant gramma-interferon. *J Neuroimmunol* 1988; **19**: 111–118.
56. Male D, Pryce G. Induction of Ia molecules on brain endothelium is related to susceptibility to experimental allergic encephalomyelitis. *J Neuroimmunol* 1989; **21**: 87–90.
57. Collart MA, Belin D, Vassalli JD. Gamma-interferon enhances macrophage transcription of the tumour necrosis factor/cachectin, interleukin-1 and urokinase genes, which are controlled by short-lived repressors. *J Exp Med* 1986; **164**: 2113–2118.
58. Duijvestijn AM, Schreiber AB, Butcher EC. Interferon-gamma regulates an antigen specific for endothelial cells involved in lymphocyte traffic. *Proc Natl Acad Sci USA* 1986; **83**: 9114–9118.
59. Sidman CL, Marshall JD, Shultz LD et al. Gamma-interferon is one of several direct B cell maturing lymphokines. *Nature* 1984; **309**: 801–804.
60. Erkman L, Wuarin L, Cadellin D et al. Interferon induces astrocytes maturation causing an increase in cholinergic properties of cultured human spinal cord cells. *Dev Biol* 1989; **132**: 375–388.
61. Vartanian T. Li Y, Zhao M et al. Interferon-gamma-induced oligodendrocyte cell death: implications for the pathogenesis of multiple sclerosis. *Mol Med* 1995; **1**: 732–742.
62. Billiau A, Heremans H, Vandekerckhove F et al. Enhancement of experimental allergic encephalomyelitis in mice by antibodies against IFN-γ. *J Immunol* 1988; **140**: 1506–1510.
63. Duong TT, St-Louis J, Gilbert JJ et al. Effect of anti-interferon-gamma and anti-interleukin 2 monoclonal antibody treatment on the development of actively and passively induced experimental allergic encephalomyelitis in the SJL/J mouse. *J Neuroimmunol* 1992; **36**: 105–115.
64. Voorthuis JAC, Uitdenhaag BMJ, de Groot CJA et al. Suppression of experimental allergic encephalomyelitis by intraventricular administration of interferon-gamma in Lewis rats. *Clin Exp Immunol* 1990; **81**: 183–188.
65. Krakowski M, Owens T. Interferon-γ confers resistance to experimental allergic encephalomyelitis. *Eur J Immunol* 1996, **26**: 1641–1646.
66. Willenborg DO, Fordham S, Bernard C et al. IFN-γ plays a critical downregulatory role in the induction and effector phase of myelin oligodendrocyte glycoprotein-induced autoimmune encephalomyelitis. *J Immunol* 1996; **157**: 3223–3227.
67. Corbin JG, Kelly D, Rath EM et al. Targeted CNS expression of interferon-γ in transgenic mice leads to hypomyelination, reactive gliosis, and abnormal cerebellar development. *Mol Cell Neurosc* 1996; **7**: 354–370.
68. Horwitz MS, Evans CF, McGavern DB et al. Primary demyelination in transgenic mice expressing interferon–γ. *Nature Med* 1997; **3**: 1037–1041.
69. Leonard JP, Waldburger KE, Goldman SJ. Prevention of experimental autoimmune encephalomyelitis by antibodies against interleukin 12. *J Exp Med* 1995; **181**: 381–386.
70. Segal BM, Shevach EM. IL-12 unmasks latent autoimmune disease in resistant mice. *J Exp Med* 1996; **184**: 771–775.
71. Robbins DS, Shiraxi Y, Drysdale BE et al. Production of cytotoxic factor for oligodendrocytes by stimulated astrocytes. *J Immunol* 1987; **139**: 2593–2597.
72. Selmaj KW, Raine CS. Tumor necrosis factor mediates myelin and oligodendrocyte damage in vitro. *Ann Neurol* 1988; **23**: 339–346.
73. Renno T, Krakowski M, Piccirillo C et al. TNF-α expression by resident microglia and infiltrating leukocytes in the central nervous system of mice with experimental allergic encephalomyelitis. *J Immunol* 1995; **154**: 944–953.
74. Baker D, O'Neill JK, Turk JL. Cytokines in the central nervous system of mice during chronic relapsing experimental allergic encephalomyelitis. *Cell Immunol* 1991; **134**: 505–510.
75. Held W, Meyermann R, Qin Y et al. Perforin and tumor necrosis factor α in the pathogenesis of experimental allergic encephalomyelitis: comparison of autoantigen induced and transferred disease in Lewis rats. *J Autoimmun* 1993; **6**: 311–322.
76. Ruddle NH, Bergman CM, McGrath KM et al. An antibody to lymphotoxin and tumor necrosis factor prevents transfer of experimental allergic encephalomyelitis. *J Exp Med* 1990; **172**: 1193–1200.
77. Selmaj K, Raine CS, Cross AH. Anti-tumor necrosis factor therapy abrogates autoimmune demyelination. *Ann Neurol* 1991; **30**: 694–700.
78. Selmaj KW, Paplerz A, Glabinski A et al. Prevention of chronic relapsing experimental

autoimmune encephalomyelitis by soluble tumor necrosis factor receptor I. *J Neuroimmunol* 1995; **56**: 135–141.

79. Klinkert WEF, Kojima K, Lesslauer W et al. TNF-α receptor fusion protein prevents experimental autoimmune encephalomyelitis and demyelination in Lewis rats: an overview. *J Neuroimmunol* 1997; **72**: 163–168.
80. Kuroda Y, Shimamoto Y. Human tumor necrosis factor-α augments experimental allergic encephalomyelitis in rats. *J Neuroimmunol* 1991; **34**: 159–164.
81. Probert L, Akassoglou K, Pasparakis M et al. Spontaneous inflammatory demyelinating disease in transgenic mice showing central nervous system-specific expression of tumor necrosis factor α. *Proc Natl Acad Sci USA* 1995; **92**: 11294–11298.
82. Frei K, Eugster H-P, Bopst M et al. Tumor necrosis factor α and lymphotoxin a are not required for induction of acute experimental autoimmune encephalomyelitis. *J Exp Med* 1997; **185**: 2177–2182.
83. Liu J, Marino MW, Wong G et al. TNF is a potent anti-inflammatory cytokine in autoimmune-mediated demyelination. *Nat Med* 1998; **4**: 78–83.
84. van Oosten BW, Barkhof F, Truyen L et al. Increased MRI activity and immune activation in two multiple sclerosis patients treated with the monoclonal anti-tumor necrosis factor antibody cA2. *Neurology* 1996; **47**: 1531–1534.
85. Cash E, Minty A, Ferrara P et al. Macrophage-inactivating IL-13 suppresses experimental autoimmune encephalomyelitis in rats. *J Immunol* 1994; **153**: 4258–4267.
86. Khoruts A, Miller SD, Jenkins MK. Neuroantigen-specific Th2 cells are inefficient suppressors of experimental autoimmune encephalomyelitis induced by effector Th1 cells. *J Immunol* 1995; **155**: 5011–5017.
87. Liblau R, Steinman L, Brock S, Experimental autoimmune encephalomyelitis in IL-4-deficient mice. *Int Immunol* 1997; **5**: 799–803.
88. Van der Veen R, Stohlman SA. Encephalitogenic Th1 cells are inhibited by Th2 cells with related peptide specificity: relative roles of interleukin (IL)-4 and IL-10. *J Neuroimmunol* 1993; **48**: 213–220.
89. Rott O, Fleischer B, Cash E. Interleukin-10 prevents experimental allergic encephalomyelitis in rats. *Eur J Immunol* 1994; **24**: 1434–1440.
90. Cannella B, Gao YL, Brosnan C et al. IL-10 fails to abrogate experimental autoimmune encephalomyelitis. *J Neurosci Res* 1996; **45**: 735–746.
91. Shull MM, Ormsby I, Kier AB et al. Targeted disruption of the mouse transforming growth factor-β1 gene results in multifocal inflammatory disease. *Nature* 1992; **359**: 693–699.
92. Schluesener HJ, Lider O. Transforming growth factor β1 and β2: cytokines with identical immunosuppressive effects and a potential role in the regulation of autoimmune T cell function. *J Neuroimmunol* 1989; **24**: 249–258.
93. Kuruvilla AP, Shah R, Hochwald GM et al. Protective effect of transforming growth factor β1 experimental autoimmune encephalomyelitis in mice. *Proc Natl Acad Sci USA* 1991; **88**: 2918–2921.
94. Racke M, Canella B, Albert P et al. Evidence of endogenous regulatory function of transforming growth factor-β1 in experimental allergic encephalomyelitis. *Int Immunol* 1991; **5**: 615–620.
95. Traugott U, Lebon P. Multiple sclerosis: involvement of interferons in lesion pathogenesis. *Ann Neurol* 1988; **24**: 243–251.
96. Hofman FM, Hintol DR, Johnson K et al. Tumor necrosis factor identified in multiple sclerosis brain. *J Exp Med* 1989; **170**: 607–612.
97. Selmaj K, Raine C, Cannella B et al. Identification of lymphotoxin and tumor necrosis factor in multiple sclerosis lesions. *J Clin Invest* 1991; **87**: 949–954.
98. Sharief MK, Hentges R. Association between tumor necrosis factor-α and disease progression in patients with multiple sclerosis. *New Engl J Med* 1991; **325**: 467–472.
99. Rieckmann P, Albrecht M, Kitze B et al. Cytokine mRNA levels in mononuclear blood cells from patients with multiple sclerosis. *Neurology* 1994; **44**: 1523.
100. Link J, Söderström M, Kostulas V et al. Optic neuritis is associated with myelin basic protein and proteolipid protein reactive cells producing IFN-γ, IL-4 and TGF-β. *J Neuroimmunol* 1994; **49**: 9–18.
101. Link J, Söderström M, Olsson T et al. Increased TGF-β, IL-4 and IFN-γ in multiple sclerosis. *Ann Neurol* 1994; **36**: 379–386.
102. Navikas V, He B, Link J et al. Augemented expression of tumor necrosis factor α and lymphotoxin mRNA in mononuclear cells in multiple sclerosis and optic neuritis. *Brain* 1995; **119**: 213–223.
103. Fogdell-Hahn A. *Human leukocyte antigens with special reference to association and linkage in multiple*

sclerosis. Academic thesis 1997, Karolinska Institute, Stockholm, Sweden.

104. Navikas V, Link J, Palasik W et al. Increased mRNA expression of IL-10 in mononuclear cells in multiple sclerosis and optic neuritis. *Scand J Immunol* 1995; **41**: 171–178.
105. Matusevicius D, Kivisäkk P, Navijas V et al. Autoantigen-induced IL-13 mRNA expression is increased in blood mononuclear cells in myasthenia gravis and multiple sclerosis. *Eur J Neurol* 1997; **4**: 468–475.
106. Johnson D, Hafler DA, Fallis RJ et al. Cell-mediated immunity to myelin-associated glycoprotein, proteolipid protein and myelin basic protein in multiple sclerosis. *J Neuroimmunol* 1986; **13**: 99–108.
107. Tournier-Lasserve E, Hashim GA, Bach MA. Human T-cell response to myelin basic protein in multiple sclerosis patients and healthy subjects. *J Neurosci Res* 1988; **19**: 146–156.
108. Ota K, Matsui M, Milford EL et al. T-cell recognition of an immunodominant myelin basic protein epitope in multiple sclerosis. *Nature* 1990; **346**: 183–187.
109. Pette M, Fukita K, Kritze B et al. Myelin basic protein-specific T lymphocyte lines from MS patients and healthy individuals. *Neurology* 1990; **40**: 1770–1776.
110. Link J, Frederikson S, Söderström M et al. Organ-specific autoantigens induce tranforming growth factor β mRNA expression in multiple sclerosis myasthenia gravis. *Ann Neurol* 1994; **35**: 197.
111. Olsson T, Sun J, Hillert J et al. Increased numbers of T cells recognizing multiple myelin basic protein epitopes in multiple sclerosis. *Eur J Immunol* 1992; **22**: 1083–1087.
112. Sun J, Olsson T, Wang W et al. Autoreactive T and B cells responding to myelin proteolipid protein multiple sclerosis and controls. *Eur J Immunol* 1991; **21**: 1461.
113. Sun J, Link H, Xiao B et al. T and B cell responses to myelin-oligodendrocyte glycoprotein in multiple sclerosis. *J Immunol* 1991; **146**: 1990.
114. Dayal AS, Jensen MA, Lledo A et al. Interferon-gamma-secreting cells in multiple sclerosis patients treated with interferon beta-1b. *Neurology* 1995; **45**: 2173–2177.
115. Rudick RA, Ransohoff RM, Peppler R et al. Interferon beta induces interleukin-10 expression—relevance to multiple sclerosis. *Ann Neurol* 1996; **40**: 618–627.
116. Andersson M, Khademi M, Wallstrom E et al. Cytokine profile interferon-beta treated multiple sclerosis patients: reduction of interleukin-10 mRNA expressing cells in peripheral blood. *Eur J Neurol* 1997; **4**: 567–571.
117. Ebers GC, Bulman DE, Sadovnik AD et al. A population-based study of multiple sclerosis in twins. *New Engl J Med* 1986; **315**: 1638–1642.
118. Williams RM, Moore MJ. Linkage of susceptibility to experimental allergic encephalomyelitis to the major histocompatibility locus in the rat. *J Exp Med* 1973; **138**: 775–783.
119. Hillert J, Olerup O. Multiple sclerosis is associated with genes within or close to the HLA-DR-DQ subregion on normal DR15, DQ6, Dw2 haplotype. *Neurology* 1993; **43**: 163–168.
120. Sawcer S, Jones HB, Feakes R et al. A genome screen in multiple sclerosis reveals susceptibility loci on chromosome 6p21 and 17q22. *Nat Genet* 1996; **13**: 464–468.
121. The Multiple Sclerosis Genetics Group. A complete genomic screen for multiple sclerosis underscores a role for the major histocompatibility complex. *Nat Genet* 1996; **13**: 469–471.
122. Ebers GC Kukay K, Bulman DE et al. A full genome search in multiple sclerosis. *Nat Genet* 1996; **13**: 472–476.
123. Sundvall M, Jirholt J, Yang HT et al. Identification of murine loci associated with susceptibility autoimmune encephalomyelitis. *Nat Genet* 1995; **10**: 313–317.
124. Lorentzen J, Andersson M, Issazadeh S et al. Genetic analysis of inflammation, cytokine mRNA expression and disease course of relapsing experimental autoimmune encephalomyelitis in DA rats. *J Neuroimmunol* 1997; **80**: 31–37.
125. Mustafa M, Vingsbo C, Olsson T et al. The major histocompatibility complex influences myelin basic protein 63-88 induced T cell cytokine profile and experimental autoimmune encephalomyelitis. *Eur J Immunol* 1993; **23**: 3089–3095.
126. Mustafa M, Vingsbo C, Olsson T et al. Protective influences on experimental autoimmune encephalomyelitis by MHC class I and class II alleles. *J Immunol* 1994; **153**: 3337–3344.
127. Issazadeh S, Kjellen P, Olsson T et al. Major histocompatibility complex-controlled protective influences on experimental autoimmune encephalomyelitis are peptide specific. *Eur J Immunol* 1997; **27**: 1584–1587.

128. Zipp F, Weber F, Huber S et al. Genetic control of multiple sclerosis: increased production of lymphotoxin and tumor necrosis factor-α by HLA-DR2+ T cells. *Ann Neurol* 1995; **38**: 723–730.
129. Wingerchuk D, Liu Q, Sobell J et al. A population-based case-control study of the tumor necrosis alpha-308 polymorphism in multiple sclerosis. *Neurology* 1997; **49**: 626–628.
130. Weinschencker BG, Wingerchuk DM, Lin Q et al. Genetic variation in the tumor necrosis factor alpha gene and the outcome of multiple sclerosis. *Neurology* 1997; **49**: 378–385.
131. Oro AS, Guarino TJ, Driver R et al. Regulation of disease susceptibility: decreased prevalence of IgE-mediated allergic disease in patients with multiple sclerosis. *J Allergy Clin Immunol* 1996; **97**: 1402–1408.
132. Conboy IM, De Kruytt H, Tate KM et al. Novel genetic regulation of T helper 1 (Th1)/Th2 cytokine production and encephalitogenicity in inbred mouse strains. *J Exp Med* 1997; **185**: 439–451.
133. Kjellén P, Issazadeh S, Olsson T et al. Genetic influence on disease course, cytokine responses and epitope spreading in relapsing experimental allergic encephalomyelitis. *Int Immunol* 1998 (in press).

16

Selection of patients for therapeutic clinical trials in multiple sclerosis

Lawrence W Myers, George W Ellison, Barbara D Leake and M Ray Mickey

INTRODUCTION

Therapeutic clinical trials are conducted for a variety of reasons.[1–3] Phase I or preliminary clinical trials are done to establish a maximum tolerated dose and to establish a dose, regimen and route of administration which is safe and tolerable. Phase II or pilot clinical trials are designed to evaluate potential efficacy. Phase III or full or pivotal clinical trials are conducted to establish efficacy in a multicentre study. Toxicity must be evaluated and risk–benefit assessments made in all phases of drug development and utilization. Further evaluation of dose, regimen and route of administration also may be done in all phases.

Multiple sclerosis (MS) therapeutic clinical trials may also be aimed at preventing or reducing the frequency and severity of relapses; preventing or reducing the residua of relapses; preventing or slowing the accumulation of impairments and disabilities or the alleviation of symptoms. All should be aimed at improving the quality of life of our patients.

All clinical trials require a protocol and one major element in the protocol is the selection of patients, which entails a listing of inclusion and exclusion criteria. The selection of patients is dependent upon several factors, including the objective or goal of the clinical trial, the feasibility of conducting the study and the extent to which the results will be applicable to a larger population, i.e. the generalizability of the results.

If the objective of a therapeutic trial is to ameliorate an MS symptom, then subjects with those symptoms are selected. If the goal of the study is to prevent or reduce the frequency and severity of relapses, then we select patients who are expected to have frequent relapses. Natural history studies and the recently completed therapeutic clinical trials of beta interferon 1a and 1b and copolymer I indicate an inverse correlation between the rate of relapses and duration of disease (Fig. 16.1).[4–6] If the goal of the study is to prevent or reduce the residua of relapses, then subjects experiencing relapses are selected for study. Given this paradigm, it would seem logical that we would select patients with progressive MS to participate in a therapeutic clinical trial designed to prevent or slow the accumulation or impairments and disabilities. However, our experience indicates that this seemingly rational approach may not be true.[7,8] In this chapter, we will describe our experiences and make some recommendations for selecting MS patients for a therapeutic clinical trial designed to prevent or slow clinical progression.

For therapeutic clinical trials in MS, we obviously will include only patients with clinically or laboratory supported definite MS. Based

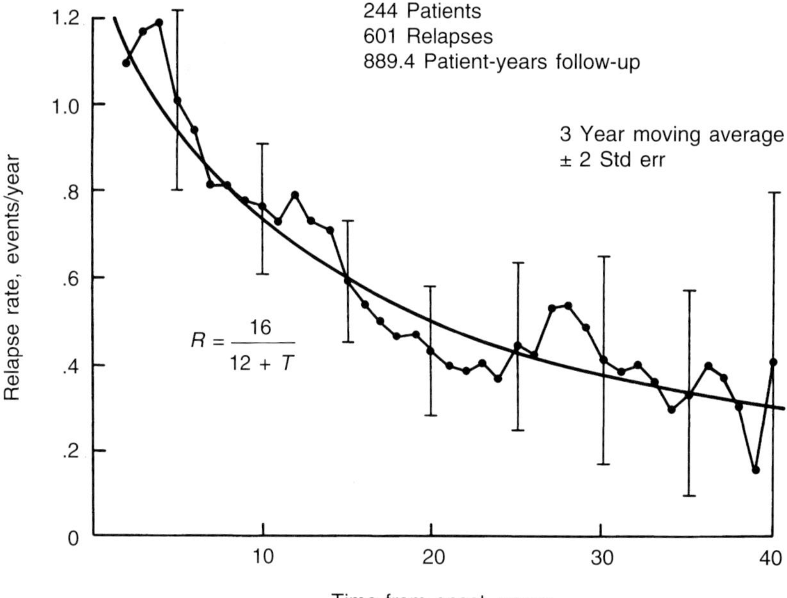

Figure 16.1 There is an inverse correlation between relapse rate (R) and duration of multiple sclerosis (T) expressed by the formula,

$$R = \frac{16}{12+T}$$

Data is from 244 patients experiencing relapses during 889.4 patient-years of follow-up in the UCLA MS Program.

upon magnetic resonance imaging (MRI) studies which indicate that patients with primary progressive MS are different than patients with secondary progressive MS we recommend selecting patients with either primary progressive MS or secondary progressive MS but not include both course types in a single study.[9,10] Because patients with secondary progressive MS are much more frequent than patients with primary progressive MS, we would envision the first therapeutic clinical trial for progressive MS would be restricted to patients with a secondary progressive course and would exclude patients with a primary progressive course or progressive–relapsing course. We would also exclude patients with a relapsing–remitting course. They are eligible for treatment with beta interferon or glatiramer acetate (formerly copolymer I).

Most recent therapeutic clinical trials for progressive MS have selected patients with an expanded disability status scale (EDSS) score[11] of 3–6 or 6.5, and we assume that will continue until there is good reason to change. Patients with an EDSS score < 3 are not likely to have secondary progressive MS. What the upper end of disability should be is somewhat arbitrary. Before the introduction of the EDSS, MS investigators thought it was more difficult to detect change in patients requiring a wheelchair, and therefore tended to exclude patients with a disability status scale (DSS)[12–14]* score ≥ 7. Patients with a DSS of 6 or greater tend to remain at those levels longer than patients with a DSS of 1–5 (Table 16.1).[15,16] However, with the EDSS, it has been found that the median staying time for half steps above 5 is approximately equal to median staying time for full steps between 1 and 5.[15,17] Therefore, it might be reasonable to enter patients with EDSS up to 7 or 7.5. Our knowledge of the course of patients with DSS or EDSS ≥ 8 is rather limited. Patients more disabled than 7.5 may be at greater risk for intercurrent problems such as urinary tract infections, decubitus ulcers, or aspiration pneumonia which could interfere with the conduct

*Integer values of the EDSS and DSS are considered equal.

Table 16.1 Comparison of distributions of DSS scores and mean and median time (years) to worsen by one step or more on the DSS in patients followed in MS clinics at UCLA and at the University of Western Ontario

Entered		Worsened		Time to worsening (years)		
DSS	Number	Number	%	Mean	SEM*	Median
UCLA:						
1	30	27	90	1.12	0.17	0.93
2	55	46	84	2.20	0.42	1.07
3	61	55	90	1.77	0.27	0.77
4	27	22	81	1.90	0.49	1.26
5	45	33	73	2.59	0.47	1.15
6	129	80	62	3.64	0.31	2.57
7	48	36	75	3.74	0.57	2.26
8	12	8	67	2.45	0.47	2.07
University of Western Ontario:						
1	1037	854	82	4.09	0.19	1.
2	829	675	81	2.80	0.14	1.5
3	662	539	82	1.95	0.11	1.
4	536	467	88	1.22	0.06	1.
5	475	444	94	1.25	0.06	1.
6	489	292	60	3.06	0.17	2.
7	306	114	37	3.77	0.32	3
8	114	32	28	2.41	0.38	2.

*Standard error of the mean.

of the therapeutic trial and therefore should be excluded. For the purpose of this chapter, we have assumed that patients will be selected with an EDSS of 3–6 or 6.5.

SHOULD WE ONLY SELECT PATIENTS IN PROGRESSION PHASE?

Nearly all the therapeutic clinical trials for progressive MS have required that patients be in progression phase. In our placebo-controlled randomized, double-masked, variable dosage, clinical trial of azathioprine with and without methylprednisolone in MS patients in progression phase, the placebo group fared substantially better than anticipated.[18,19] This has been a common experience and has been ascribed to placebo effect[20] or regression to the mean.[21] Historically it has been assumed that once a patient entered the progression phase of MS, the patient would continue to progress inexorably. Recent natural history studies and clinical trial data indicate that this is not correct.[7,16,22] Patients with a primary or secondary progressive course fluctuate in their rate of progression, sometimes progressing rapidly and at other times slowly or not at all. If one selects patients who have progressed in the last 1–2 years, there is a high probability many of these patients will not progress in the subsequent 1–3 years, i.e. they regress to the mean.

To better describe the natural history of MS, George Ellison and I (LWM), in 1971, instituted uniform criteria for evaluating and classifying patients in terms of the probability of having MS,[23] the type of clinical course and phase of disease[24] and extent of impairment and disability.[12–14,25] With the introduction of evoked potentials and MRI we adopted the criteria of the Poser Committee to define the probability of having MS.[26]

The course of MS describes the overall pattern of the patient's disease from onset to the time of classification. We classified all patients into one of three course types. Relapsing course is characterized by periods of worsening lasting more than 24 hours and less than 6 months. Progressive course is characterized by periods of continuous worsening lasting 6 months or more. This is now referred to as primary progressive MS.[27] Relapsing and progressive course is characterized by periods of relapsing disease and progressive disease. Recently it has been recommended that this course be divided into secondary progressive course and progressive–relapsing course.[27] The secondary progressive course begins with a relapsing course and is followed by a progressive course. The progressive–relapsing course begins with a progressive course and eventually has superimposed relapses.[27]

The phase of MS describes the current activity of the patient's disease determined clinically.

We classified each patient into one of seven disease phases at each visit.[24] The definitions are as follows:

(a) relapse phase—a period of worsening of > 24 hours and less than 6 months and not due to intercurrent problems such as fever, infection or emotional distress
(b) plateau phase—a period from the end of the relapse phase until either improvement or 6 months have elapsed without change
(c) remission phase—a period of improvement for 1 month or more following a relapse or plateau phase
(d) stationary phase—a period of no change for 1 month or more following either a remission phase, a 6-month plateau phase, or a progression phase
(e) progression phase—a period of gradual continuous worsening of > 6 months
(f) temporary worsening phase—a period of worsening of < 24 hours or worsening due to intercurrent problems in which the worsening disappears when the intercurrent problem disappears
(g) temporary improvement—a period of improvement of < 1 month.

At each patient visit, a semi-quantitative standard neurological examination (SNE) was performed by scoring each neurologic function as normal or mildly, moderately or severely abnormal.[25] Following the SNE, we recorded scores for functional systems (FS) and DSS.[12–14] We recorded the SNE, FS and DSS without reference to prior scores to maintain independence of data points. After these scores were recorded, we reviewed prior records and scores to determine the phase and course classifications.

Between 1971 and 1991, we completed 6913 evaluations on 569 patients using the preceding described procedures. We have used this database to help describe the natural history of MS and to plan and organize clinical trials, including the selection of patients for therapeutic clinical trials—the topic of this chapter.

IS THIS DATA REPRESENTATIVE OF MS?

Between 1972 and 1974, our colleagues in the Division of Epidemiology, School of Public Health at UCLA conducted an epidemiologic study of MS in which they attempted to identify all patients with MS who resided in Los Angeles County, California in 1970.[28] They identified 1764 cases of clinically definite or probable MS of which 82 cases were registered in our clinic at the time. We compared the cohort of patients in our clinic to the entire cohort, excluding our patients, and found no significant differences in 25 demographic or clinical features including gender, symptoms at onset, duration of disease, disability status, migration history, or family size, etc. Our patients tended to be slightly younger with earlier onset of MS symptoms, to be more often never married, and to be better educated. Overall, our patients appear to be fairly representative of MS patients as a whole.

We have also compared our natural history data to that from the London, Ontario MS Center (Table 16.1).[16] The distribution of DSS scores shows the same bimodal pattern in both cohorts. More importantly for this report, the mean and median time to worsen by one or more steps on the DSS is quite similar for each step on the DSS. We therefore conclude that our data are reasonably representative to describe the natural history of MS and can be used to help plan therapeutic clinical trials in MS.

HOW SHOULD WORSENING OR PROGRESSION OR TREATMENT FAILURE BE DEFINED?

Weinshenker et al.[22] have made a cogent argument for requiring an increase ≥ 1 step on the EDSS for patients entering the study with an EDSS ≤ 5.5 and an increase of ≥ 0.5 step on the EDSS for patients with an entry score of ≥ 6.0. The worsening should be sustained for 3 months.[22] Goodkin previously proposed an increase ≥ 1 step on the EDSS for those entering with an EDSS ≤ 5.0 and an increase of ≥ 0.5 step for those with an entry EDSS of 5.5 to 6.5 with the worsening sustained ≥ 2 months.[29]

Failure to confirm worsening may be due to a relapse followed by remission or due to lack of reproducibility (reliability, precision) in the scoring using the DSS or EDSS. Interrater reproducibility in scoring the EDSS is reported to be 49–69%,[30–32] whereas intrarater reproducibility was reported to be 95%.[31] Reproducibility was reported to be better for EDSS ≥ 5.0.[31,33] Investigators in these studies scored patients on the same day. The examinations were conducted specifically to test the reproducibility of scoring. This is an artificial situation. Instead we have evaluated the reproducibility of scoring with the DSS by comparing scores given for patients in our clinic on two successive visits occurring within 90 days of each other and in which the neurologists had concluded that the patient was in stationary phase at both visits. DSS scores varied by one step or more between visits 22–28% of the time.[34] Most of the scoring was by the same neurologist at both visits, i.e. intrarater.

For the clinical trial of beta interferon-1b (IFN-β1b), a one-point worsening on the EDSS gave a statistically significant proportion of patient worsening on placebo (39%) versus IFNβ-1b at 8 MIU (27%) (p = 0.043).[4] If the worsening had to be confirmed ≥ 90 days later, the results were not statistically significant; placebo 28% versus IFN-β1b at 20% (p = 0.161). For the clinical trial of intramuscular IFN-β1a, a one-point worsening on the EDSS either unconfirmed or sustained for 6 months demonstrated a delay in the time to treatment failure and a decreased proportion of patients worsening with the experimental treatment compared to placebo.[5]

We recommend a full step increase on the EDSS from 1 to 5. We agree with Goodkin's proposal to make the cut between 5 and 5.5 rather than 5.5 and 6.0 because the difference between 5 (walking 200 m without aid or rest) and 5.5 (walking 100 m without aid or rest) are 'easily discernible'.[29] We prefer to require the worsening to persist ≥ 3 months to define the worsening as sustained or confirmed. To compare study outcomes, it would be of some benefit if investigators would either use a uniform definition of treatment failure or report results using the multiple definitions described by Weinshenker et al.[22]

For the analysis of the natural history data collected by us between 1971 and 1991, we have defined worsening as an increase ≥ 1 step on the DSS sustained ≥ 90 days (or 3 months). Using this definition, we found that the probability of worsening over 2 or 3 years was not significantly different for patients who were classified as being in progression phase as compared to patients in stationary phase within 2 years of entering our study (Table 16.2).[7] For that analysis the definition of progression was based upon the neurologists' (GWE, LWM) overall analysis of the clinical course of the patients and was not confined to the use of DSS scores. However, we have also found that a worsening ≥ one step on the DSS sustained ≥ 90 days in the preceding 1 or 2 years also is not predictive of sustained worsening in the subsequent 1–3 years (Table 16.3).[8]

In 1995, we submitted an abstract to the American Neurological Association in which we reported that sustained worsening on the DSS is a useful criterion for selecting patients for MS clinical trials. We subsequently discovered errors in the analysis of the data and withdrew the abstract. Unfortunately, the abstract was published.[35] The information in that abstract should not be used and we apologize to anyone who may have been misled by the publication.

For this chapter, we have conducted further analysis of our data attempting to identify patients who are at greater risk of progressing during a therapeutic clinical trial lasting 1–3 years. We found that patients with no worsening over 1–5 years are at no greater risk of having sustained worsening in the next 1–3 years compared to those who have had any worsening (sustained or unsustained) in the preceding 1–2 years (Table 16.3). Furthermore, patients who have had a two-step worsening on the DSS in the preceding 1–2 years are at no greater risk of having sustained worsening in the next 1–3 years (Table 16.3).

A comparison of the percentage of patients worsening by ≥ 1 step on the DSS sustained for 3 months with an initial DSS of 1–7 shows no significant difference for patients selected because of progression before the study[22] or for patients in our clinic unselected for progression (Table 16.4).[15]

We conclude that requiring evidence of recent worsening, either as defined by the study investigator or as defined by a documented worsening on the DSS or EDSS, should not be used as a criterion for selecting patients for a trial to slow or stop progression.

Table 16.2 Number worsening/at risk and percentage (in parentheses) of patients worsening ≥ 1 step on DSS sustained for 3 months within 2 years or 3 years of entering the UCLA MS Program in patients in progression phase compared to patients in stationary phase

DSS	Phase: Progression		Phase: Stationary	
Two years follow-up:				
1–7	104/257	(41)	146/324	(45)
1–5	49/82	(60)	84/169	(50)
3–5	45/77	(58)	52/101	(52)
3–7	85/255	(38)	100/226	(44)
Three years follow-up:				
1–7	128/221	(58)	160/264	(61)
1–5	65/84	(77)	98/151	(65)
3–5	60/79	(76)	58/87	(67)
3–7	123/216	(57)	120/200	(60)

WHAT PREDICTS PROBABILITY OF WORSENING?

Gender, age of onset, duration of disease, and progression index are not predictive of worsening over the next 2–3 years.[22] Weinshenker et al. found that patients with a brainstem function system score ≥ 2 had an increased risk of worsening.[22] How much this increased the risk of worsening is unclear, and this needs to be defined before it is accepted as an inclusion criterion. Cerebellar and cerebral function system scores correlated with brainstem function scores but in themselves did not contribute to the probability of worsening.

Table 16.3 Comparison of number and percentage (in parentheses) of patients worsening by one or more steps on the DSS sustained for 3 months during 1–3 years of follow-up in patients with sustained worsening in the preceding 1–2 years, unsustained worsening in the preceding 1–2 years, worsening by ≥ 2 steps on DSS in the preceding 1–2 years or no worsening in the preceding 1–5 years. Patients are from the UCLA MS Program

	Duration of follow-up (years)					
	1		2		3	
Sustained worsening in preceding:						
1 year	16/106	(15)	32/83	(39)	41/78	(53)
2 years	19/126	(15)	37/102	(36)	47/97	(49)
Unsustained worsening in preceding:						
1 year	11/164	(7)	44/134	(33)	53/117	(45)
2 years	12/168	(7)	45/137	(33)	54/119	(45)
Worsening ≥ 2 steps on DSS in preceding:						
1 year	7/106	(7)	23/87	(26)	28/78	(36)
2 years	6/110	(6)	23/90	(26)	29/81	(36)
No worsening in preceding:						
1 year	24/172	(14)	56/157	(36)	75/130	(58)
2 years	14/118	(12)	37/95	(39)	45/90	(50)
3 years	7/71	(10)	16/65	(25)	23/61	(38)
4 years	6/57	(11)	15/54	(28)	22/49	(45)
5 years	7/52	(14)	19/48	(40)	21/48	(44)

Pyramidal function was highly associated with EDSS and therefore is not a useful selection criterion.

Patients remain at DSS or EDSS 6 or 7 significantly longer than at lower scores (Table 16.1). By defining treatment failure stratified by entry DSS (≥ 1 step for entry EDSS 1–5.5 and ≥ 0.5 step for entry EDSS ≥ 6) one increases the probability of worsening in the placebo group from approximately 31% to 45%.[22] This minimizes the effect of the longer staying time (lower progression rate) for patients who enter the study with a DSS or EDSS score of 6–7. The longer one follows patients, the greater the probability of worsening (Table 16.3). However, the longer the trial the more difficult it becomes to keep subjects in the study. The minimum duration should be 2 years; 3 years would be better, but more than 3 years may not be practical.

SUMMARY

The authors recommend the following criteria for selecting subjects for a therapeutic clinical trial

Table 16.4 Comparison of the number worsening (*n*), at risk (*N*), and percentage (in parentheses) of patients worsening by one or more steps on the DSS sustained for 3 months within 2 years in patients selected for antecedent progression (A) or unselected for antecedent progression (B). Patients in A received placebo while participating in one of four randomized clinical trials.[22] Patients in B are from the UCLA MS Program.

DSS	*N*	*n* Worse (%)
A. Selected for antecedent progression:[22]		
2	5	2 (40)
3	56	17 (30)
4	51	24 (47)
5	75	32 (43)
6	337	63 (19)
7	38	17 (45)
B. Unselected for antecedent progression:[15]		
2	55	25 (45)
3	61	27 (44)
4	27	13 (48)
5	45	20 (44)
6	129	28 (22)
7	48	13 (27)

aimed at finding a treatment which will stop or slow progressive accumulation of impairments, disabilities and handicaps in people with MS. The authors anticipate such trials will be multicentre, placebo-controlled, double-masked and the interventions randomly assigned; the primary outcome will be time to sustained progression, i.e. an increase in the EDSS score of one step or more for patients entering with an EDSS of 3–5 or a half step or more for patients entering with an EDSS of 5.5.–6.5; the increase in the EDSS must be sustained for at least 90 days.

(a) inclusion criteria:
  (1) definite diagnosis of MS[26]
  (2) secondary progressive course[27]
  (3) EDSS 3–6.5
  (4) age 18–65
  (5) mentally and emotionally competent, able and willing to give informed consent, and to understand and comply with the study protocol

(b) exclusion criteria:
  (1) people unable to fulfil the inclusion criteria
  (2) females who are pregnant or plan to become pregnant during the next 3 years
  (3) females who are breast-feeding
  (4) people who have any other serious medical condition (cardiac, pulmonary, renal, gastrointestinal, hepatic, immunologic, infections, neoplastic, or dermatologic)
  (5) people with other conditions that would interfere with assessing neurologic dysfunction such as deforming arthritis or a major amputation
  (6) patients who have experienced a relapse in the 90 days preceding enrolment
  (7) patients who have received adrenocorticotrophin (ACTH), glucocorticosteroids (GCS), interferon, glatiramer acetate, intravenous immunoglobulin (IVIG), or plasma exchange (PE) in the 90 days preceding enrolment
  (8) patients who have received immunosuppressive agents such as azathioprine, cyclophosphamide, methotrexate, mitoxatrone, cyclosporin, tacrolimus, or experimental therapy in the 6 months preceding enrolment
  (9) patients who have been treated with total lymphoid irradiation, monoclonal antibody or bone marrow transplantation
  (10) people who have antibodies to HIV-1, HIV-2, or HTLV-I
  (11) people who have clinical evidence of Lyme disease.

REFERENCES

1. Friedman LM, Furberg CD, DeMets DL. *Fundamentals of Clinical Trials*, 2nd edn. Littleton, MA: PSG Publishing, 1985: 23–32.
2. Spilker B. *Guide to Clinical Trials*. New York: Raven Press, 1991: 147–158.
3. Brown JR, Beebe GW, Kurtzke JF et al. The design of clinical studies to assess therapeutic efficacy in multiple sclerosis. *Neurology* 1979; **29(2)**: 3–23.
4. The IFNB Multiple Sclerosis Study Group. Interferon beta-1b is effective in relapsing–remitting multiple sclerosis. I. Clinical results of a multicenter, randomized, double-blind, placebo-controlled trial. *Neurology* 1993; **43**: 655–661.
5. Jacobs LD, Cookfair DL, Rudick RA et al. Intramuscular interferon beta-1a for disease progression in relapsing multiple sclerosis. *Ann Neurol* 1996; **39**: 285–294.
6. Johnson KP, Brooks BR, Cohen JA et al. Copolymer 1 reduces relapse rate and improves disability in relapsing–remitting multiple sclerosis: results of a phase III multicenter, double-blind, placebo-controlled trial. *Neurology* 1995; **45**: 1268–1276.
7. Myers LW, Ellison GW, Leake BD. Progression phase of multiple sclerosis not a useful entry criterion for therapeutic trials. *Ann Neurol* 1993; **34**: 312 [abstract].
8. Myers LW, Leak BD, Ellison GW. Worsening on DSS is not a useful entry criterion for multiple sclerosis clinical trials to prevent progression. *Ann Neurol* 1996; **40**: 552 [abstract].
9. Thompson AJ, Kermode AG, MacManus DG et al. Patterns of disease activity in multiple sclerosis: clinical and magnetic resonance imaging study. *BMJ* 1990; **300**: 631–634.
10. Thompson AJ, Kermode AG, Wicks D et al. Major differences in the dynamics of primary and secondary progressive multiple sclerosis. *Ann Neurol* 1991; **29**: 53–62.
11. Kurtzke JF. Rating neurologic impairment in multiple sclerosis: an expanded disability status scale (EDSS). *Neurology* 1983; **33**: 1444–1452.
12. Kurtzke JF. On the evaluation of disability in multiple sclerosis. *Neurology* 1961; **11**: 686–694.
13. Kurtzke JF. Further notes on disability evaluation in multiple sclerosis with scale modifications. *Neurology* 1965; **15**: 654–661.
14. Kurtzke JF. A proposal for a uniform minimal record of disability in multiple sclerosis. *Acta Neurol Scand* 1981; **64 (suppl 87)**: 110–129.
15. Ellison GW, Myers LW, Leak BD et al. Design strategies in multiple sclerosis clinical trials. *Ann Neurol* 1994; **36**: S108–S112.
16. Weinshenker BG, Rice GPA, Noseworthy JH et al. The natural history of multiple sclerosis: a geographically based study. 4. Applications to planning and interpretation of clinical therapeutic trials. *Brain* 1991; **114**: 1057–1067.
17. Ellison GW, Myers LW, Leake BD et al. Revised recommendations for therapeutic trials for multiple sclerosis. *Ann Neurol* 1993; **34**: 312 [abstract].
18. Ellison GW, Myers LW, Mickey MR et al. A placebo-controlled, randomized, double-masked, variable dosage, clinical trial of azathioprine with and without methylprednisolone in multiple sclerosis. *Neurology* 1989; **39**: 1018–1026.
19. Ellison GW, Myers LW, Mickey MR et al. Clinical experience with azathioprine: the pros. *Neurology* 1988; **38 (suppl 2)**: 20–23.
20. Myers LW, Ellison GW, Leake BD et al. Placebo effect in multiple sclerosis (MS). *Can J Neurol Sci* 1993; **20 (suppl 4)**: S158.
21. Ebers GC, Paty DW. Natural history studies and applications to clinical trials. In: Paty DW, Ebers GC, eds. *Multiple Sclerosis*. Philadelphia: FA Davis, 1998; 222–223.
22. Weinshenker BG, Issa M, Baskerville J. Meta-analysis of the placebo-treated groups in clinical trials of progressive MS. *Neurology* 1996; **46**: 1613–1619.
23. Rose AS, Ellison GW, Myers LW et al. Criteria for the clinical diagnosis of multiple sclerosis. *Neurology* 1976; **26(2)**: 20–22.
24. Schumacher GA, Beebe G, Kibler RF et al. Problems of experimental trials of therapy in multiple sclerosis: report by the panel on the evaluation of experimental trials of therapy in multiple sclerosis. *Ann NY Acad Sci* 1965; **122**: 552–568.
25. Rose AS, Kuzma JW, Kurtzke JF et al. Co-operative study in the evaluation of therapy in multiple sclerosis; ACTH vs placebo in acute exacerbations, preliminary report. *Neurology* 1968; **18(2)**: 1–20.
26. Poser CM, Paty DW, Scheinberg L et al. New diagnostic criteria for multiple sclerosis: guidelines for research protocols. *Ann Neurol* 1983; **13**: 227–231.
27. Lublin FD, Reingold SC. Defining the clinical course of multiple sclerosis: results of an international survey. *Neurology* 1996; **46**: 907–911.

28. Visscher BR, Detels R, Coulson AH et al. Latitude, migration, and the prevalence of multiple sclerosis. *Am J Epidemiol* 1977; **106**: 470–475.
29. Goodkin DE. EDSS reliability. *Neurology* 1991; **41**: 322 [editorial].
30. Amato MP, Groppi C, Siracusa GF et al. Inter- and intra-observer reliability in Kurtzke scoring systems in multiple sclerosis. *Ital J Neurol* 1987; **8 (suppl 6)**: 129–132.
31. Amato MP, Fratiglioni L, Groppi C et al. Interrater reliability in assessing functional systems and disability on the Kurtzke scale in multiple sclerosis. *Arch Neurol* 1988; **45**: 746–748.
32. Noseworthy JH, Vandervoot MK, Wong CJ et al. The Canadian Cooperative MS Study Group. Interrater variability with the Expanded Disability Status Scale (EDSS) and Functional Systems (FS) in a multiple sclerosis clinical trial. *Neurology* 1990; **40**: 971–975.
33. Goodkin DE, Cookfair D, Wende K et al. Inter- and intrarater scoring agreement using grades 1.0 to 3.5 of the Kurtzke Expanded Disability Status Scale (EDSS). *Neurology* 1992; **42**: 859–863.
34. Myers LW, Ellison GW, Leake BD. Reliability of the Disability Status Scale (DSS). *Neurology* 1993; **43**: A204.
35. Myers LW, Leake D, Ellison GW. A useful entry criterion for multiple sclerosis clinical trials to prevent progression. *Ann Neurol* 1995; **38**: 339 [abstract].

17

Placebo-controlled trials: are they still needed or indeed ethical in multiple sclerosis?

Xavier Montalban

INTRODUCTION

Although a universal definition of placebo does not exist, we can say that 'placebo' is an intervention which is believed to lack a specific effect on the condition in question.[1] Nevertheless, in most cases placebo effect is positive or at least less negative (progressive disorders) than no intervention. Controlled clinical trials are designed to show whether a product has a pharmacological effect. Some trials seek evidence by using historical controls, some by comparing the product with no treatment, and others by showing a dose–response relation for the new drug. But, the gold standard in clinical research is the randomized placebo-controlled, doubled-blind clinical trial.

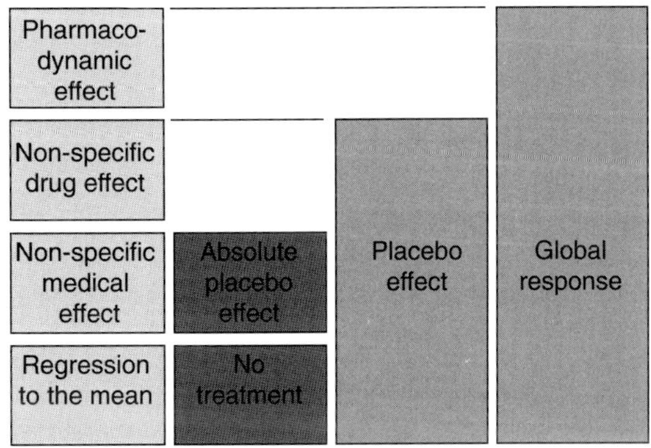

Figure 17.1 Response to a treatment.

The placebo group in a clinical trial should reflect the behaviour of the natural history of the disease in the wider population. However, there is always an inevitable deviation as a result of selection, greater supervision during the trial and the placebo effect itself. Placebo group behaviour may differ between multiple sclerosis (MS) trials to a greater extent than the observed treatment effect. One example is that a higher proportion of the control group in the interferon-beta 1a (IFN-β1a) trial did worse than in the interferon 1b (IFN-β1b) trial.[2,3] Likely this variation is due to the different clinical outcomes measured and differences in entry criteria. Nevertheless, the placebo effect might influence results, not only in the control group but also in the active group. Most active treatments have also a placebo effect in most patients (see Fig. 17.1).

The first of the modern codes of ethics in medical research is the Nuremberg Code, promulgated following the Second World War. This was followed by the 1964 Helsinki World Medical Association's Declaration stating that 'in any medical study, every patient—those of a control group included, if any, should be assured of the best-proven diagnostic and therapeutic method.'[4] Therefore, an essential ethical condition for using placebo is whether an already approved treatment of proved or accepted value is available. From this point of view the use of placebo when efficacy has already been established would almost certainly be regarded as unethical. Incidentally, it also seems to preclude study of active experimental drugs since proof of their efficacy cannot come until the trial is completed.

Obviously, there is no consensus of opinion. Other authors believe that if a new drug has only been compared to an active control (without a placebo-controlled trial) this is not convincing proof of efficacy (even if equivalence can be demonstrated).[5] Collier stated that the Helsinki recommendations which undermine the use of placebos generally need revision.[6]

In principle, no scientific rule requires the comparison in trial to involve a placebo instead of, or in addition to, an active treatment. Why, then, are placebo controls considered important? There are some requirements.[7]

1. Establishing a reference point. Even if a new treatment is worse than an existing one, it may still be 'effective' in that it is better than no treatment. But, as Bradford Hill suggested,[8] who cares whether the new treatment is more or less effective than nothing?

   Very few drugs, if any, have a universal effect on all subjects with a given disease. This fact is even more valid in MS. Clinical and prognostic heterogeneity between individuals in MS is so important that, theoretically, it would not be surprising that a drug effective in a subgroup of MS patients were statistically inferior in terms of efficacy compared to another drug on the whole of MS population, which is mainly effective in a completely different subgroup of MS patients.
2. Avoiding difficult decisions about comparison drugs. Apart from efficacy, one should take into account other factors such as side-effects, drug interactions, posology and route of administration, and cost. For some patients there may be advantages to a treatment that is inferior to a current standard with regard to efficacy but better with respect to quality of life.
3. Increasing the power of statistics. Although it is important to understand that statistical results do not give guaranteed results, and that a statistically significant treatment effect may not be of clinical significance, official drug agencies heavily rely on statistical significance in finding the efficacy of new drugs. To estimate comparative efficacy or to show equivalence there is no escape from designing studies that are much larger than the usual placebo-controlled studies. If placebo is not used, sample size must be increased between 30% and 40% to detect a treatment effect. Cost of the trial is of course much higher.
4. Difficulty in designing trials. If we do not use the 'gold standard' placebo versus experimental drug trials, which is the best trial? Should we use only a two arm trial comparing the 'active' versus the experimental drug alone, or should we add a third placebo arm? See Fig. 17.2 for some possibilities; each one has some advantages and disadvantages. There are other factors that complicate the design of the trial if the putative experimental agent is also a parenteral drug, do we need two separate injection programs? Issues of cooperation between various funding agencies (possibly involving two drug companies) will present considerable confounding factors.

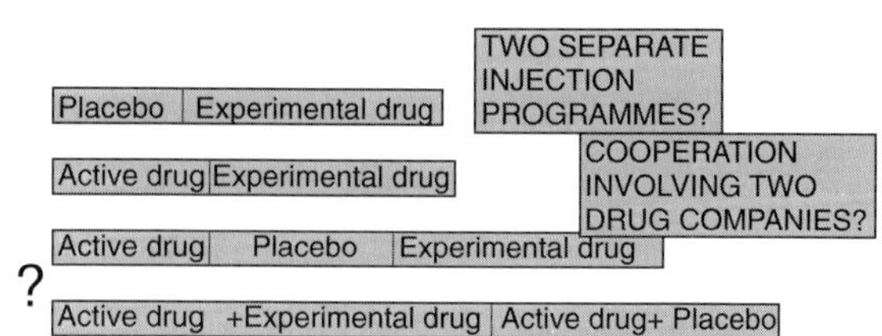

Figure 17.2 Difficulty in designing the trial.

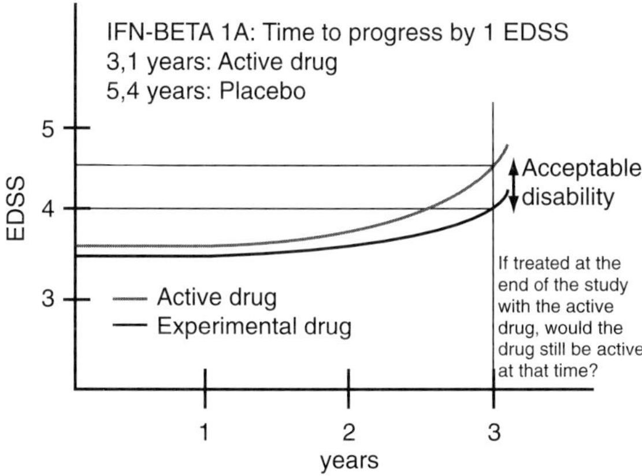

Figure 17.3 A hypothetical case.

5. Ethical arguments. One can argue that not using an accepted treatment may lead to serious harm. This concedes to individual investigators and to institutional review boards the right to determine how much discomfort or temporary disability patients should tolerate for the purpose of research. We can show a couple of examples. If IFN-β1a decreases the rate of sustained disability by 75% and increases the time to progress by one point in the EDSS score (3.1 years in the treated group vs. 5.4 years in the placebo group); a patient enroled in a 3-year trial with an entry EDSS score of 3.5 will increase his disability by one point, that is he will finish the trial with a 4.5 score. Meanwhile an active treated patient will do so with an EDSS score of 4.0. Is this 0.5 difference acceptable for the patient? In the case of IFN β1b it reduces the relapse rate by one-third. It protects individuals from about one relapse every 3 years. Is the risk of one attack with incomplete recovery acceptable? Even in the absence of residual disability, is one attack still acceptable? (see Fig. 17.3).

The second argument is the informed consent. Patients are fully informed about the risks of entering a trial. Nevertheless, despite the best efforts to inform patients, they will rarely, if ever, be as well informed about their treatment options as their physicians. It may be more desirable to a patient to be a part of the trial than to decline to participate. Patients are not given any other choice—trial or nothing. Therefore, even informed consent, important though it is, is not enough protection, because of the asymmetry in knowledge and authority between researchers and their subjects.

After reviewing these arguments and sharing all my concerns and doubts, I would say that an acceptable statement is that only if there was a genuine doubt about the benefits of treatment would a placebo group be ethically justified. What is the current evidence of 'effective' treatment in MS? In February 1998, there is a lack of effective treatment in the first attack of demyelinating disease, secondary progressive MS and primary progressive MS. Therefore, the answer

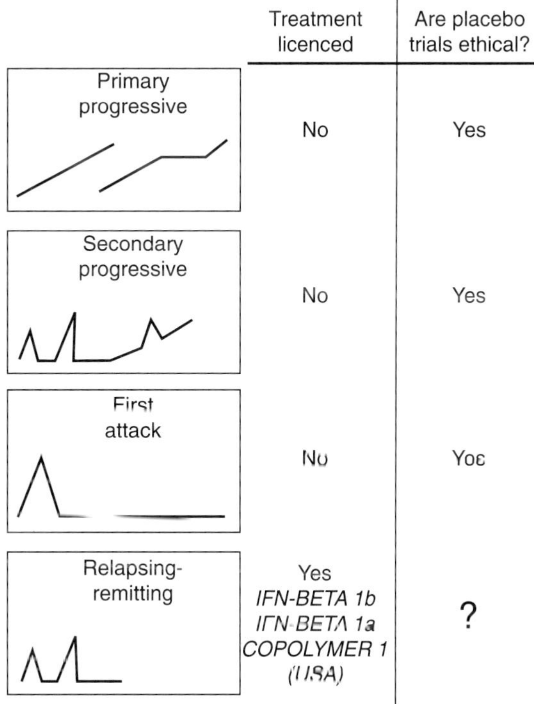

Figure 17.4 Clinical trials in MS populations.

to the ethical issue about performing clinical trials in those MS populations is clear—it is ethical to perform a double-blind, placebo-controlled, randomized trial. There are, however, several ongoing trials that will conclude soon. If such trials are positive, in fact, it seems that the IFN-β1b secondary progressive trial has been positive, other ongoing trials at that moment studying the same population of MS will have to be reviewed from an ethical point of view.

Phase III randomized, controlled clinical trials have now provided support that patients relapsing–remitting (RR) MS treated with either IFN-β1b (Betaferon®), IFN-β1a (Avonex®) or copolymer-1 (Copaxone®) fare better than placebo-treated patients in terms of relapse frequency (all agents), MRI activity (both interferons) and possibly the rate of clinically determined disability progression (IFN-β1a).[2,3,9] Recently, we have been told that another IFN-β1a (Rebif®) is also effective in improving all three parameters (relapse rate, progression of clinical disability and MRI activity). Theoretically, each of those agents could be employed as the control limb in future trials of RRMS.

Are these treatments effective enough and free of significant short- and long-term side effects to be offered to all study subjects as the control limb against which future therapies are to be measured? Surely an understanding of the positive results will determine what constitutes a RRMS future trial design.

Since 1993, two forms of recombinant interferon beta (IFN-β1b, Betaferon® and IFN-β1a, Avonex®, later approved by the EC) have been approved by the FDA for patients with RRMS and copolymer 1 (Copaxone®).

EFFECT ON RELAPSE RATE

Treatment with Avonex® and the higher dose of Betaferon® reduced the relapse rate by one-third (32% and 34%, respectively). The reduction in the relapse rate for all randomized patients in the Avonex® study was 18%. Copaxone® decreased the relapse rate by 29% and Rebif®, where results still await for peer review, by 32% (28.9% for patients on 6MUI). There has been much debate on whether a modest effect on relapse rate is useful for MS patients. Placebo trials defenders may argue that relapses are distressing but usually self-limiting, although they cause disability if recovery is poor. Furthermore, these results are only meant to protect individuals from about one relapse every 3 years. In most natural history studies, relapse frequency has not emerged as a factor which predicts disability, but in the North American study, the number of relapses in the first 2 years, and the time to the first relapse after presentation, both correlated with eventual disability.

Another distressing problem is the presence of neutralizing antibodies (NAB) formation, mainly in IFN-β1b treated patients. NAB+ influence in IFN-β therapy must be better understood.

EFFECT ON DISABILITY

In the treatment of MS, the most effective strategy, short of a complete cure, is to prevent accumulation of disability. To date, however, very few treatments have been reported to show the accumulation of disability. None has consistently and repeatedly demonstrated a long-term shift in the natural history of MS.

Avonex® treatment resulted in a significantly lower probability of developing disability progression compared with placebo recipients ($p = 0.024$). Although there was a trend in high-dose IFN-β1b patients to show favourable slowing of EDSS progression, these findings did not reach statistical significance ($p = 0.096$). No convincing reduction of disability progression was shown by the copolymer 1 (glatiramer acetate) study. Rebif® seems to have a positive impact on EDSS progression, although data are still preliminary.

It seems likely that the favourable effect on disability progression during the short-term clinical trial will result in less severe disability over longer follow-up intervals, but this remains to be demonstrated. In fact, predictors of short-term and long-term outcome were shown to differ.

EFFECT ON MRI

Betaferon® has shown a reduction in lesion load (T2) during the first 4 years ($p = 0.0055$) and in the rate of active lesions during the first 2 years (no gadolinium (Gd) was used). Avonex® reduced the rate of active lesions measured with Gd but a reduction in T2 lesion load was not observed. There is limited MRI data available of Copaxone®. MRI data from the Rebif® study seem also to be very impressive. Nevertheless, the correlation between MRI changes and long-term disability needs to be understood better. Also the discrepancy between clinical and MRI behaviour of the patients receiving 1.6 MIU of Betaferon® needs to be clarified.

CONCEPT OF EQUIPOISE

Noseworthy reminded us of the concept of 'equipoise' introduced by Freedman in 1987.[10] As such, the investigator should be 'equally poised' with respect to his preference for either treatment A or B. If these two treatments (one of which may be placebo) are not equivalent, ethical practice requires that the superior treatment be given. As Compston wrote, each position has its strengths and weaknesses, but the hopes and fears of individual patients must not be manipulated either for reasons of commercial interest or through professional rigidity.[11]

In my opinion, after reviewing our own experience with IFN and if Rebif's results are confirmed by a peer review, it is rather hard to accept a trial on RRMS patients using a placebo control. This is of course a personal, and perhaps temporary, opinion.

REFERENCES

1. Gøtzsche PC. Is there any logic in the placebo? *Lancet* 1994; **344**: 925–926.
2. Jacobs LD, Cookfair DL, Rudick RA et al. Intramuscular interferon beta-1a for disease progression in relapsing multiple sclerosis. *Ann Neurol* 1996; **39**: 285–294.
3. The IFNB Multiple Sclerosis Study Group and the University of British Columbia MS/MRI Analysis Group. Interferon beta-1b in the treatment of multiple sclerosis: final outcome of the randomized controlled trial. *Neurology* 1995; **45**: 1277–1285.
4. Declaration of Helsinki IV, WMA, 41st World Medical Assembly, Hong Kong, September 1989. In: Annas GJ, Grodin MA, eds. *The Nazi Doctors and the Nuremberg Code: Human Rights in Human Experimentation.* New York: Oxford University Press, 1992; 339–342.
5. Spriet A, Dupin-Spriet T, Simon P. Choice of the comparator: placebo or active drug? In: *Methodology of Clinical Drug Trials.* 2nd edn. New York: Karger, 1994.
6. Collier J. Confusion over use of placebos in clinical trials. *BMJ* 1995; **311**: 821–822.
7. Rothman KJ, Michels KB. The continuing unethical use of placebo controls. *New Engl J Med* 1994; **331**: 394–398.
8. Hill AB. Medical ethics and controlled trials. *BMJ* 1963; **1**: 1043–1049.
9. Johnson KP, Brooks BR, Cohen JA et al. Copolymer 1 reduces relapse rate and improves disability in relapsing–remitting multiple sclerosis. *Neurology* 1995; **45**: 1268–1276.
10. Noseworthy J. Are placebo controlled clinical trials still ethical in MS? In: *Treatment and Management of Multiple Sclerosis.* Thompson AJ, Polman C, Hohlfeld R, eds. London: Martin Dunitz, 1997.
11. Compston A. Beta-interferon and multiple sclerosis: not a final solution to the problem. *Br J Hosp Med* 1995; **53**: 547–553.

18

Interferon beta—responders versus non-responders

Fred D Lublin

INTRODUCTION

The clinical effectiveness of interferon beta (IFN-β) for the treatment of multiple sclerosis (MS) has been documented by three double-blind, placebo-controlled, randomized clinical trials; one with interferon beta-1b (IFN-β1b)[1] and two with interferon beta-1a (IFN-β1a),[2,3] as well as several smaller studies. Although each study had unique features and differences that make it impossible to compare the results between the studies, one can view the aggregate results as a clear affirmation of the effectiveness of IFN-β, albeit partial. The design of these studies was to compare treatment group(s) to a placebo group, looking for differences in one of the populations, using various outcome measures (Table 18.1). Gauging the effect of IFN-β on the course of MS is much easier when viewing data on populations of patients. Determining individual responsiveness is a much more challenging task. It is extremely difficult to track individual responses using current clinical outcome measures as they tend to fluctuate in non-predictable ways, and often, the nature of the endpoint is such that repetitive measures over time are impractical because the outcome is either too infrequent (e.g. relapse rate) or too insensitive to subtle, graded change (e.g. Kurtzke expanded disability status scale (EDSS)) to allow intra-individual assessment. The absence of accepted surrogate markers of disease activity further hampers the task. Magnetic resonance imaging (MRI) activity and lesion load, when sequentially measured, may provide evaluable

Table 18.1 Potential markers of interferon responsiveness

Clinical
Reduction in relapse rate
Percentage of patients relapse-free
Time to define sustained disability level
Percentage of patients reaching a defined disability level
Integrated disability status score
MRI
Reduced lesion load accrual
Measure of activity—new/enlarging lesions, gadolinium enhancements
Biologic response markers
Neopterin
β-2 microglobulin
Kappa light chains
Neutralizing antibodies

data on an individual response to therapy, but have not yet been universally accepted as surrogates for clinical disease activity and provide only modest correlation with the clinical outcome measures utilized in current clinical trials in MS.

The clinical outcome measures used in these clinical trials included relapse rate (primary outcome measure for the interferon beta-1b study[1] and one of the IFN-β1a,[2,3]) confirmed change in the Kurtzke EDSS (primary outcome measure in the other IFN-β1a study), proportion of patients exacerbation-free at the end of a given time, time to first (and subsequent) exacerbation, number of moderate of severe relapses, percentage better-same-worse, steroid use, and hospitalizations. A new scale, the integrated disability status score, which integrates the time and extent of disability (as measured by the EDSS), including time during exacerbations, was employed in a recent trial.[3]

The MRI assessments included measures of activity, such as new or enlarging lesions or number or volume of gadolinium (Gd) enhancing lesions, and measures of lesion burden, such as T2 lesion load, using manual or automated systems.

The first study to demonstrate the effectiveness of systemically administered IFN-β was the North American IFN-β1b (Betaseron) study which started in 1988.[1] This study utilized a double–blind, placebo-controlled design. The inclusion criteria were patients with relapsing–remitting disease, Kurtzke EDSS scores of 0–5.5 and two or more exacerbations in the prior 2 years. Data were obtained from 372 patients randomized to receive either placebo, 1.6 MIU IFN-β, or 8 MIU IFN-β, subcutaneously, every other day. The primary outcome measures were reduction in annual exacerbation rate and proportion of exacerbation-free patients. At the end of the planned 2 year study, patients were offered re-enrollment for an additional year to assess progression of disease, as assessed by change in EDSS.

The results of this study, after 2 years, were that patients who received 8 MIU of IFN-β had a significant reduction of one-third in the annual exacerbation rate, as compared to placebo-treated patients (0.84 vs. 1.27; $p = 0.0001$). More importantly, the degree of reduction in exacerbation rate was most impressive, almost 50%, in those exacerbations rated as moderate or severe. The other primary endpoint—proportion of patients remaining exacerbation-free—also showed a significant difference, favouring IFN-β (8 MIU IFN-β = 36, placebo = 18, $p = 0.007$). The median time to first exacerbation was significantly prolonged, nearly twice as long in the 8 MIU group as compared to placebo ($p = 0.015$). Further, there were significant reductions in the number and days of hospitalization and need for steroids in the IFN-β treated group. The IFN-β 1.6 MIU group demonstrated a dose–response effect, with clinical values between that of the 8 MIU group and the placebo group in most outcome measures.

The patients in this study had baseline and yearly MRI scans which were analysed in a blinded fashion at one study site. MRI activity was assessed by measuring new or enlarging lesions in a subset of 52 patients who had scans every 6 weeks for 2 years. MRI activity was reduced in the IFN-β 8 MIU treatment group by 80% compared to the placebo group ($p = 0.0062$). The rate of new lesions, active lesions and number of patients free of new lesions all significantly favoured the IFN-β 8 MIU group. MRI lesion burden, measured on T2 weighted images, was significantly less 2 years in the treatment group ($p < 0.001$).[4,5]

By the time all enrolled patients had completed 3 years on the protocol, the total data set for the blinded, placebo-controlled study included patients with a median time on the study of almost 4 years and a few patients who had completed 5 years. The analysis of the 3-year data and that for the entire data set (all patients, all time on study) shows a continued significant decrease in the relapse rate of about 30% ($p = 0.006$, pooled data, all patients, all time points on study). The same holds true for each individual year, although significance was achieved individually only for the first 2 years, probably owing to loss of power from successive drop-outs in the later years. Progression of disease—assessed by the proportion of patients with a sustained worsening by one point on the EDSS—showed a trend, but not a significant difference, in favour of IFN-β. The study was not powered to show a change in EDSS, but rather to assess the change in relapse rate. The MRI data for all patients over the course of the study continued to show a dramatic effect from treatment with IFN-β, with no significant increase in lesion burden through year five. The placebo group increased their T2 burden by about 10% per year. This data demonstrates a persistence of effect in the group response to IFN-β.

A double-blind, placebo-controlled multicentre trial of IFN-β, using recombinant IFN-β1a (Avonex), reported results in March of 1996.[2] This study differed from the IFN-β1b study in several important ways. The drug was administered intramuscularly, weekly at a dose of 6 MIU (the measure of activity, in MIU, was not directly comparable between these studies). The inclusion criteria were relapsing MS, EDSS scores of 1.0–3.5, and two or more exacerbations in the previous 3 years. The primary outcome measures was time to onset of sustained increase in disability, as measured by a worsening of the Kurtzke EDSS score by at least one point. The study demonstrated a significant effect of IFN-β on delaying disability (p = 0.02). Also seen were significantly fewer exacerbations (p=0.03) and a significant reduction in MRI activity in patients receiving IFN-β, as measured by the number and volume of Gd-enhancing lesions on MRI scans. The effect on T2 burden was not as impressive, a significant difference at the end of 1 year, but no significant difference at 2 years.

Another clinical trial of IFN-β1a (Rebif) from a different company recently presented results of a multicenter placebo controlled study of 560 patients with relapsing–remitting MS and Kurtzke scores of 0–5.0, who were randomized into a placebo group, 6 MIU or 12 MIU IFN-β1a, administered subcutaneously three times weekly for 2 years. The results of this study were that patients in both treatment groups performed significantly better than placebo-treated patients in respect to reduction in relapse rate, percentage of patients relapse-free, time to first relapse, number of moderate or severe attacks, steroid use and hospitalizations. Time to confirmed progression of disability by an increase in one point on the Kurtze scale was also better in the treated groups. Analysis of MRI scans in the groups revealed decreased activity and lesion burden in the IFN-treated patients. Although the higher dose group did better, there were no significant differences in the major clinical outcome measures between the two dosing groups. The results of this study are not yet published.

Additional evidence for the effectiveness of IFN-β comes from studies of its effect on Gd-enhanced MRI scans, where IFN-β produced a marked reduction in the number of enhancing lesions,[6] suggesting an effect on the breakdown of the blood–brain barrier that occurs as an early manifestation of new lesions in MS.[7] The use of serial Gd-enhanced scans provides a very sensitive, and to date the best, method of assessing individual response to a therapy. New lesions seen on Gd-enhanced scans occur 5–10 times more frequently than discernible clinical events. Therefore, one can look at the effect of a therapy on serial enhanced MRI scans as a screening method for promising new agents. As there can be considerable variation from scan to scan, one must employ a frequent scanning paradigm to obtain accurate results. Using such a paradigm, studies have shown that the level of detectable enhancement seen on frequent scans is dramatically decreased in nearly all patients when therapy with IFN-β is instituted. Similarly, in some patients there is a return of Gd when interferon antibodies are detected, while in others there is little effect of antibodies (H. McFarland, personal communication). The use of frequent MRI scans with Gd is the only well-defined marker of individual response to IFN-β, but the clinical relevance of this observation is unclear. While reduction in Gd-enhancing activity is a sensitive indicator, it is not a very specific indicator of clinical effect. Use of corticosteroids can also decrease Gd-enhancement without any lasting effect on disease course. Further, in the IFN-β1b study, the low dose group had a significant decrease in Gd-enhancements without any effect on disability. Using a cohort of patients that were followed for at least 6 months before the start of IFN-β1b with monthly MRI scans with Gd and then monthly scans for another 6 months on IFN therapy, Stone et al.[8] were able to discern individual response rates in 29 patients. They found a degree of heterogeneity in the response to IFN therapy over the 6-month treatment period. All but two of the patients had a reduction in lesion frequency. Based on their natural history study cohort, a reduction of 60% in total contrast enhancing lesion frequency was considered a 'responder'; 83% of the treated group met this criteria. Another definition of 'responder' was a reduction in new lesion frequency of 67%; in the treated group, 91% of the patients were responders by this definition. Stone et al. were not able to identify any disease demographic or baseline MRI characteristic that predicted the MRI response to therapy with IFN. The MRI response was seen to occur within the first 3 months on therapy. Thus, serial assessment of Gd-enhancement on MRI is a sensitive indicator of individual therapeutic response to IFN therapy. However, it is not yet clear how well the MRI response will predict a clinically meaningful response to therapy, as the current measures of clinical response are not sensitive enough to employ in a similar natural history, frequent measurement paradigm. Further, these MRI studies required monthly scans for long periods to obtain valid results. In practice, this would be extremely costly (even when measured against the cost of IFN-β) and would place a severe burden on MRI resources.

Therefore, we can determine a group response to IFN-β use, e.g. 30% reduction in relapse rate in IFN-treated groups or significant slowing of disability compared to placebos, but we are unable to discern which patients will achieve a clinically significant response (as opposed to MRI) to therapy and to what extent an individual will respond.

The usefulness of IFN-β may be mitigated by the development of neutralizing antibodies, suggesting that IFN antibodies could alter the responsiveness pattern of IFN-β. Although these antibodies were found in patients in all IFN-β studies, a detailed analysis has only been published for the IFN-β1b population.[9] This analysis revealed that 35% of patients treated with IFN-β developed neutralizing antibodies after 3 years exposure, and the vast majority of these antibodies by the end of the first year. In those patients developing neutralizing antibodies, the relapse rate approximated that seen in placebo patients, suggesting a loss of efficacy. Conversely, in the 65% of treated patients who did not develop these antibodies, the relapse rate reduction was approximately 50%, strengthening the evidence for the clinical efficacy of IFN-β. Additional analysis of the study data is underway to determine the long-term effect of the antibodies and their persistence. Not all patients who developed antibodies lost efficacy. Further, in both IFN-β studies, patients who developed antibodies tended to have less progression of disease as measured by the change in EDSS than those without antibodies. A recent analysis of this data using a new assay for IFN-β1b antibodies and a different statistical paradigm—longitudinal analysis rather than cross-sectional analysis—did not show as significant an effect of antibody. Also, there is evidence that a significant percentage of patients lose their antibodies over time. More data will be needed to better understand the full implications of this phenomenon.

More recently. Rudick et al. reported that in the IFN-β1a (Avonex) study, the sub-group of patients that best responded to therapy was a group that had little in the way of Gd-enhancement on MRI scans and lower levels of kappa light chains in the cerebrospinal fluid.[10] This is a rather surprising result that will need confirmation in other studies, as the response to IFN-β on Gd-enhancements was so dramatic. Also, this result will cast some doubt on the value of using reduction in Gd-enhancement as a clinically relevant marker of IFN response.

Analysis of variables such as age, sex, body mass, and disease severity has yielded little in the way of discriminant data as to responder status. In the IFN-β1b study, the degree of IFN-related side-effects was inversely related to body mass, but the response to therapy was not. In the IFN-β1a (Avonex) trial, most of the therapeutic effect was seen in those patients with an EDSS of 2.5–3.5, with less effect seen in the lower (1–2) EDSS patients. In the IFN-β1b study, there was no difference in the effect in patients whose EDSS was either greater than or less than 3. Although interferon can induce a change in a variety of biologic response modifiers, such as levels of circulating neopterin and β2 microglobulin, these do not appear to be predictive of therapeutic effect.

In two of the major studies,[1,3] and an additional study of IFN-β1a by Pozzilli et al.,[11] there were comparisons of two different IFN doses. While a dose–response effect was seen in favour of higher doses, the magnitude varied depending on the outcome measure and was not predictive of individual response.

To date, all the IFN studies have been on relapsing–remitting patients. It is not yet known whether a similar effect will be seen on other forms of MS. Studies are underway in secondary progressive MS, with a preliminary report that IFN-β1b is effective for that form of the disease. Additional data analysis and the results of other studies will answer this question. The issue of primary progressive MS is more problematic. Few trials have been conducted on this form of MS, in which patients often show less impressive changes on MRI scans. If the clinical effect of IFN-β is directly related to its effect on MRI scans, one might not expect a very robust effect on primary progressive disease.

Thus, although the grouped data shows a consistent therapeutic effect of IFN-β on reduction in measures of relapse rate, time to development of disability, percentage of patients progressing and a variety of MRI measures, we have little data yet to guide us in determining whether a given individual will obtain a clinical benefit from this therapy. Further, we do not yet have the tools to follow an individual clinical response easily or to know when an individual is no longer a responder to therapy. Using a frequent Gd-enhanced MRI scanning paradigm provides an MRI definition of 'responder', but the cost, drain on resources and absence of clear clinical correlation mitigate against its usefulness in general practice. The development of neutralizing antibodies, although initially thought to be predictive of loss of biologic activity, does not now appear to be reliable as a sole indicator of responsiveness, and may be a transient phenomenon. This absence of reliable markers of individual efficacy is rather problematic when one considers the high cost of IFN-β. Hopefully, ongoing research will reveal a simple biological indicator of responsiveness.

REFERENCES

1. IFNB MS Study Group. Interferon beta-1b is effective in relapsing–remitting multiple sclerosis. I. Clinical results of a multicenter, randomized, double-blind, placebo-controlled trial. The IFNB Multiple Sclerosis Study Group [see comments]. *Neurology* 1993; **43**: 655–661.
2. Jacobs LD, Cookfair DL, Rudick RA et al. Intramuscular interferon beta-1a for disease progression in relapsing multiple sclerosis. The Multiple Sclerosis Collaborative Research Group (MSCRG). *Ann Neurol* 1996; **39**(3): 285–294.
3. PRISMS (Prevention of Relapses and Disability by Interferon-beta 1a Subcutaneously in Multiple Sclerosis) Study Group. Randomized double-blind placebo-controlled study of interferon-beta 1a in relapsing–remitting multiple sclerosis. *Lancet* 1998; **352**: 1498–1504.
4. Paty DW, Li DK, UBC MS, IFNB Multiple Sclerosis Study Group. Interferon beta-1b is effective in relapsing–remitting multiple sclerosis. II. MRI analysis results of a multicenter, randomized, double-blind, placebo-controlled trial. *Neurology* 1993; **43**: 662–667.
5. IFNB Multiple Sclerosis Study Group and the University of British Columbia MS/MRI Analysis Group. Interferon beta-1b in the treatment of multiple sclerosis: final outcome of the randomized controlled trial. The IFNB Multiple Sclerosis Study Group and the University of British Columbia MS/MRI Analysis Group. *Neurology* 1995; **45**: 1277–1285.
6. Calabresi PA, Stone LA, Bash CN et al. Interferon beta results in immediate reduction of contrast-enhanced MRI lesions in multiple sclerosis patients followed by weekly MRI. *Neurology* 1997; **48**(5): 1446–1448.
7. Kermode AG, Thompson AJ, Tofts P et al. Breakdown of the blood–brain barrier precedes symptoms and other MRI signs. *Brain* 1990; **113**: 1477–1489.

8. Stone LA, Frank JA, Albert PS et al. Characterization of MRI response to treatment with interferon beta-1b: contrast-enhancing MRI lesion frequency as a primary outcome measure. *Neurology* 1997; **49** (3): 862–869.
9. IFNB Multiple Sclerosis Study Group and The University of British Columbia MS/MRI Analysis Group. Neutralizing antibodies during treatment of multiple sclerosis with interferon beta-1b: experience during the first three years. *Neurology* 1996; **47**: 889–894.
10. Rudick R, Cookfair D, Simon J et al. CSF kappa light chains and gadolinium-enhancing brain lesions as predictors of response to therapy with interferon beta 1a (Avonex) in patients with relapsing multiple sclerosis. *Neurology* 1998; **50 (suppl)**: A342.
11. Pozzilli C, Bastianello S, Koudriavtseva T et al. Magnetic resonance imaging changes with recombinant human interferon-beta-1a: a short term study in relapsing–remitting multiple sclerosis [see comments]. *J Neurol Neurosurg Psychiatry* 1996; **61(3)**: 251–258.

19

Treatment alternatives in relapsing–remitting multiple sclerosis

Oluf Andersen

INTRODUCTION

The milestones in the history of multiple sclerosis (MS) include the clinicopathological definition of the disease by Cruvelhier and Carswell, the description of the variable symptomatology by Charcot, the discovery of the intrathecal immunoglobulin production by Kabat, the epidemiological observation of significant previous infections, the magnetic resonance imaging (MRI) revelation of the 'never sleeping' focal activity, the confirmation of a hereditary predisposition, and, during the last 5 years, the advent of the first treatments that reduce the relapse frequency in relapsing–remitting MS (RRMS). The purpose of this chapter is to:

(1) Discuss the indication for interferon-beta (IFN-β) and copolymer-1 treatment in subgroups of RRMS patients
(2) Search for possible differences between these agents
(3) Discuss whether other treatment alternatives, not least cheaper alternatives, are relevant
(4) Point out the moderate dimension of the effect, our lack of knowledge on the individual response to different doses, and the continued need for development of our therapeutic arsenal against MS.

THE TREATMENT ALTERNATIVES WITH AND WITHOUT SCIENTIFIC PROOF, AND THE 'WAIT-AND-SEE' OPTION

Primary alternative: the drugs with proven effect in relapsing–remitting MS: the beta-interferons and Copaxone

Betaseron® (IFN-β1b), Avonex® (IFN-β1a) Rebif® (IFN-β1a) and Copaxone® (copolymer 1)

At the time of writing, Betaseron® and Avonex® were approved by the FDA (Food and Drug Administration) and by the EMEA (European Medicines Evaluation Agency) for the treatment of RRMS. Copaxone® was approved by the FDA and Rebif® by the EMEA. These agents were also approved by other national authorities. With additional solid and peer-reviewed data from the Rebif® (IFN-β1a) study[1] we have proof that IFN-β has therapeutic effect in RRMS. The main results of the trendsetting Betaseron®,[2] Avonex®[3] and Copaxone®[4] trials are summarized in Table 19.1, along with the corresponding data from the Rebif® (IFN-β1a) trial in RRMS (as presented at the 1997 AAN and ECTRIM congresses).[1] Examination of the Rebif® trial results is required as it is a recent and large study. With its 560 randomized patients it is the largest trial in RRMS until now. According to preliminary results impressive proportion of

Table 19.1 Dosage, inclusion criteria and main results from the four major recent trials of IFN-β1a, IFN-β1b and copolymer-1

	Trial			
	Betaseron[2]	Avonex[3]	Rebif[1]	Copaxone[4]
Proprietary name	Interferon beta-1b	Interferon beta-1a	Interferon beta-1a	Copolymer 1
Dose	1.5 or 8 MIU s.c. each other day	30 μg once a week	22 or 44 μg s.c. three times a week	20 mg s.c. daily
Indication, MS course	RRMS	RRMS	RRMS	RRMS
Indication, EDSS range	0–5.5	1–3.5	0–5	0–5
Reduction of relapse rate over 2 years	8% or 34%	18%	28% or 32%	29%
Reduction of moderate–severe* relapse rate over 2 years	29% or 49%	n.a.	28% or 37%	n.a.
Criterion for reduced progression 1 EDSS step	Not sustained or 6 months sustained	6 months sustained	3 months sustained	Not sustained or 3 months sustained
Progression retarded?	8 MIU: yes (not sustained) no (3 months sustained)	Yes	Yes	Yes (not sustained) No (3 months or not sustained)
MRI lesion volume after 2 years	Placebo +16.5% 1.5 MIU + 11.4% 8 MIU – 0.8%	n.s.	Placebo +11% 6 MIU –1% 12 MIU –4%	n.a.

*NRS decrease of 8 or more.
n.a., data not available; n.s., not significant.
†6-week interval.
‡, 1-month interval.

Table 19.2 Frequency of exacerbations in the Rebif® trial in RRMS with three parallel arms; 29–31% reduction during 2-year trial in the low and high dose groups.[1]

Treatment group	Annualized rate	Group comparisons
Placebo	1.33	
22 μg	0.94	$p = 0.0002$
44 μg	0.92	$p < 0.0001$

95.2% of patients randomized were available with complete data at 24 months. The primary endpoint was exacerbation count per patient. A reduction was observed in Rebif® receivers of 28.9% for the lower dose (22 μg 3 times a week) and 32.4% for the high dose (44 μg 3 times a week) (Table 19.2). The reduction was of the same magnitude as in the high dose group of the Betaseron® trial.[2]

The reduction in moderate and severe exacerbations (with Scripp's score decrease > 7 points) was 37% in the high dose group (Fig. 19.1). Time to progression in disability, as defined by a 1 point increase in EDSS confirmed at one further examination 3 months later, was significantly delayed in Rebif® receivers (Fig. 19.2).

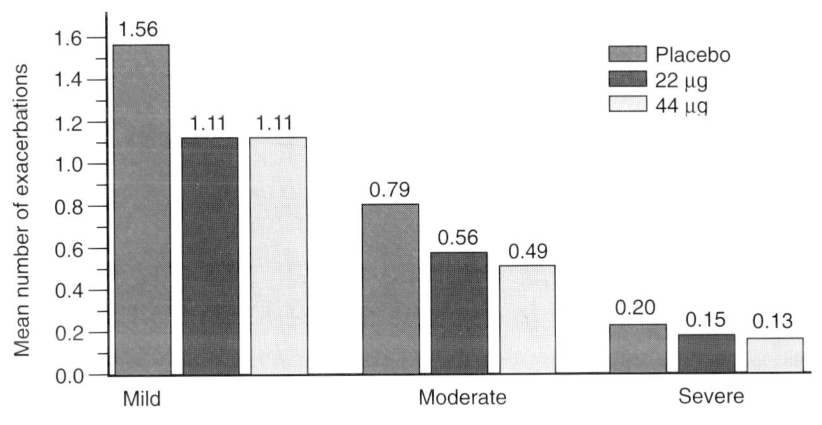

Figure 19.1 The mean number of exacerbations per patient during the 2-year trial in the placebo, 22 μg and 44 μg Rebif® receivers. The treatment effect was seen in both mild, moderate and severe relapses. There was no significant difference between the low and high dose groups.[1]

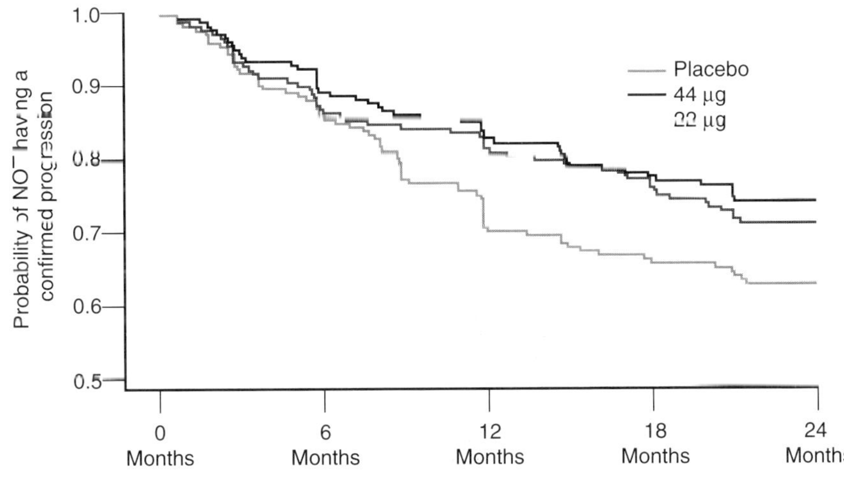

Figure 19.2 Kaplan–Meier analysis of the probability to escape progression in the placebo and the IFN β1a 22 and 44 μg receivers, showing a delay in the time to progression in the patients who received Rebif®.[1]

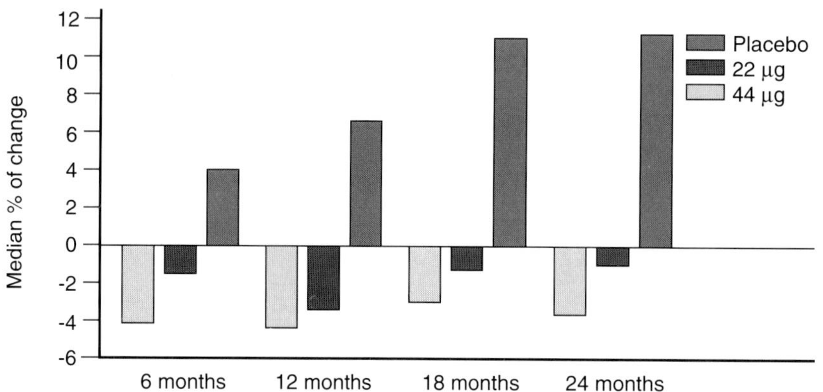

Figure 19.3 The Rebif® trial. The MRI burden shows a progressive change, while the high dose group shows an initial and sustained improvement, and the low dose group shows little change.[1]

Table 19.3 Adverse events in the Rebif® trial in RRMS. Percentage patients reporting adverse events at least once.[1]

		Rebif dose (μg)	
Adverse event	Placebo	22	44
Headache	62.6	64.6	70.1
Flu-like symptoms	51.3	56.1	58.7
Injection site inflammation	15.0	65.6	65.8
Fatigue	35.8	32.8	41.3
URTI	32.6	36.0	29.3
Fever	15.5	24.9	27.7

MRI burden of disease, assessed by biannual scans, showed significantly less increment, actually a reduction, in the two treatment groups compared with placebo (Fig. 19.3). Also, in 205 patients who underwent 11 monthly MRI, the median number of T2 active lesions per month was definitely lower in the treatment groups, particularly in the high dose group. The adverse effects of Rebif® included frequent injection site reactions. Influenza-like reactions occurred as frequently among placebo as IFN-β1a receivers (Table 19.3). However, crucial information on the severity of these reactions and their time relation to injections was not presented. IFN-α therapy often leads to lassitude, and suicides were more frequent in the IFN-β receivers in the Betaseron® trial. However, in the Rebif® trial depression tended to be less frequent in the patients receiving Rebif®. There was one suicide in the placebo group.[1]

Equivalent dose

Are the differences between study results (Table 19.1) due to dose, route of administration, or different characteristics and preparations of the IFN-β? A prerequisite for discussing dose is knowledge of pharmacological equivalents between the different agents.

Avonex® and Rebif®, both IFN-β1a, were found to be equivalent per weight unit in antiviral assays using two viruses and a standard IFN-β (F Antonetti, M Mascia, M Terlizzese, K Hardy, A Eshkol, unpublished material presented at the 7th Meeting of the European Neurological Society (ENS), 14–17 June, Rhodes, Greece). However, the assays used by the two companies differ, so 6 million units of Avonex is 30 μg of IFN-β1a, while 6 million units of Rebif is 22 μg of IFN-β1a. IFN-β1a was found to be 10-fold more potent per weight unit than IFN-β1b.[5] Using biological response markers (such as β2-microglobulin and neopterin, representing increased turnover of the human leukocyte antigen (HLA) molecules and macrophage activation) it was found that IFN-β1a is approximately 25% more active per unit than IFN-β1b. A single dose of 22 μg Rebif and 8 MIU Betaseron are almost equivalent.

Route of administration

Compared to an intravenous injection of IFN-β1b, the total bioavailability measured as the area under the curve (AUC), was 50% after an intramuscular injection and 30% after a subcutaneous injection in monkey experiments. Studies in healthy human volunteers showed that subcutaneous (s.c.) or intramuscular (i.m.) IFN-β injections have an effect on the biological response markers equivalent to an intravenous (i.v.) injection in spite of higher blood IFN concentrations after the i.v. injection. The biological response to both IFN-β1a and IFN-β1b, as measured by several IFN-induced proteins, was significantly increased for 2–3 days and slightly elevated for up to 1 week. The duration of these effects was essentially the same after s.c. and i.m. injections. The route of administration seemed to be of minor importance. Injection two or more times per week sustained biological markers more than injection once per week.[6] Recent reports provided divergent results on the pharmacokinetics of two brands of IFN-β1a. In one study, no difference was found between intramuscular and subcutaneous injections.[7] In the other study, the AUC for serum IFN activity was two- to threefold higher after intramuscular injections than after subcutaneous ones,[8] but pharmacodynamic parameters showed a much less marked difference of 30% or less.

Neutralizing antibodies

Neutralizing antibodies (NAB) develop during IFN therapy, dependent on dose, duration and type of disease. In IFN-α treatment of chronic myeloid leukaemia, the patients who developed high (>400 INU/ml) titres of NAB became unresponsive to the therapy.[9] Reported incidences of NAB were very variable, and one factor contributing to this variability was the lack of a standard assay system.[10] Studies on the Betaseron® in MS trial data[11] revealed that in the group where NAB occurred, usually in the first year, the exacerbation rates after 18 months resembled placebo rates, while the annual exacerbation rates in IFN-β-treated NAB-negative patients were 50% of those seen in untreated patients. This suggests that there is a higher than average efficacy in the NAB-negative group. On the other hand, there was a trend against development of less deficit in the NAB+ patients. One possible explanation is that the NAB were predetermined to occur in a subgroup with a high degree of inflammatory activity. Further data analysis, which took into account confounding factors like the expected overall decrease in relapse frequency with time, showed that there was a significant reduction of efficacy on relapse frequently associated with the transition to the NAB+ status in the low dose arm and a similar but non-significant trend in the high dose arm (evaluated by 95% confidence intervals). The change to NAB+ status was associated with statistically nonsignificant increases in expanded disability status scale (EDSS) scores for both doses but, on the contrary, the change to the NAB+ status was associated with a nonsignificant improvement in the percentage change per year in MRI lesion burden for both doses.[12] The proportion of patients with neutralizing antibodies in the Rebif® study was higher in the 22 μg

Table 19.4 Patients with neutralizing antibodies with titre 20 NU/ml or higher occurring at least once in the Rebif® trial in RRMS.[1]

Rebif dose (μg)	Total no. positive patients (%)	No. patients lost antibodies	No. patients positive at 24 months (%)
22	49 (25.9)*	4/49	44 (23.8)*
44	32 (17.4)	9/32	23 (12.5)

*Incidence significantly lower in the 44 μg group.

1 Placebo patient positive at 24 months.

than in the 44 μg group (Table 19.4).[4] A study in patients treated with 1.6 or 8 MIU IFN-β1b showed that NAB developed in 11 of 31 patients by the second year, but had disappeared in every case by 102 months.[13] Data support that the NAB+ status is associated with higher relapse frequency (indicating diminished effectiveness of IFN-β) in some dose intervals, but the results in different subgroups are confusing. Further individual prospective studies with standardized assays on the relationship between IFN-β dose, type of IFN, subtype of MS and ultimate therapeutic efficacy on deficit are essential.

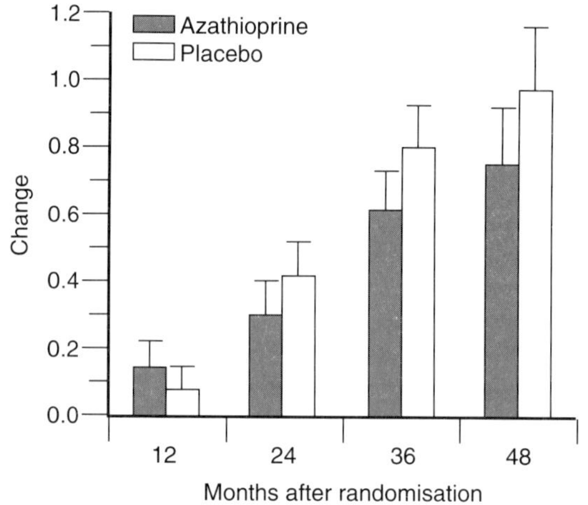

Figure 19.4 Mean changes in EDSS for patients on azathioprine and placebo. Horizontal bars = SEM. Reproduced with kind permission.[17]

Relative efficacy

No study shows that any one of the three IFN-β agents, or Copaxone®, is generally superior for RRMS therapy. This is at least partly owing to the complexity of these large trials studies with their somewhat deviating design (Table 19.1) with intervention groups differing both in their clinical characteristics and in the IFN-β agent used. A preliminary meta-analysis using odds ratios for some clinical events (in the active drug receivers compared to the placebo receivers) in the Betaseron®, Avonex® and Copaxone® trials showed no statistical differences, apart from the proportion of withdrawals due to side-effects, which was smaller in the Copaxone® treated patients. Based on the relapse frequency reduction in the three large IFN trials (Table 19.1), a small dose-finding study,[14] and supported by experimental findings,[6] it is tempting to conclude that there is a dose–effect relationship in favour of the higher dose interval, levelling out within the high dose interval of 22–44 μg IFN-β1a used in the Rebif® study (Table 19.1). A further dose-finding study for Avonex® is expected. Recently, a 1–11 month extension of the Copaxone® trial was published,[15] which revealed a 32% reduction of the relapse rate but no significant effect on sustained progression, as in the core 24-month study (Table 19.1). Thus, the effect of Copaxone® is largely comparable to IFN-β, but no extensive dose-finding data are available for Copaxone®.

Alternative drugs traditionally used in long-term therapy of relapsing–remitting MS—but without definite scientific proof

The quality and efficiency of multicentre clinical trials in MS developed immensely during the last decade, by the use of computerized handling of large amounts of data, double masking techniques and substitute parameters. The previous generation of drugs used in MS therapy, notably azathioprine, was not evaluated by equally efficient techniques. The increase in cancer risk was found to be 4.4 (95% confidence intervals 0.9–20.9) after more than 10 years of azathioprine treatment.[16] Although the large Dutch–British study showed clear trends in favour of azathioprine compared with placebo with the statistical method used (95% confidence intervals), the difference in EDSS change between treatment and placebo groups never reached significance (Fig. 19.4).[17] Also a meta-analysis showed a tendency towards a therapeutic effect of azathioprine that only approached the level of significance.[18] Similar data sets were retrieved from the three IFN-β studies and the Copaxone® study. In the

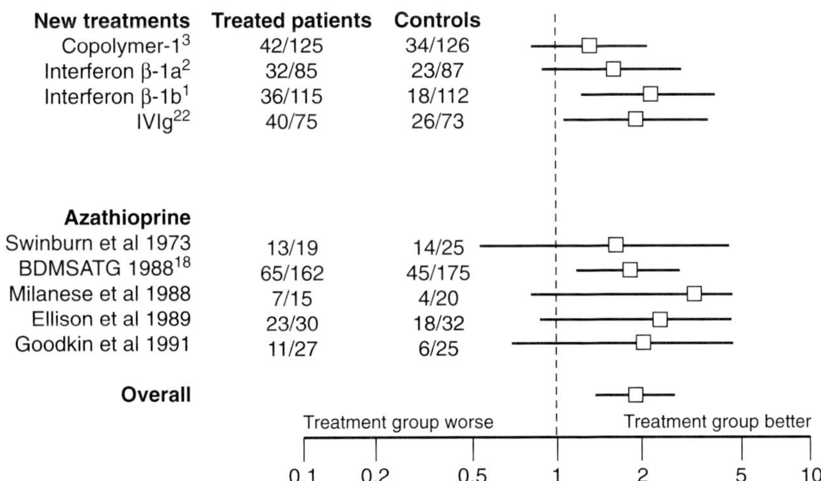

Figure 19.5 Odds ratio of being relapse-free at 2 years. Comparison of new treatments with azothiaprine. Reproduced with kind permission.[19]

Betaseron® trial there was no significant difference in the proportion EDSS stable (3 months sustained) between the Betaseron® and placebo groups.[1] In the Avonex®[2] and Rebif®[4] studies, a significant therapeutic effect was obtained, using life-table statistics or analysis of variance to evaluate the time to a confirmed one-step increase in EDSS. These are different methods, but in a second analysis of the Avonex® data, EDSS data were presented in a simpler way, rather similar to the azathioprine trial presentation, with the Mann–Whitney test showing numerically small but significant differences between IFN-β1a and placebo receivers after 2 years. As the study was terminated before the time stated by the protocol, contained no secondary progress MS (SPMS) patients (some were included in the azathioprine study), and data were not evaluated in quite the same way as in the azathioprine study, with 95% confidence intervals,[17] the results cannot be compared directly. To further improve comparability, two Oxford researchers calculated the odds ratios of being relapse-free at 2 years for Copaxone®, Betaseron® and Avonex®, i.v. immunoglobulin (IVIG), and azathioprine receivers, compared with their placebo groups. They obtained raw data from the publications and also by personal communication with the authors. Using these odds ratios, azathioprine seemed to be as efficient as the four newer therapies in increasing the proportion of relapse-free patients after 2 years trial (Fig. 19.5).[19] Although these meta-analyses suggest that azathioprine was never given a fair trial, this of course is not a substitute for a new trial (or a comparative trial with IFN-β) and does not change our conclusion on the four agents available with proven therapeutic effect on the relapse rate in RRMS.

New treatments that showed promise in RRMS, in phase II studies, with restricted use according to local traditions

IVIG

In a small double-blind, cross-over study of 25 randomized RRMS or relapsing–progressive MS patients, high-dose IVIG tended to reduce the exacerbation rate. With the IVIG pulse used (1 g/kg daily for 2 days), there was a high number of adverse effects, including palm or generalized eczema in 10 patients.[20] A randomized 2-year study of IVIG was performed in 150 Austrian RRMS patients. According to their report, the treating neurologist was aware of the treatment allocation. The EDSS score (not confirmed at a later visit) decreased on average with 0.23 in the patients who received IVIG and

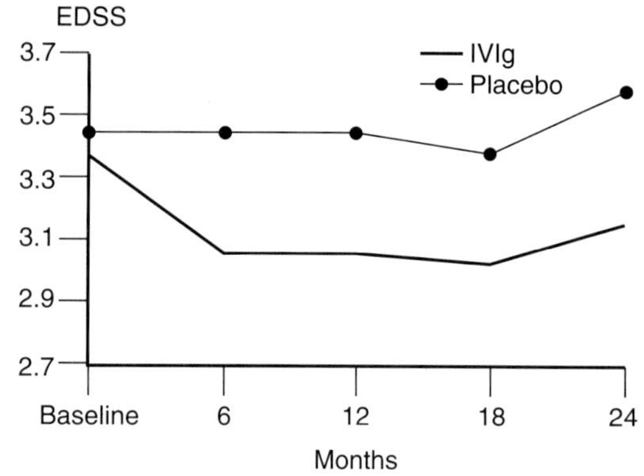

Figure 19.6 Effects of IVIG on EDSS. Reproduced with kind permission.[22]

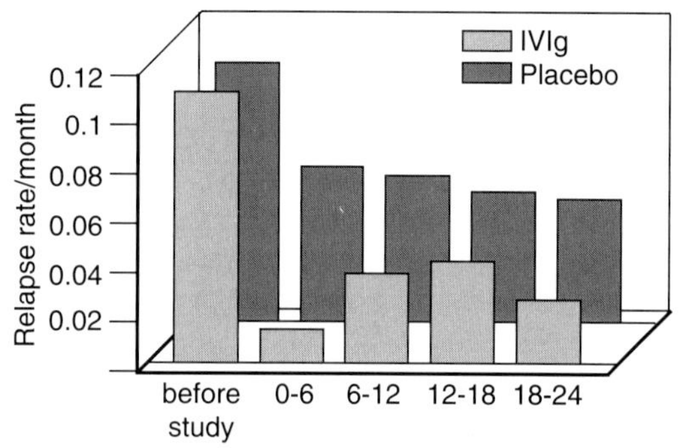

Figure 19.7 Effects of IVIG on release rate. Reproduced with kind permission.[22]

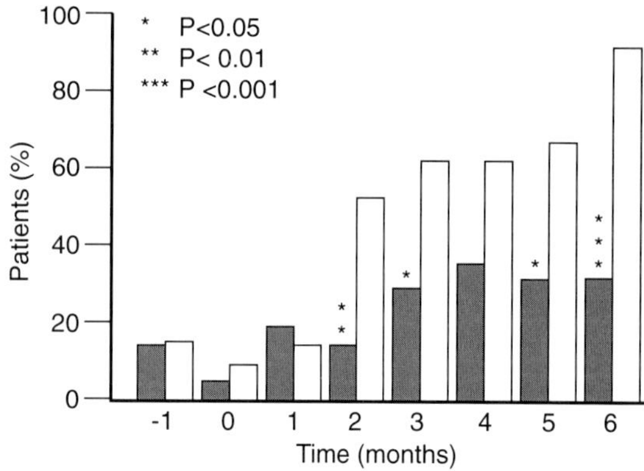

Figure 19.8 Mitoxantrone trial. Proportion of patients with no enhancing lesions. Reproduced with kind permission.[23]

increased by 0.12 in the placebo group. The annual relapse rate was 0.52 in the IVIG-treated patients and 1.26 in the placebo-treated group. Both differences were significant, in favour of IVIG.[21] The improvement of deficit in the IVIG group occurred during the first 6 months of the trial and was sustained during the remaining 18 months (Fig. 19.6). Also, the difference between IVIG-treated and placebo patients, expressed as a monthly relapse rate, peaked during the first 6 months (Fig. 19.7).[22]

IFN-α

In a Norwegian multicentre study, 97 RRMS patients were randomized to receive placebo, 4.5 MIU IFN-α2a, or 9.0 MIU IFN-α2a three times a week. There was significant efficacy measured as fewer new gadolinium (Gd)-enhancing MRI lesions during the treatment period. The median number of enhancing lesions at the end of the treatment period was lower in the IFN-α2a receivers, but the difference disappeared during the follow-up (K Myhr, personal communication).

Mitoxantrone

A French centre selected 42 patients with very active MS disease, implicating either two relapses with sequelae or a two points EDSS progression within the last 12 months. A randomized trial was performed with either monthly i.v. methylprednisolone alone, or monthly i.v. methylprednisolone combined with i.v. mitoxantrone. In the mitoxantrone group there was a month by month decrease of patients with no new enhancing lesions, the primary outcome variable. For study month 6 this proportion amounted to 90%, as compared to 31% in the placebo group (Fig. 19.8). A statistically significant reduction of relapses occurred in patients receiving mitoxantrone, but regrettably this clinical assessment was unblinded. Severe side-effects occurred, including transient pronounced leukopenia approximately 2 weeks after the injections, as well as nausea and mild alopecia. The mitoxantrone dose was 20 mg i.v., which is less than that used for malignant diseases. In this study no mitoxantrone cardiotoxicity was observed.[23] The authors conclude that a long-term, double-blind study is necessary.

However, owing to its bone marrow effects and its potential for producing asymptomatic left ventricular lesions, some have contended that mitoxantrone for MS should be limited to short-term therapy.[24] A 2-year double-blind trial of mitoxantrone in 51 RRMS patients showed that the drug reduced the relapse rate, but produced no consistent results on the EDSS or on the T2-weighted MRI lesions.[25]

Drugs extensively used for the treatment of acute relapses, with inconclusive evidence for long-term effects

Previous studies of adrenocorticotropic hormone (ACTH) and high-dose methylprednisolone in RRMS were short term. A significant effect was found at 1 and 4 weeks after i.v. methylprednisolone in a double-blind study including 22 RRMS patients.[26] The best data source on the long-term effect of one corticosteroid pulse therapy in RRMS is the optic neuritis study. The predictive value of optic neuritis does not differ from that of other MS onset bouts.[27] The optic neuritis study had three arms, i.v. methylprednisolone, oral prednisone and oral placebo (but, notably, no i.v. placebo). At the 2-year follow-up, the rate of new episodes was significantly higher in the oral prednisone group than in the placebo group, and slightly lower in the i.v. methylprednisolone group.[28] However, by the end of the third year of follow-up, the cumulative incidence of definite MS in each arm was similar: 17.3% in the i.v. methylprednisolone group, 21.3% in the placebo group and 24.7% in the oral prednisone group.[29] Consequently, there are no long-term effects of a single early pulse of corticosteroid therapy in RRMS. A randomized trial of 80 patients in acute relapse showed no clear advantage of i.v. as compared to oral methylprednisolone pulse when evaluated at 1, 4 and 24 weeks. Therefore, it was considered preferable to use oral rather than i.v. steroids.[30] Is continued intermittent corticosteroid pulse therapy effective in RRMS? No long-term trial was performed with this regimen in RRMS. Recently, preliminary negative results were reported in a trial of repeat corticosteroid pulse treatments in progressive MS. Our experience is that in RRMS there is no postponement of deterioration to the end of the interval (e.g. 6-week interval) between pulses, as we see in intermittent steroid pulse therapy for sensitive diseases like myasthenia gravis. Recurrent high doses of methylprednisolone were used during 3 years in RRMS, but this was an open uncontrolled study.[31] It may be anticipated that the incitement to perform a large controlled trial of long-term repeat corticosteroid pulses in RRMS will be less robust following the negative report in progressive MS and the negative 3-year results from the optic neuritis study.

No immediate alternative: some disappointing results during the last year

Sulfalazine

In a nine-centre trial of sulfalazine, conducted in Canada and the USA, 155 RRMS and 44 SPMS patients were randomized, seen at 3-monthly intervals and followed for a mean of 3.8 years. A subset of the patients had MRI with 6 months intervals. At 18 months, there was considerable evidence of a positive effect with apparent slowing of EDSS progression, and fewer clinically active quarters. These effects did not last to 36 months and beyond. Eventually, there were no EDSS effects (J Noseworthy, personal communication).

Cladribine

The recent essentially negative report on cladribine in SPMS is discussed in another chapter. Cladribine may also, according to a congress report on a cross-over study, have some effect on relapses but not on progression in RRMS.[32] Cladribine induces a defect also in normal resting lymphocytes, which may lead to prolonged lymphopenia predominating in T cells, especially in the CD4 subset.[33] Although trials of cladribine continue, its general use in RRMS does not seem warranted if its beneficial effect in RRMS is mainly restricted to a reduction in relapse frequency, an effect which can be obtained by less toxic drugs.

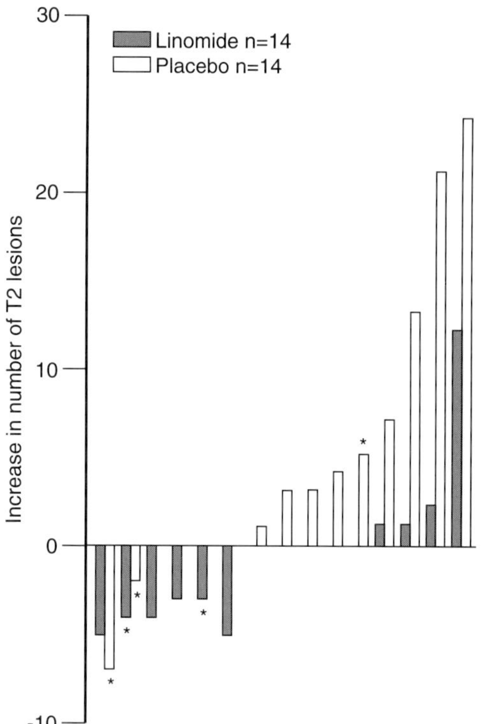

Figure 19.9 Linomide trial. Net result of new and disappeared T2 lesions (no. at week 24 minus no. at baseline). Asterisks indicate patients with more than one contrast-enhancing lesion at baseline. Reproduced with kind permission.[34]

Linomide

The synthetic immunomodulator linomide, a quinoline-3-carboxamide, had a profound inhibitory influence in several experimental autoimmune diseases, including acute and chronic experimental allergic encephalomyelitis (EAE). In a double-blind trial in Göteborg, 31 patients with relapsing–remitting multiple sclerosis were randomized to oral doses of 2.5 mg linomide or placebo once a day for 6 months. The mean number of active (new and enlarged T2-weighted) lesions per monthly MRI scan was significantly reduced in the patients receiving linomide. The total number of T2 lesions (new minus disappearing) increased in the placebo group but was, on average, stable in the linomide treated patients (Fig. 19.9). When neurological deficit was assessed by the regional functional scoring system (RFSS), the linomide group showed an improvement of 1% of the maximal RFSS range and the placebo group a deterioration of 0.2%. However, the trends in clinical results were not significant. A severe adverse event of pleuropericarditis occurred in one of the linomide-treated patients but eventually resolved. The most frequent adverse event in the Göteborg study was musculoskeletal pain, of mild to severe degree, characteristically in the jaws.[34] In a parallel linomide study on SPMS performed in Israel, there were similar effects on active MRI lesions and a tendency towards inhibition of the progression evaluated by the EDSS.[35] The main results in the Göteborg study were based upon number of active T2 lesions, which should be an adequate parameter in rather benign cases. A subsequent phase III trial in RRMS and SPMS patients was terminated after eight cases of myocardial infarction occurred in addition to two instances of sudden unexplained death. No risk factors were found for the myocardial infarctions in cases investigated with coronary angiography. In additional linomide toxicology studies in Beagle dogs, necrotic lesions were sometimes found in the myocardium (Pharmacia-Upjohn, personal communication). The mechanism of action of linomide is not clear. Analysis of lymphocyte subgroups did not support previously reported linomide-induced enhancement of natural killer (NK) cells.

Oral myelin basic protein (MBP)

Oral administration of self-antigens can induce organ-specific immune tolerance. After a double-blind pilot study with positive effects in subgroups,[36] a phase III trial was performed with oral cow myelin (Myloral), involving 515 individuals with RRMS at 14 centres. The results were presented at the 1997 ANA meeting, but this study failed to show that the treatment as administered could reduce the frequency of relapses, which was the primary endpoint. However, new trials using other doses or preparations of orally dispensed

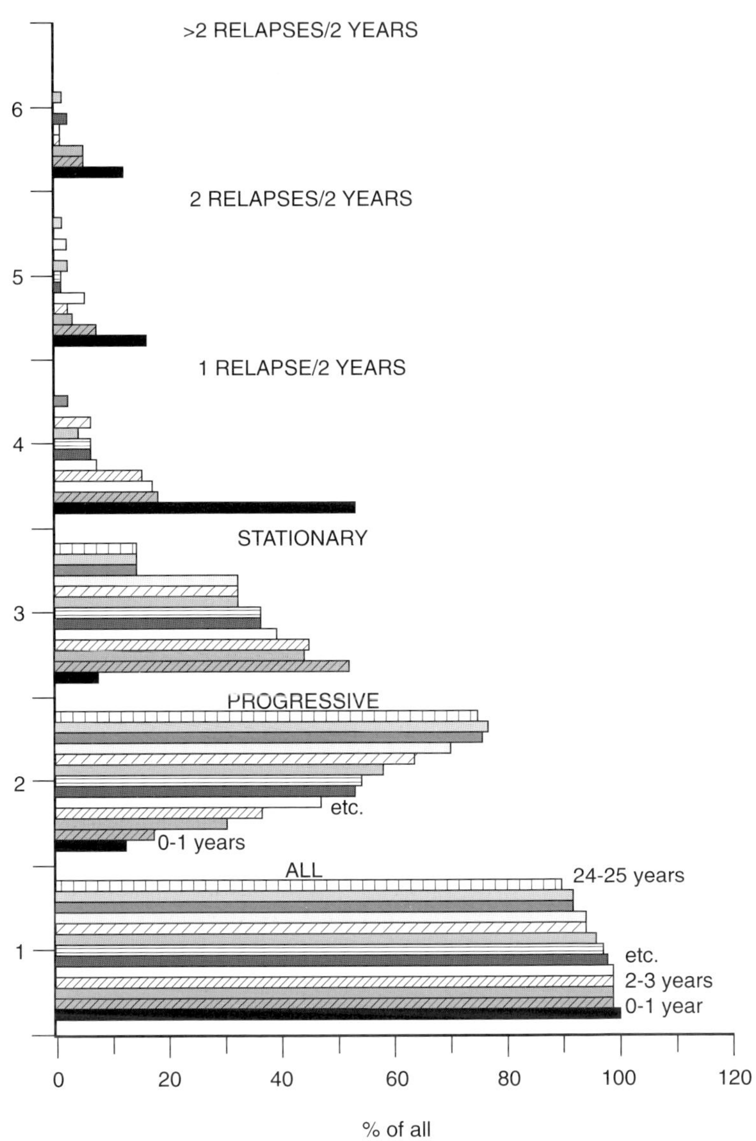

Figure 19.10 100 patients were selected from the Göteborg incidence cohort by an unbiased procedure. Each horizontal bar represents the number of patients surviving and having a particular type of course in a particular 2-year period after onset. The small reduction from year 0–1 to 24–25 in the group of bars named 'all' represents the mortality. The area in each type of course compared with the area in 'all' shows the proportion of MS patients in this representative material up to 25 years of follow-up having a particular type of course. The proportion of patients having two or more relapses per 2-year period is 5%.

myelin antigen are planned (Howard Weiner, personal communication).

The 'wait-and-see' option

Population-based studies reveal that a large proportion of MS cases are inactive. Authorities in Sweden and other countries recommend that the use of IFN-β in RRMS is restricted to patients who had two or more relapses and no progression during the previous 2 year period, thus conforming to the standard inclusion criteria used in three of the trials described in Table 19.1. However, only 5% of the MS population fulfil these criteria (Fig. 19.10, unpublished data from the Göteborg epidemiological database). Although 5% is strictly non-progressive, a number of bouts occur in the progressive phase. It is probably easier to diagnose a relapse than to verify an insiduous progression, and this may not least apply to patients in the complicated 'transition phase' between remitting and progressive course. The total proportion of patients with two or more relapses during the previous two-year period is less than 10%. However, this 10% limitation of indication for therapy means the time when medication is instituted. It is less defined when therapy should be terminated, and there is no doubt that therapy very often is continued during periods of, for example, stationary course where the institution of new therapy had not been indicated, thus increasing the proportion of the MS patients on treatment. None the less, many patients with very benign MS, including essentially stationary patients with intervals of several years between relapses, belong to a group that was never evaluated in a trial. Without any safe knowledge on long-term benefits and risks, continued observation without therapy is reasonable in a large proportion of benign MS patients.

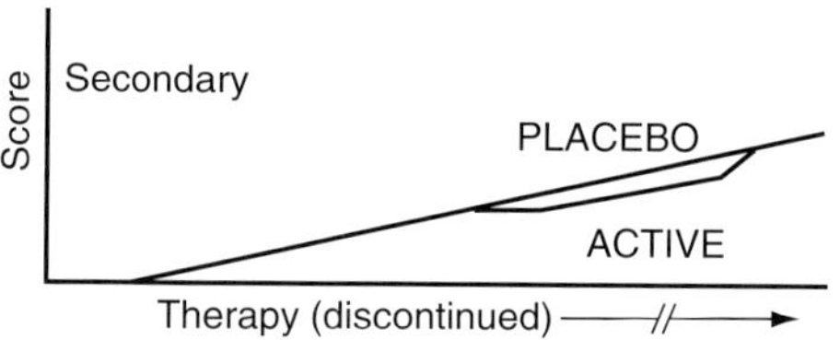

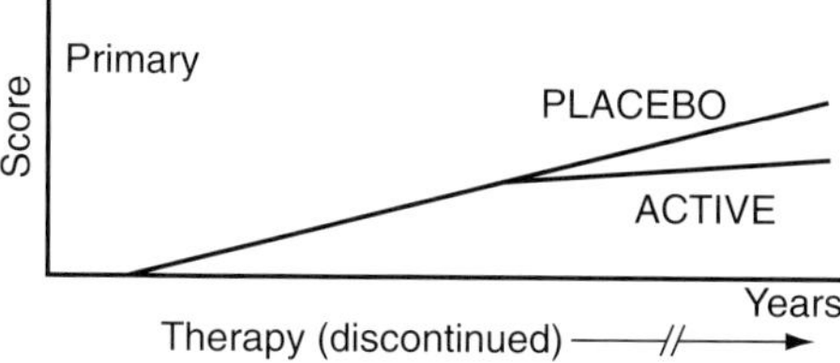

Figure 19.11 Theoretical outcome of intervention against a secondary or primary pathogenetic process, with different shapes of the deficit–time curve.

EXTENDING THERAPY OUTSIDE THE SHORT-TERM CONDITIONS OF THE PIVOTAL TRIALS?

The 'shape' of the treatment effect on the deficit–time curve

A question which will be more pertinent as more patients are being treated with IFN-β and Copaxone® is what 'shape' the treatment effect has, when expressing the MS-associated deficit as a function of time. In Fig. 19.11, one curve describes the deficit of patients receiving the active treatment, and another curve describes the untreated patients (ideally receiving placebo). The continued behaviour of the deviation of the treatment group from the placebo group (or the AUC) may reveal the nature of the therapeutic effect. Theoretically, a successful treatment of a secondary (e.g. inflammatory) phenomenon would produce an initial and sustained effect disappearing with the discontinuation of therapy, while a successful treatment of a primary pathogenetic process could elicit an increasing effect, sustained after discontinuation. Taking the data on MRI burden from the 5-year extension of the Betaseron® trial as an example (Fig. 19.12), it

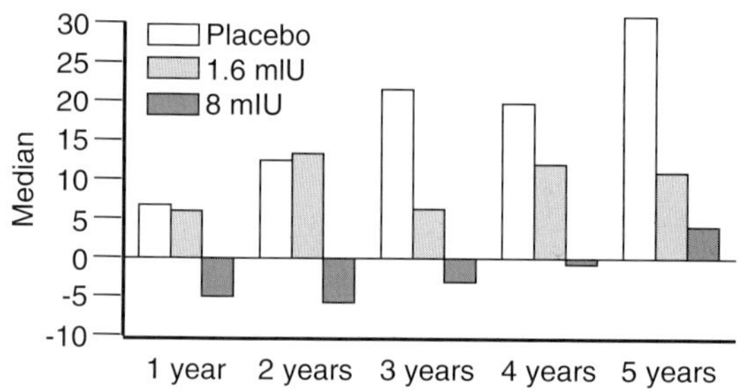

Figure 19.12 Cumulative MRI lesion burden median change after baseline, by treatment arm, in 217 patients having at least a fourth-year annual scan. Reproduced with kind permission.[37]

would not be unreasonable to consider this to be a set of curves of the 'primary' type, emphasizing the steady increase of MRI burden in the placebo group and the small changes in the high dose group.[37] However, there is also a tendency from the third year towards a parallel increase in the intervention groups after the initial treatment

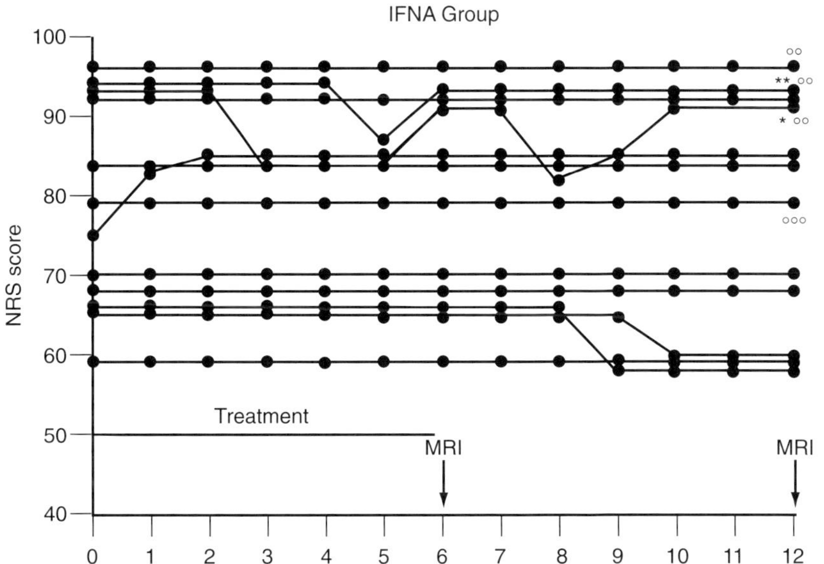

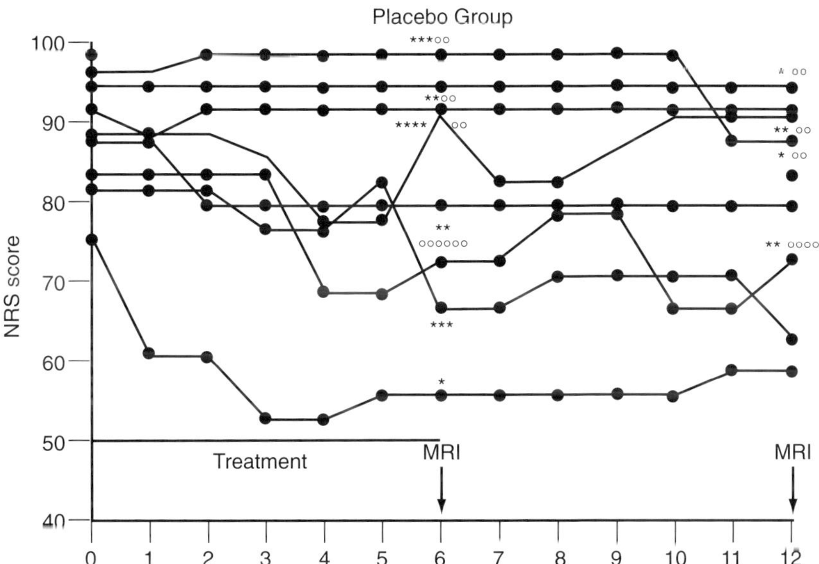

Figure 19.13 IFN-α treatment. Serial Scripps (NRS) scores and occurence of new (asterisk) or enlarging (circle) lesions at the 6-month MRI. Follow-up continued 6 months after treatment. Note, MRI rebound at 12 months. Reproduced with kind permission.[38]

effect. This cannot be settled at this stage, but there is a need for trial designs allowing groups of patients to be followed for extended periods, perhaps as very long-term cross-over studies. One immediately important side of this question is whether there will be a rebound of MS disease activity, and even of the degree of MS disability, when the treatment is terminated. There is a need for 'stop trials'. No IFN-β or Copaxone® trial was devoted to this issue, but the study of IFN-α in MS by Durelli et al. revealed a significant rebound of MRI activity and a tendency towards clinical deterioration when the IFN-α treatment was interrupted after 6 months (Fig. 19.13).[38]

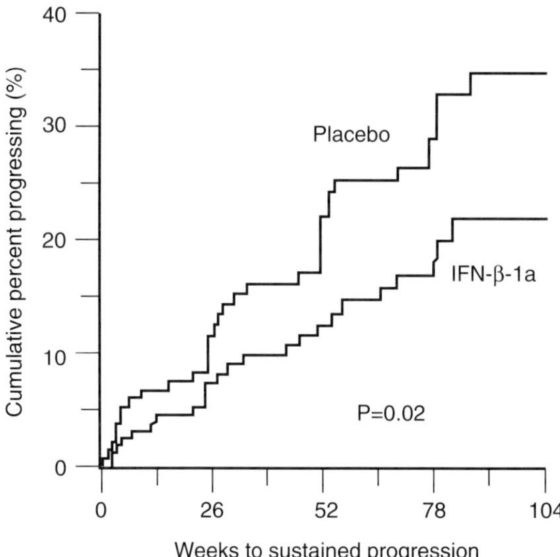

Figure 19.14 Kaplan–Meier failure–time curve showing the cumulative percent progressing according to number of weeks to beginning of sustained disability progression. Reproduced with kind permission.[3]

Signs of an 'initial and sustained' effect were distinctly observed and discussed in the IVIG study.[22] Tendencies to pursue this pattern can be found in many trials, for instance the IFN-α2a trial and the Rebif® trial in RRMS[4] where the effect on relapse frequency and the time to first exacerbation seemed to be larger during the first year. However, if IFN-β prevents the residuals after a few devastating bouts, this may justify prophylactic treatment of a larger number of patients.

The predictive value of the results in RRMS

A related issue is the predictive value of the therapeutic results obtained in RRMS, usually in the early stages of the disease. In the Avonex® trial the drug produced a significant delay in the time to a confirmed one-step progression in the EDSS (Fig. 19.14).[3] The delay of the 'sustained' progression mean was the main outcome of the Avonex® study. The proportion of subjects progressing, estimated from the Kaplan-Meier curves, was 34.9% for placebo recipients and 21.9% for IFN β-1a recipients (Fig. 19.14). The occurrence of sequele after early relapses is one major determinant for long-term disability. This was demonstrated by 25 year life-table analysis in the Göteborg incidence cohort: the occurrence of complete or incomplete remission after the onset relapse significantly influences the risk of being in a progressive course 25 years after onset. The curve suggests an initial and sustained effect (Fig. 19.15). The graph shows life-table analysis with the start of a progressive course as an endpoint. All probable and definite MS cases with relapse onset from the 15-year incidence cohort were included. Prognosis in patients with complete remission after first relapse was compared with those with incomplete remission. There is a better prognosis with complete remission after 15 years (p <0.01) and 25 years (p <0.05). This means that sequele after early relapses, which would be recorded as 'sustained' progression in the Avonex® study, could have important future consequences, much more than immediately appears from the

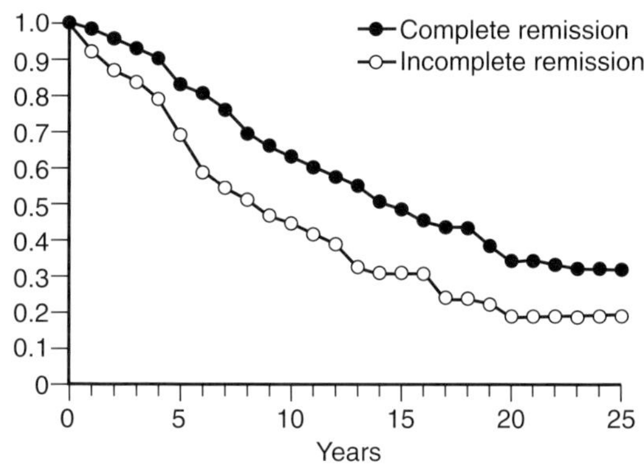

Figure 19.15 Impact of onset bout: chance for a non-progressive course after onset bout with complete or incomplete remission. Reproduced with kind permission.[44]

small increments recorded in EDSS. However, the life-table curves shown describes the natural course of MS.[38] It is not known whether the predicitive effect will be the same when the difference in initial events is a result of modification by therapy. The criterion for 'confirmed' progression was a sustained EDSS result at a further neurological examination after a 6 months interval. This could be due to:

1) relapses with slow or incomplete remission
2) sequele after relapses
3) insidious progression during the relapsing-remitting stage
4) new relapses.

The occurrence of a relapse increases the risk of a subsequent relapse after a short time interval, in other words: relapses tend to occur in groups.[39] Furthermore, some relapses are protracted, with new symptoms occurring during several weeks or months so frequent that no new relapse can be recorded according to the one month free interval criterium, but eventually remits. In the Göteborg incidence material, 220 such protracted or migrating relapses were recorded among 247 patients with relapse onset. The probability that a patient returns to baseline after one EDSS step progression according to this 6 months criterion will persist was approximately 11%.[40] The neuroanatomic details of the EDSS progression in the Avonex® study gives the impression that this sustained progression may have a stronger relationship to relapse phenomena than to genuine progression, as it mainly occurs in relapse-related systems (sensory, visual, brain stem), and to a lesser degree in pyramidal or cerebellar systems that are progression-related.[41]

The emergence of efficient therapies for MS—and more powerful statistics

Repeated measures and the area under the curve (AUC)

New statistical methods may be much more powerful to demonstrate a therapeutic effect. These include the repeated measures used in the Copaxone® study[3] and related methods using the AUC. One ingenious but simple method was proposed by Lance Blumhardt, Nottingham, UK for further evaluation of the Rebif® study results (the investigators made it clear that these methods were not in the trial protocol). The potential for more powerful analysis is evident from Fig. 19.16. Using a more powerful method makes good sense, as a means of securing valuable partial effects in small patient samples and evading troublesome problems of definition concerning type of course. One should bear in mind, however, that addition of the AUC may contribute to the quality of data if observations are added, but it may also make the significance level easily approachable in much the same way as using a one-sided test. Comparisons with reconstructions of the natural course of MS[33] suggest that the AUC produced by examinations at 3-month intervals exaggerates the effects of relapses. Reconstructions of the deficit curve during relapses make a much more slim and peaky outline (Fig. 19.17) than those obtained by the AUC polygon (Fig. 19.16). It was stated that little is gained by including more than around five pre- and postrandomization visits in a clinical trial.[42]

Number of methods and variant scales

A more basic and serious problem is the number of methods used. It is not always completely explained whether powerful methods such as the repeated measures were in the original trial protocol.[3] Definitions of steps in scoring systems may have the effect of increasing the quantity of change in the part of the scale where most patients are scored. In the design of the Avonex® study, the Kurtzke '3' was a slighter deficit (e.g. paraparesis 4/5 of muscle score, or loss of vibration up to the knee) than probably intuitively used by most clinical researchers. This was clearly defined before the trial[43] and may have had the effect of increasing the power of the evaluation. Sensitive and well-defined scoring systems like the regional functional scoring system (RFSS)[34]

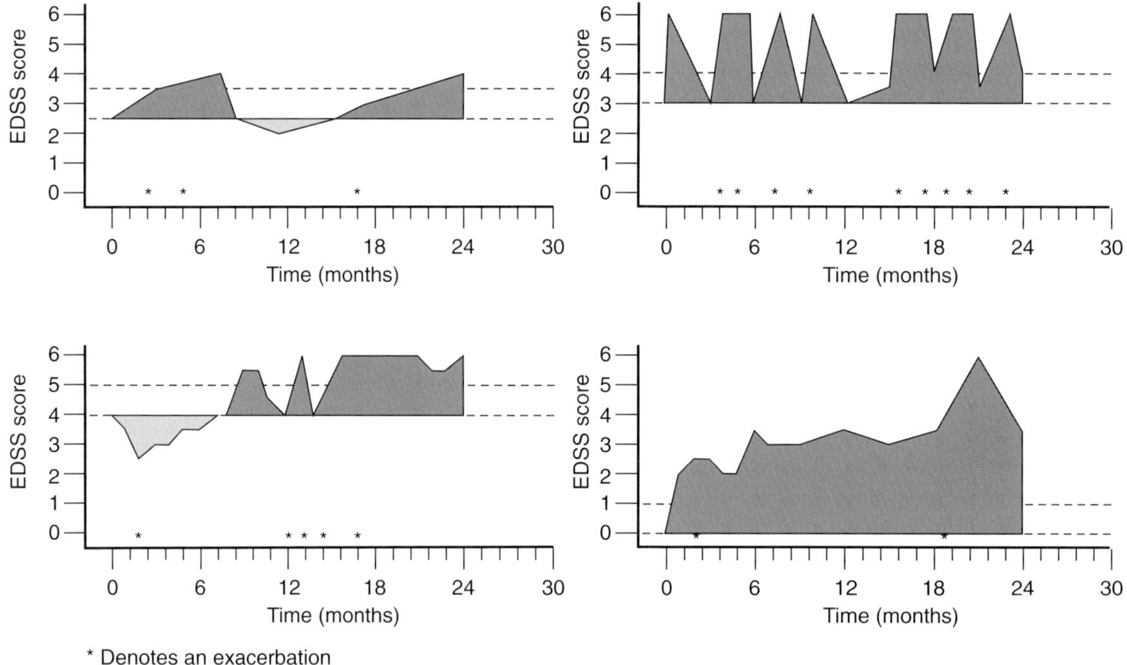

Figure 19.16 The integrated disability status score (IDSS) is simply the area under the curve (AUC) representing the EDSS as a function of time, with the EDSS at baseline corrected to be zero, IDSS in four MS patients.[1]

should be useful in phase I–II trials, tending to reduce variability and increase power. Recommendations of composite scores were given by a task force.[44] After the first report on the Avonex® study, a further analysis demonstrated that the capability of Avonex® to reduce the proportion of MS patients that progressed in their EDSS was at least as convincing and clinically meaningful when more stringent definitions for sustained progression were used (such as two or more EDSS steps, and sustained increase for 1 year).[41] While this survey certainly provides answers to many questions, showing that the significance obtained was largely independent of the details of the outcome parameters chosen, additional analysis will also add to the problem of multiple, mutually correlated methods. Some have contended that readers of scientific articles on trials should have the right to require the original trial protocol (and its amendments) simply by a number provided in the article.[45]

Other examples of variable definitions

Why use '3 months sustained' data to verify that progression occurred? From previous studies[40] it can be inferred that the 'not sustained' data are less informative than the '6 months sustained' data. The reasons for introducing '3 months sustained' data are not clear, but could be that 6 months sustained data were not available, or less straightforward to use when patients were examined at 3-month intervals. A very common situation where a statistical task force could be useful for standardization is the evaluation of the differences between two slopes (e.g. EDSS values

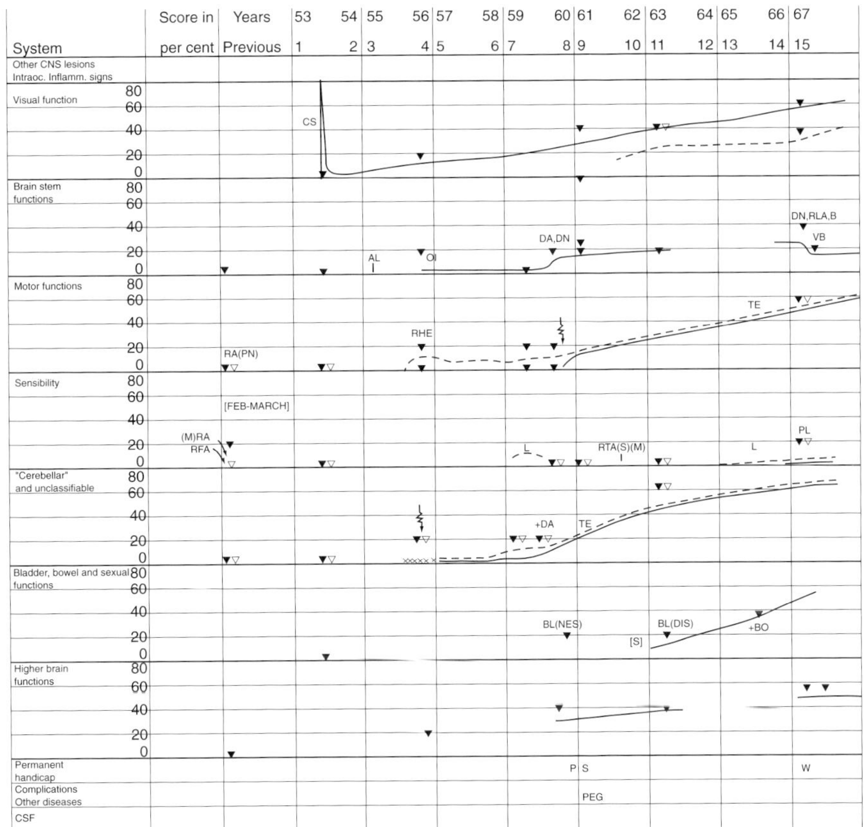

Figure 19.17 This graph is one of 308 reconstructions, one for each of the patients in the Göteborg incidence cohort, based upon complete neurological examinations (triangles) and intervening history, of the course in each of the 7 Kurtzke functional systems, divided into right and left side of the body where feasible. The numbers 0–80 for the rows is percentage of total RFSS deficit score in each system and side, and each column (1-2,3-4,...) represents 2 years. This and most other graphs suggest that the area under the curve is many times smaller in the RR phase than in the subsequent SP phase. Reproduced with kind permission.[34]

for the treated and placebo groups) in order to use more deficit data than the life-table methods, without confining the analysis to endpoint data. Possibilities include: group analysis (or 95% confidence intervals) between the groups at predetermined time points, including the end of the study; or regression analysis of slopes or group analysis of the regression coefficients of the individuals in the two groups. A statistical taskforce is needed for standardization.

Coding of adverse events

The coding is usually performed in a standardized way that may efface new characteristic side-effects. The consequence is that the frequency of typical side-effects in the active drug receivers does not stand out much against the frequency in the placebo receivers. For example, to retrieve the high frequency of myalgia, concentrated in the jaw region, in the linomide trial, original data had to be retrieved.[34] The IFN-β trials do not specifically account for the group of acute intermittent adverse effects that importantly occur rather constantly a certain time (a few hours) after the IFN-β injections. The spectrum of adverse events is large, from practically no side-effects to severe injection site reactions and general influenza like reactions including increased spasticity and paresis. In some patients, particularly in the progressive phase, these influenza-like reactions do not clear completely before the next injections (for agents dispensed at 2-day intervals). These side events abate after a few months in some patients, but in some they persist, unpredictably, and eventually lead to dose reduction or treatment discontinuation.

The trial as experiment

There may be one further reason for a critical analytical attitude. While there is consensus on the pathogenesis of MS in the very broadest sense—an immunological process in the CNS damaging myelin more than axons in genetically disposed individuals, and probably triggered by early viral infections—the essential antigens and chain of events are unknown. However, clinical trials are also scientific experiments as long as their methodology is solid enough to produce supportive evidence for or against their rationale. For instance, a number of trials with oral MBP that suppresses immunoreactivity against MBP, could ultimately control enough sources of error to evaluate the theory that MBP is an important antigen in MS. Therapeutic efficacy could become the ultimate proof of an aetiologic theory.

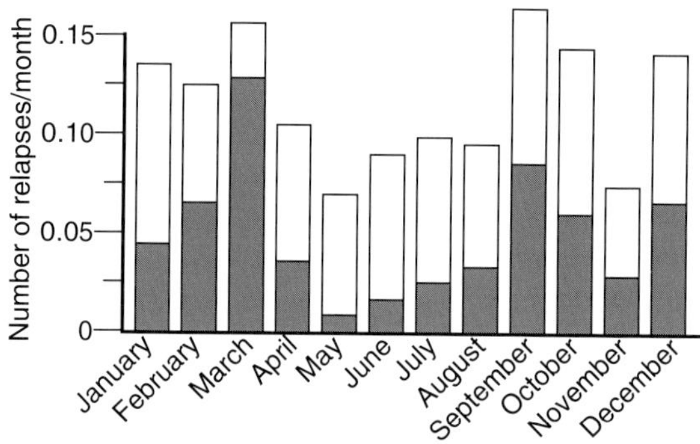

Figure 19.18 Total number of relapses (bars) and at risk (AR) relapses (shaded-area) per month using 7-week AR periods, showing the trough level during summer and more relapses during the winter. (□: NAR relapses; □: AR relapses, 7 weeks). Reproduced with kind permission.[47]

Further results on the presently 'proven' drugs will appear in the near future. Also, results from a number of phase I–II studies will appear

Systemic immunoactivation

The clinical effect of the new therapies is at best moderate, until now. Is the paradigm right? Probably, there needs to be a systemic immunoactivation to explain the initiation of the immune response in MS, and indeed its persistence (whereas the intrathecal immune response after other CNS lesions may be protracted but not life-long). The theory of molecular mimicry is still relevant, and new suspected viral agents have emerged.[46] Some trivial upper respiratory infections, including adenovirus, increase the risk for a subsequent relapse in manifest MS, with a maximum risk approximately 2 weeks after the infection, and thereby influence the periannual distribution of relapses (Fig. 19.18).[47] There are rationales for the involvement of some of the herpes viruses (HSV, EB and HHV-6) in MS. The antiviral agent acyclovir was used in a 2-year double-blind trial in 60 RRMS. The acyclovir receivers had 34% fewer exacerbations than the placebo receivers, but this result was not significant in the group analysis. A categorical analysis gave significantly positive results in the same material, but this was not predicted in the study protocol. A significantly positive effect was also found in a subgroup with at least 2 years of disease before the study (Fig. 19.19).[5,48] This study is presently followed by a two-centre trial of valaciclovir—which gives better tissue concentration than acyclovir—in 70 RRMS patients using monthly MRI. Results from this valaciclovir study are expected during 1998.

Ongoing trials

Tens of cited clinical trials in MS are ongoing. Many of these are phase I, others are closely related to the treatments described in the first section of this chapter, such as dose-finding studies, or studies in other types of course. For example, the first results of the large ongoing trials of IFN-β in the progressive phase of MS (Betaseron®, Rebif®, Avonex®) are expected during 1998–99. A more individualized dose of IFN-β is desirable, due to obvious individual

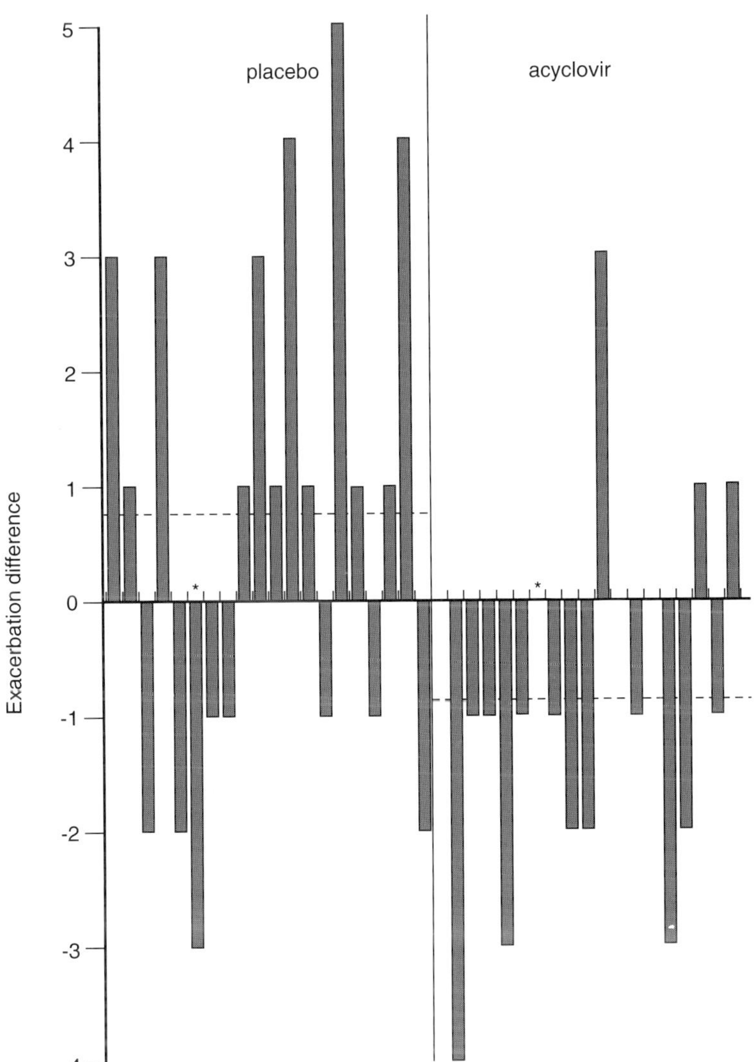

Figure 19.19 Exacerbation differences in MS patients between the 2 pre-study years and during the 2-year trial. A subgroup consisting of 20 placebo and 19 acyclovir patients, with a duration of MS of at least 2 years before entry, was selected. Positive bars indicate increased and negative bars indicate reduced number of exacerbations. Dotted lines indicate mean exacerbation differences per 2 years. Patients whose disease course changed to progressive during the study are indicated by an asterisk. Reproduced with kind permission.[48]

difference in sensibility, and corroborated by a large individual variability in the production of IFN-responsive proteins.[6,7,49,50] In recent phase II studies, IVIG treatment reduced the number of gadolinium enhancing MRI lesions[49] and reduced the exacerbation rate[50] in RRMS. No phase III study of IVIG was performed in RMSS. While Austrian insurance has accepted IVIG for MS, no application for IVIG was filed to the EMEA (F. Fazekas, personal communication). Also combination therapies are planned. The ERAZIMUS study, a French single centre study, evaluates the safety of the combination IFN-β1a with azathioprine.[51] If this is positive, a multicentre study is planned to compare this combination with IFN-β1a alone. A considerable number of cytokine and anticytokine therapies as well as T-cell/T-cell receptor vaccinations are in the pilot or phase I trial stage. A monoclonal anti-CD4 antibody was used in a double-blind phase II trial in 71 RRMS and SPMS cases, but was not able to reduce MS activity as measured by the number of active lesions in monthly Gd-enhanced MRI during 9 months, and a statistically significant reduction in relapse rate was not considered reliable by the authors due to physician unblinding.[53] The potential for new therapies based on proliferating immunological knowledge are described elsewhere in this book.

CONCLUSION

Currently there is no high quality evidence that any drug is equivalent to the IFNs or Copaxone® in the treatment of selected RRMS patients. The essential point is that IFN-β is capable of preventing future relapses, particularly severe relapses. Unfortunately, trials did not specifically examine whether treatment prevents residuals from disastrous relapses using long-term predictors, controlled trials of IFN-β or Copaxone® in RRMS regarding the risk of transition to the progressive phase should be feasible. Far from all RRMS patients fulfil the relapse rate criteria for IFN-β therapy used in the large trials and by national authorities. While many RRMS patients will probably hesitate to continue therapy once started during subsequently long latent intervals the efficacy of IFN-β in benign cases with sporadic activity remains to be established. Probably the 'wait-and-see' option should be preferred in periods of latency. The issue of placebo is complicated and depends on the relative toxicity of the drugs to be tested, but it could be argued that RRMS patients with low or moderate disease activity should still be eligible for placebo-controlled trials.

REFERENCES

1. PRISMS (Prevention of Relapses and Disability by Interferon beta-1a Subcutaneously in Multiple Sclerosis) Study Group. Randomized double-blind placebo-controlled study of IFN-β1a in relapsing–remitting Multiple Sclerosis. *Lancet* 1998; **52**: 1408–1504.
2. The IFNB Multiple Sclerosis Study Group. Interferon beta-1b is effective in relapsing–remitting multiple sclerosis, 1. *Neurology* 1993; **43**: 655–661.
3. Jacobs LD, Cookfair DL, Rudrick RA et al. Intramuscular interferon beta-1a for disease progression in relapsing multiple sclerosis. *Ann Neurol* 1996; **39**: 285–294.
4. Johnson KP, Brooks BR, Cohen JA et al. Copolymer 1 reduces relapse rate and improves disability in relapsing–remitting multiple sclerosis: results of a phase 3 multicenter, double-blind, placebo-controlled trial. *Neurology* 1995; **45**: 1268–1276.
5. Runkel L, Meier W, Pepinsky B et al. Structural analysis of human interferon beta (IFN-beta): studies addressing the activity differences between IFN-beta-1-a and IFN-beta-1b. *Multiple Sclerosis* 1997; **3(5)**: 337.
6. Witt PL. Pharmacokinetics of interferon-beta and the biological markers it induces. In: Reder AT, ed. *Interferon Therapy of Multiple Sclerosis*. New York: Marcel Dekker, 1997: 77–93.
7. Munafo A, Trinchard-Lugan I, Nguyen T et al. Comparative pharmacokinetics and pharmacodynamics of recombinant human interferon β-1a after intramuscular and subcutaneous administration. *Eur J Neurol* 1998; **5**: 187–193.
8. Alam J, McAllister A, Scarmamucci J et al. Pharmacokinetics and pharmacodynamics of interferon β-1a (IFN-β1a) in healthy volunteers after intravenous, subcutaneous or intramuscular administration. *Clin Drug Invest* 1997; **14**: 35–43.
9. Von Wussow P, Jakschies D, Freund M et al. Treatment of anti-recombinant interferon-alpha 2 antibody positive CML patients with natural interferon-alpha. *Br J Haematol* 1991; **78**: 210–216.
10. Schellekens H, Ryff J, van der Meide P. Assays for antibodies to human interferon-alpha: the need for standardization. *J Interferon Cytokine Res* 1997; **17 (suppl 1)**: S5–S8.
11. The IFNB Multiple Sclerosis Study Group. Neutralizing antibodies during treatment of multiple sclerosis with interferon beta-1b: experience during the first three years. *Neurology* 1996; **47**: 889–894.
12. Petkar J, White R. Neutralizing antibodies and the efficacy of interferon beta-1b in relapsing–remitting multiple sclerosis. *Mult Scler* 1997; **3**: 402.
13. Rice GP. The evolution of neutralizing antibodies in patients taking beta interferon 1b. *Multiple Sclerosis* 1997; **3 (5)**: 344.
14. Knobler R, Greenstein J, Johnson K et al. Systemic recombinant human interferon-beta treatment of relapsing–remitting multiple sclerosis: pilot study

analysis and six-year follow-up. *J Interferon Res* 1993; **13**: 333–340.

15. Johnson K, Brooks B, Cohen J et al. Extended use of glatiramer acetate (Copaxone) is well tolerated and maintains its clinical effect on multiple sclerosis relapse rate and degree of disability. *Neurology* 1998; **50**: 701–708.
16. Confavreux C, Saddier P, Grimaud J et al. Risk of cancer from azathioprine therapy in multiple sclerosis: a case-control study. *Neurology* 1996; **46**: 1607–1612.
17. British and Dutch Multiple Sclerosis Azathioprine Trial Group. Double-masked trial of azathioprine in multiple sclerosis. *Lancet* 1988; **2**: 179–183.
18. Yudkin PL, Ellison GW, Ghezzi A et al. Overview of azathioprine treatment in multiple sclerosis. *Lancet* 1991; **338**: 1051–1055.
19. Palace J, Rothwell P. New treatments and azathioprine in multiple sclerosis. *Lancet* 1997; **350**: 261.
20. Soelberg Sørensen P, Wanscher B, Schreiber K et al. A double-blind, cross-over trial of intravenous immunoglobulin G in multiple sclerosis: preliminary results. *Multiple Sclerosis* 1997; **3**: 145–148.
21. Fazekas F, Deisenhammer F, Strasser-Fuchs S et al. Randomised placebo-controlled trial of monthly intravenous immunoglobulin therapy in relapsing–remitting multiple sclerosis. *Lancet* 1997; **349**: 589–593.
22. Fazekas F, Deisenhammer F, Strasser-Fuchs S et al. Treatment effects of monthly intravenous immunoglobulin on patients with relapsing–remitting multiple sclerosis: further analyses of the Austrian immunoglobulin in MS study. *Multiple Sclerosis* 1997; **3**: 137–141.
23. Edan G, Miller D, Clanet M et al. Therapeutic effect of mitoxantrone combined with methylprednisolone in multiple sclerosis: a randomised multicentre study of active disease using MRI and clinical criteria. *J Neurol Neurosurg Psychiatry* 1977; **62**. 112–118.
24. Gonsette R. Mitoxanthrone immunotherapy in multiple sclerosis. *Mult Scler* 1996; **3**: 269.
25. Millefiorini E, Gasperini C, Pozzilli C et al. Randomized, placebo-controlled trial of mitoxantrone in relapsing–remitting multiple sclerosis: 24-month clinical and MRI outcome. *J Neurol* 1997, **244**. 153–159.
26. Milligan NM, Newcome R, Compston DAS. A double-blind controlled trial of high dose methylprednisolone in patients with multiple sclerosis: 1. Clinical effects. *J Neurol Neurosurg Psychiatry* 1987; **50**: 511–516.
27. Runmarker B, Andersen O. Prognostic factors in a multiple sclerosis incidence cohort with twenty-five years of follow-up. *Brain* 1993; **116**: 117–134.
28. Beck EW, Cleary PA, Anderson MM et al. A randomized, controlled trial of corticosteroids in the treatment of acute optic neuritis. *New Engl J Med* 1992; **326**: 581–588.
29. Beck RW, Trobe JD. The optic neuritis treatment trial. Putting the results in perspective. *J Neuro-Ophthalmol* 1995; **15**: 131–135.
30. Barnes D, Hughes R, Morris R et al. Randomized trial of oral and intravenous methylprednisolone in acute relapses of multiple sclerosis. *Lancet* 1997; **349**: 902–906.
31. Bosco A, Cazzato G, Antonello RM et al. Recurrent high doses of methylprednisolone in patients with RRMS. 3 years follow-up. *Multiple Sclerosis* 1997; **3(5)**: 352.
32. Stelmasiak Z, Solski J, Nowicki J et al. Cladribine (2-CDA) in treatment of remitting–relapsing multiple sclerosis: 2 year double-blind crossover placebo-controlled study. *Multiple Sclerosis* 1997; **3(5)**: 348.
33. Dighiero G. Adverse and beneficial immunological effects of purine nucleoside analogues. *Hematol Cell Ther* 1996; **38 (suppl 2)**: S75–S81.
34. Andersen O, Lycke J, Tollesson PO et al. Linomide reduces the rate of active lesions in relapsing–remitting multiple sclerosis. *Neurology* 1996; **47**: 895–900.
35. Karussis DM, Meiner Z, Lehmann D et al. Treatment of secondary progressive multiple sclerosis with the immunomodulator linomide: a double blind, placebo-controlled pilot study with monthly magnetic resonance imaging evolution. *Neurology* 1996; **47**: 341–346.
36. Weiner HL, Mackin GA, Matsui M et al. Double-blind pilot trial of oral tolerization with myelin antigens in multiple sclerosis. *Science* 1993; **259**: 1321–1324.
37. The IFNB Multiple Sclerosis Study Group, The University of British Columbia MS/MRI analysis group. Interferon beta-1b in the treatment of multiple sclerosis: final outcome of the randomized controlled trial. *Neurology* 1995; **45**: 1277–1285.
38. Durelli L, Bongioanni MR, Ferrero B et al. Interferon alpha-2a treatment of relapsing–remitting multiple sclerosis: disease activity resumes

after stopping treatment. *Neurology* 1996; **47**: 123–129.

39. Andersen O. Restricted dissemination of clinically defined attacks in an MS incidence material. *Acta Neurol Scand* 1980; **62 (suppl 77)**: 34–41.
40. Ellison GW, Myers LW, Leake BD et al. Design strategies in multiple sclerosis clinical trials. *Ann Neurol* 1994; **36**: S108–S112.
41. Rudick R, Goodkin D, Jacobs L et al. Impact of interferon beta-1a on neurologic disability in relapsing multiple sclerosis. *Neurology* 1997; **49**: 358–363.
42. Ogenstad S. Analysis and design of repeated measures in clinical trials using summary statistics. *J Biopharm Stat* 1997; **7(4)**: 593–604.
43. Jacobs L, Cookfair D, Rudick R et al. A phase III trial of intramuscular recombinant interferon beta as treatment for exacerbating–remitting multiple sclerosis: design and conduct of study and baseline characteristics of patients. *Multiple Sclerosis* 1995; **1**: 118–135.
44. Rudick R, Antel J, Confavreux C et al. Recommendations from the National Sclerosis Society Clinical Outcomes Assessment Task Force. *Ann Neurol* 1997; **42**: 379–382.
45. Mulrow R. Rationale for systemic reviews. *BMJ* 1994; **309**: 597–599.
46. Steinman L, Oldstone MB. More mayhem from molecular mimics. *Nat Med* 1997; **3**: 1321–1322.
47. Andersen O, Lygner P-E, Bergström T et al. Viral infections trigger multiple sclerosis relapses: a prospective seroepidemiological study. *J Neurol* 1993; **240**: 417–422.
48. Lycke J, Svennerholm B, Hjelmqvist E et al. Acyclovir treatment of relapsing–remitting multiple sclerosis. A randomized, placebo-controlled, double-blind study. *J Neurol* 1996; **243**: 214–224.
49. Sorensen PS, Wauscher B, Jensen CV et al. Intravenous immunoglobulin G reduces MRI activity in relapsing multiple sclerosis. *Neurology* 1998; **50**: 1273–1281.
50. Achiron A, Gabbay U, Gilad R et al. Intravenous immunoglobulin treatment in multiple sclerosis. Effect on relapses. *Neurology* 1998; **50**: 398–402.
51. Moreau T, Blanc S, Grimaud J et al. ERAZIMUS: early azathioprine versus interferon in multiple sclerosis. *Multiple Sclerosis* 1997; **3(5)**: 339.
52. Van Oosten B, Lai M, Hodgkinson S et al. Treatment of multiple sclerosis with the monoclonal anti-CD4 antibody cM-T412. *Neurology* 1997; **49**: 351–357.

20

How to treat progressive multiple sclerosis

Dimitrios M Karussis and Oded Abramsky

INTRODUCTION

Multiple sclerosis (MS) is a chronic inflammatory disease of the central nervous system (CNS) characterized histologically by focal lymphocyte and macrophage infiltrates and demyelination and, clinically, by multifocal neurological signs.[1,2] The disease follows a relapsing and remitting or a chronic progressive course. In 50% of the patients the initial relapsing disease reverts to a secondary progressive one. However, in about 11–18% of the MS patients, a progressive course is seen from the onset of the disease, without any clear remission periods.[3–5] This form of MS is defined as, primary progressive (PP) and differs from secondary progressive (SP) in various aspects: (a) its clinical onset usually appears at a later age than in SP[3,6] and there is less—if any—female predominance;[4,7] (b) it more frequently involves the spinal cord (chronic myelopathy) and less often the visual tract or cognitive functions;[8] (c) it is less 'inflammatory', as shown in pathological studies;[9] and (d) it exhibits less 'activity' in the magnetic resonance imaging (MRI) (less new gadolinium (Gd-DTPA)-enhancing lesions)[10–15] (Table 20.1). Furthermore, data from our laboratory, as well as previous studies, indicate that a human leukocyte antigen (HLA) profile different from that in relapsing disease may be associated with the PP type of MS.[16–19] Some investigators have suggested that PP disease has a distinct immunopathogenesis and,

Table 20.1 Differences between primary and secondary progressive MS

Primary progressive	Secondary progressive
(1) Later age of onset	(1) Earlier age of onset
(2) No female predominance	(2) Female predominance
(3) More chronic myelopathy; less cognitive impairment	(3) More cognitive impairment
(4) Less active lesions in MRI	(4) More active lesions in MRI
(5) Less immunologic (less inflammatory lesions in pathology)	(5) More immunological activity
(6) HLA: DQB1, DR4	(6) HLA: DR2

therefore, in most of the recent clinical trials, patients with PPMS, were excluded.

Extensive studies have been performed in the last 20 years in an effort to elucidate the immunopathogenetic mechanisms involved in MS. It is now widely accepted that the putative autoimmune (immune-mediated) process in MS is initiated in the peripheral immune system. Following activation by macrophages/antigen-presenting cells (APCs), lymphocytes, mainly of the helper (CD4)-subtype, expressing myelin antigens-specific T-cell receptor (TCR), proliferate and begin to express on their surface, adhesion molecules/markers of activation, which help them to extravasate the vessel endothelium and reach the site of inflammation in the CNS.[20–28] Following clonal expansion, T-helper (Th) cells differentiate, becoming either Th1 helpers that provide help to cytotoxic or CD4 T cells (positive feedback), producing interleukin (IL)-2, IL-12, tumor necrosis factor (TNF)-α and IFN-γ (pro-inflammatory cytokines), or Th2 helpers which assist mainly B-cells and secrete IL-4, IL-6 and IL-10.[29–33] The lymphocytes involved in the inflammatory process in MS brain lesions are predominantly of the Th1 phenotype.

In acute MS plaques, activated T cells secreting regulatory cytokines (mainly of the Th1 subtype) and expressing growth factor receptors for IL-2, as well as activated class II major histocompatibility complex (MHC) positive macrophages, are present. There are two main explanations for the CNS inflammation: the white matter (possibly the oligodendrocytes that produce myelin) is infected by a virus or other infectious agent against which the infiltrating cells are targeted. Alternatively, the infiltrating cells are primarily of an autoimmune nature and attack normal myelin proteins, such as myelin basic protein (MBP), proteolipid protein (PLP), or membrane oligodendrocyte glycoprotein (MOG). Although either hypothesis reasonable, it appears more conceivable that the role of any putative infectious agent is to trigger/drive the autoimmune process, rather than to serve as the primary target of infiltrating cells.

Experimental autoimmune encephalomyelitis (EAE) is an animal model for immune-mediated demyelination. It is induced by injecting whole spinal cord homogenate or the myelin proteins MBP and PLP. The pathologic picture of EAE, especially in the chronic relapsing form, is very similar to MS. EAE is mediated by T cells, mainly of the CD4 phenotype, that react to myelin proteins.[34–50] Although it is arguable whether EAE is a good model for MS, owing to their immunologic and pathologic similarities EAE is widely used in the investigation of various treatments for MS.

Based on the immunological model for the pathogenesis of MS, therapeutic approaches to control the progression of the disease imply anti-inflammatory, immunosuppressive and immunomodulating treatments, aimed to suppress the immune-mediated process. However, although significant progress has been made in recent years in the treatment of relapsing–remitting MS and several immunomodulating treatments have been introduced (Betaseron, Avonex, Copaxone), results with such treatments in progressive MS are either not satisfactory or pending. Unfortunately, in most of the clinical trials in progressive MS, no distinction was made between primary and secondary progressive patients and this further complicates interpretation of the results. In this review we classify and described the various groups of immunotherapeutic approaches, focusing on their efficacy in progressive disease.

ANTI-INFLAMMATORY DRUGS

The most widely used treatment, especially during an acute relapse of MS, is *methylprednisolone or other corticosteroid preparations*.[51-59] Steroids have various effects on the immune system, such as inhibition of immune activation and T-cell proliferation,[51] reduction of antibody production and of adhesion molecule expression. Most importantly, intravenously administered steroids appear to reduce the permeability of the blood–brain barrier[52,53] as evidenced by the reduction in Gd-DTPA enhancement of acute lesions in the MRI. However, this effect is short-lived and new enhancing lesions reappear within weeks following treatment with steroids.[52] Results from the National Cooperative ACTH study, revealed that adrenocorticotropin hormone (ACTH) may hasten recovery at 1 month after treatment.[56] Other studies have shown comparable or superior results with methylprednisolone.[54,55,57] More recent data from the Optic Neuritis Treatment Trial, show that intravenous methylprednisolone is superior to oral prednisone for the treatment of acute optic neuritis.[58,59] However, the long-term effect or both treatment regimens on the visual acuity was marginal and there was no significant 'protection' against later development of definite MS.[58,59] In one study, in patients with primary progressive MS, treatment with high dose intravenous (i.v.) methylprednisolone, followed by oral (p.o.) prednisone, induced a statistically significant clinical improvement, as evidenced in a 3-month follow-up period.[60] Short-term improvement with high dose methylprednisolone in PPMS, was also reported in another trial.[61] However, both studies stressed that these effects were short-lived; even repeated i.v. infusions of methylprednisolone failed to inhibit disease progression in another study.[62] This indicates that although steroids may exert a transient beneficial effect, they do not significantly alter the natural history of the disease. Therefore, the extensive use of steroids in progressive MS does not appear to be justified. Moreover, chronic steroid administration may induce several adverse effects, like osteoporosis, aseptic bone necrosis, hypertension, hyperglycaemia, cataracts and psychotic events.

IMMUNOSUPPRESSIVE TREATMENTS

Cytotoxic/cytostatic drugs

As for other autoimmune diseases, the conventional therapeutic strategies used to control chronic MS are based on immunosuppressive modalities aimed at reducing the proliferation of autoreactive lymphocytes.[63–67] However, most of the immunosuppressive treatments have only shown moderate efficacy in halting the progression of the disease (Table 20.2). In addition, they are usually associated with cumulative and toxic side-effects.[68,69]

Table 20.2 Efficacy of immunosuppressive drugs in progressive MS

Drug	Clinical effect	MRI effect
Azathioprine	+	?/+*
Cyclophosphamide	+	?
Cyclosporine-A	+	–
Mitoxantrone	–/+/++*	–/++/+++*
Cladribine	++/–*	+++*
Methotrexate	+	+
Deoxypergualin	–	–

?: no data; +: mild efficacy; ++: moderate efficacy; +++: strong efficacy; –: no efficacy.
*Variable results in different studies (see text).

Several immunosuppressive (cytotoxic or cytostatic) drugs have been tried in the last decade, but with only marginal efficacy. Azathioprine, an antimetabolite with broad spectrum immunosuppressive effects, was tested in several clinical trials.[65,70–75] In the largest controlled trial,[74] it was shown to reduce the rate of progression during a 3-year follow-up period; in this study, the worsening in the expanded disability status scale (EDSS) score was 0.62 in the azathioprine group as compared with 0.80 in the placebo-treated patients. A meta-analysis of the seven randomized controlled blinded trials with azathioprine, showed a mild beneficial effect (reduction in the worsening of EDSS score by 0.22 points)[76] after 2 years of treatment. In all the above trials patients with both relapsing and progressive disease were included, and this may further complicate interpretation of the results. Moreover, no study has tested the efficacy of azathioprine treatment in prevention of MRI activity. A more recent small single-blind trial showed some efficacy of azathioprine in combination with plasmapheresis, in inhibiting the activity of the disease, in SPMS patients, as reflected in the reduced lesion load in the MRI follow-up.[77] However, there was no detectable effect on the Gd-DTPA-enhancing lesions.

Cyclophosphamide, an alkylating agent, was also tested in several studies.[78–85] The Northeastern Cooperative Treatment Group reported a benefit from cyclophosphamide 'boosters'. However, the difference in stabilization rates (38 vs. 24% in 24 months) was small and disappeared by 36 months.[85] MRI data were not available in this trial. On the other hand, the Canadian Cooperative Multiple Sclerosis Study failed to show any beneficial effect of cyclophosphamide on disease progression rate.[81] In the same study, plasmapheresis also did not reveal any beneficial effect on MS. Therefore, the use of cyclophosphamide for the treatment of progressive MS has remained controversial.

Methotrexate, an antimetabolite, was recently reported to have a mild beneficial effect at a low dose, on the progression of disability in patients with chronic progressive MS, as revealed by the nonconventional '9-hole test' for dexterity of the upper extremities.[86] However, the effect of this treatment was less pronounced when changes in EDSS score and Ambulation Index were used as outcomes.[86] The effect of methotrexate on the MRI activity was also marginal.[87] Another trial with methotrexate[88] showed some reduction in the relapse rate but no benefit in patients with progressive disease.

Cyclosporine-A was studied in a multicentre double-blind clinical trial involving 547 patients with chronic progressive MS[89] and was found to mildly reduce the progression rate and to delay the 'wheelchair-bound' state. However, the high rate of hypertension and impaired renal function resulting from this treatment limits its use.[68] Recently reported MRI data from 163 patients from the MS study group treated with cyclosporine, failed to show any effect of this treatment in reducing total lesion load (burden of disease) during 2-years of treatment.[90]

Another immunosuppressive agent, cladribine, has shown some promising results in progressive MS patients,[91,92] but these remain to be confirmed by a recently completed phase III trial. Preliminary data from this study show only a marginal clinical effect (partially owing to the low progression rate in the control group—which included both primary and secondary progressive patients), but an impressive effect on the MRI activity, with a considerable inhibition of the Gd-DTPA-enhancing lesions.[93]

The cytostatic agent mitoxantrone (at a low dose) was tested in a randomized double-blinded placebo-controlled, multicentre trial, on 25 patients with relapsing–remitting MS. The results showed a mild reduction in relapse rate, but there was no effect on disability status. Serial Gd-DTPA-enhanced MRI did not reveal any significant difference between the mitoxantrone-treated and placebo groups.[94] In another, open, study, 10 MS patients with a rapid deteriorating/progressive disease profile, were treated with 12 mg/m^2 mitoxantrone, administered every 3 months. In all treated patients deterioration was halted following the initial dosage and eight out of nine patients showed improvement after 1 year compared to their enrolment status. The MRI results from this study were more significant: at admission, this group of patients presented with a total of 169 Gd-DTPA-enhancing lesions, whereas only 10 enhancing lesions were detected in nine patients 12 months after initiation of treatment.[95,96] However, another open trial with mitoxantrone (8 mg/m^2 every 3 weeks) failed to show any significant clinical or MRI effect in patients with progressive MS.[97] In a more recent study,[98] 42 patients with very active disease according to clinical and MRI criteria were treated with a higher dose of mitoxantrone (20 mg i.v. monthly) in combination with methylprednisolone (1 g i.v. monthly) or methylprednisolone alone over 6 months. Analysis of the MRI data revealed significantly more patients with no new enhancing lesions in the mitoxantrone group, compared with the number in the steroid alone group. In the mitoxantrone-treated group there was a month by month decrease, in the number of new enhancing lesions, and in the total number of enhancing lesions, whereas both remained high in the steroid alone group. There was also a significant clinical effect, but the assessments were performed in this trial in an unblinded way.[98]

All of the above-mentioned immunosuppressive treatments are associated with considerable side-effects, mainly owing to the induction of bone marrow suppression, resulting in greater risk of infections and thrombocytopenia and development of malignancies. Therefore, in light of their marginal efficacy (Table 20.2), caution should be practiced in their application to MS.

Other immunosuppressive modalities

Total lymphoid irradiation (TLI), a radical immunosuppressive modality, was previously reported to inhibit the progression of MS.[99] However, a more recent trial conducted by the same group showed that only the combination of TLI with steroids had some beneficial effect, preventing the rate of deterioration in progressive MS.[99] This treatment is associated with substantial risk owing to the extensive immunosuppression it engenders. Low dose *total body irradiation* (TBI) was shown in one study to prevent progression of disability for 1 and 2 years, as compared with sham irradiation.[100] However this trial was small and no data were provided for the inhibition of MRI activity.

Treatment of progressive MS with the humanized monoclonal antibody CAMPATH-1H (anti-CDw52) was also evaluated to assess the effect of systemic lymphocyte depletion on disease activity. Seven patients received a 10-day i.v. course of CAMPATH-1H, and indications for the efficacy of the treatment were obtained by MRI follow-up. The difference in lesion incidence rate before and after treatment varied and the rate ratio was significantly reduced in only three patients.[101] Such treatment is associated with the risk of generalized immunosuppression. In addition, the first infusion of the antibodies induced a significant exacerbation or reawakening of pre-existing symptoms, lasting for several hours, due to elevated levels of TNF-α and interferon (IFN)-γ.[102]

Treatment with the anti-CD3 antibody Muromonab-CD3 (Orthoclone OKT3) in an open trial[103] including 16 patients with progressive MS induced acute severe T-cytopenia in all of them. At the conclusion of follow-up, only four patients had deteriorated by 1.0 or more points according to the EDSS scale (73% stabilization rate) and no new MRI activity was detected in the treated patients. Side-effects were common and severe, and included hypotension, nausea and vomiting, diarrhoea, fever, and myalgia. The attendant toxicity of OKT3 makes it unlikely that it will play a major role in the treatment of MS.

In another open trial, 21 patients with active MS (16 with progressive and 5 with relapsing course) were treated with murine monoclonal anti-T CD4/BF5 antibodies. Tolerance was relatively good. Nine months after initiation of treatment, no relapse had occurred in any of the five patients with the recurrent form and improvement was observed in three patients with the progressive form. At the end of the treatment period, there was a clear drop in the number of CD3+ cells and particularly in CD4+ cells. All the patients who had side-effects had an increased level of serum IL-6 and TNF-α. These findings demonstrate that this type of long-term treatment is feasible in patients with MS, but larger controlled studies should be performed to access the efficacy of such treatment.[104]

An even more radical approach to the treatment of progressive MS is autologous bone marrow transplantation (BMT). Based on results from EAE, where syngeneic BMT was able to reverse the paralytic signs and to induce long-term tolerance[105–108] such treatment protocols have been applied in patients with severely progressive MS.[109] In this study, peripheral blood stem cells (PSC) instead of bone marrow cells were used as a source of multipotential immune progenitors. The EDSS score of patients treated according to this protocol improved significantly and no major toxicity was observed. Recently, a committee was established in Europe for the evaluation of BMT or PSC treatment in several autoimmune diseases. Preliminary results in patients with systemic lupus erythematosus (SLE) and rheumatoid arthritis seem to be very promising. However, due to the radical immunosuppressive conditioning protocols used, such treatment is still highly risky for most MS patients.

The use of immunosuppressive treatments that mainly affect antibody production, like *plasmapheresis*, is also controversial. Two controlled studies failed to reveal any efficacy of plasmapheresis.[81,110] and a meta-analysis of the studies with plasma-exchange in the literature did not show any beneficial effect of this modality in chronic progressive MS.[111]

IMMUNOMODULATORY APPROACHES

Due to the limited efficacy of the immunosuppressive modalities in MS, the focus of research over recent years has been targeted towards the development of treatments that do not induce generalized suppression of the immune cells, but rather specific downregulation of potentially harmful cells and a parallel upregulation of naturally existing suppressor cells, i.e. immunomodulation.

This approach has been strengthened by recent studies advocating the importance of immune networks for the preservation of an intact 'self', which have provided a new insight into the pathogenesis of autoimmune diseases. According to these theories autoreactive cells and antibodies present, even in healthy individuals, are prevented from inducing autoimmunity by downregulatory circuits.[112,113] Disruption of these delicate balances, or defects in the normal immunoregulatory mechanisms, may be involved in the pathogenesis of autoimmunity. Several reports of defective natural killer (NK) cell activity and reduced proportions of suppressor or suppressor-inducer cells in patients afflicted with autoimmune diseases[114–126] lend support to this theory. Therefore, alternative immunomodulating approaches to the treatment of MS (and autoimmunity in general) may be preferably directed towards activation of normal downregulatory circuits or towards induction of specific unresponsiveness (tolerance/anergy) of myelin-reactive T cells.

The following sections describe paradigms of immunoregulation, and indicates the levels at which it is possible to interfere with the development of the autoimmune process in MS. It should be noted that most of the following treatments are still in the experimental stages.

Antigen presentation

An autoimmune inflammatory process is initiated after the presumed autoantigen (MBP, PLP or MOG) is presented to T-lymphocytes by macrophages that act as APCs (Fig. 20.1). For full activation/immunization, the lymphocyte has to receive two signals: (a) one provided by

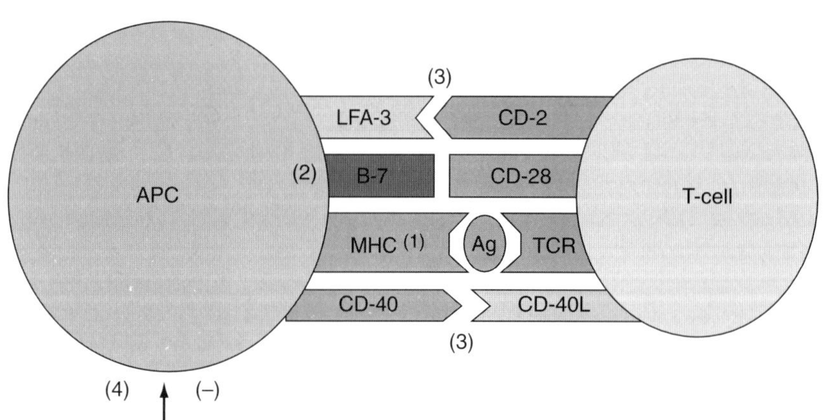

Figure 20.1 Antigen presentation to T cells: possible sites of immune intervention (1: Antigen-TCR specific intervention; 2: Level of secondary signal (B-7/CD28); 3: Secondary pathway/adhesion molecules; 4: Cytokines that downregulate APC).

the MHC–antigen complex, which binds to the specific TCR; and the second (b) supplied by the B7–CD28 (adhesion molecule) complex. In the absence of the secondary costimulatory signal, the lymphocytes fail to produce the T-cell growth factor, IL-2 and, therefore, antigen presentation leads to anergy of the lymphocytes towards the specific antigen.[127] There are also other accessory molecules, like the LFA-3/CD2 complex, that enhance lymphocyte reactivity in a nonspecific manner. The latter represent a second pathway (independent of the TCR pathway) for T cell-activation.[128]

At this level, therapeutic intervention can be induced in various ways.

Tolerization towards the specific myelin autoantigens

This can be achieved by oral tolerization techniques[129–133] immunization with peptides/parts of the specific TCR (as for example those that react against MBP or PLP),[134–136] T-cell vaccination,[112,137–142] immunization with altered myelin antigen epitopes[143] and blockage/antagonism of the MHC–TCR complex (by proteins mimicking myelin antigens or equivalent polymers, such as copolymer-1 (COP-1)).[144–149]

The results of a phase II study, showing the therapeutic potential of oral tolerization with myelin antigens (Myloral) in patients with relapsing–remitting MS have already been published.[132] In this trial, 6 out of 15 patients treated with oral myelin had at least one major exacerbation of MS, as compared with 12 of patients 15 in the placebo group. A larger phase III trial with oral myelin was recently completed but the preliminary data do not seem promising. This approach represents an antigen-specific therapeutic modality, where the antigen-driven peripheral immune tolerance is acquired by mechanisms inducing deletion, inactivation (anergy) or active suppression of the antigen-reactive clones.

Attempts have also been made to induce tolerance to myelin antigens by immunization with TCR peptides/parts of those TCRs usually found with greater frequency (e.g. the Vb-8.2, Vb-5.2 and Vb-6.1 TCR)[136,150] in the encephalitogenic lines in the EAE model and in some MS patients. Thus, neutralizing antibodies or anti-idiotypic T cells are induced which, in turn, block the APC–myelin antigen complex. This treatment succeeded in inhibiting EAE in the Lewis-rat model and has already been applied to some MS patients.[136] In patients immunized with Vb-5.2 peptides, a reduction in the frequency of MBP-reacting cells and amplification of anti-TCR-reacting cells was observed. However, this approach has certain drawbacks, since there is a great heterogeneity of TCRs among myelin-reactive T cells in MS patients[151–154]

To overcome this obstacle, Cohen and Ben-Nun in their seminal work[138,139] on T-cell vaccination, attempted to vaccinate EAE-animals with attenuated (by irradiation) encephalitogenic T-cell lines and showed that this treatment effectively suppressed EAE. Phase I clinical trials have recently shown that this treatment is technically feasible.[141,142,155] According to this protocol, a sample of T cells is removed, irradiated and reinjected into the patients. Thus, an anti-idiotypic reaction can be induced that may be specific to each individual. However, even in the same patient different T-cell clones bearing variable TCRs may be activated/expanded at various stages of the disease, during MS relapse and, therefore, vaccination should be repeated several times in order to obtain wide-scale tolerance.

Another approach, aimed at blocking/antagonizing the MHC/TCR complex, is to use analogues of myelin antigens. Preliminary data indicate that immunization with modified MBP or PLP-peptides protects mice from developing EAE.[143,156] This modality is still within the experimental realm.

COP-1 (Copaxone, Teva, Israel) is a synthetic copolymer, composed of alanine, glutamine, lysine and tyrosine, with some immunologic similarities to the MBP molecule (as well as to other myelin antigens), without itself being encephalitogenic. After finding that it inhibits EAE,[144,146] COP-1 proved successful in two double-blind trials in patients with relapsing–remitting MS.[147,149] In a recently completed 2-year double-blind trial carried out in the USA, and involving 251 patients with relapsing–remitting MS, COP-1 induced a 29% reduction in relapse rate (1.19/2 years vs. 1.68 in the placebo group). There was no difference between the two groups in the proportion of patients free of relapse or progression of disability at 2 years, or in the time to first relapse. MRI activity, which was monitored in one of the centres by monthly scans, showed only marginal (statistically) inhibition of disease activity, in the COP-1-treated patients. Adverse effects were usually mild, including localized, injection-site reactions (at least once in 90% of the patients) and a systemic reaction occurring within moments of COP-1 administration (associated with chest pain, palpitations or dyspnoea lasting up to 30 min) in 15% of the patients. COP-1 is presumed to block the MHC–TCR complex and to downregulate the presentation of antigens, such as MBP, PLP and MOG, to T cells.

However COP-1 failed to show any clear beneficial effect in chronic progressive MS in a double-blind trial involving 106 patients in two centres.[157] In this study, the major endpoint, confirmed progression of 1.0 or 1.5 units (depending on baseline disability) on the Kurtzke EDSS was observed in 9 (17.6%) treated and 14 (25.5%) control patients. The differences between the overall survival curves were not significant. Progression rates at 12 and 24 months were higher for the placebo group (p = 0.088) with 2-year probabilities of progression of 20.4% for the COP-1 and 29.5% for the placebo group. A significant difference at 24 months between the two groups was observed at only one centre. Two-year progression rates for two secondary endpoints, unconfirmed progression and progression of 0.5 EDSS units, were significant (p = 0.03).

Blocking/inhibition of the secondary signal and induction of anergy

This can be achieved by using antibodies that bind to adhesion molecules, especially B7 and CD28.[158,159] It was shown in a diabetic model in transgenic mice, that only those animals expressing the B-7.1 subtype on the pancreatic islet cells and having T cells expressing a TCR that recognizes antigens of pancreatic islet cells, fully developed diabetes. Early upregulation of B-7.1 expression was demonstrated in plaques of patients with MS.[160]

Blocking of accessory signals

This can be accomplished with the aid of antibodies that bind to the CD2 molecule[161] and thereby inhibit the alternative-bystander T-cell activation pathway. Phase I studies are already underway in this direction. However, this approach has certain drawbacks since it induces nonspecific lymphocyte suppression. Moreover, repeated injection of monoclonal (mouse) antibodies induces the production of human anti-mouse antibodies that may neutralize the effect of the anti-CD-2 monoclonal antibodies.

Antibodies against intercellular adhesion molecule-1 (ICAM-1) or leukocyte function associated antigen-1 (LFA-1) also proved effective in suppressing EAE[162,163] and may represent an alternative—though still experimental—nonspecific immunosuppressive modality for MS. Finally, blocking of CD40L was shown to downregulate the proliferation of autoreactive T cells isolated from patients with MS, and the production of IL-12, which is one of the major Th1 cytokines involved in the pathogenesis of this disease.[164] However, the later treatments are nonspecific and may induce generalized immunosuppressive effects.

Downregulation of macrophages/APC

This can be achieved through utilization of cytokines or substances that downregulate antigen processing and presentation, such as IFN-β,[165–172] IL-10[173] TGF-β,[174] prostaglandin (PGE)-2[175] and free radicals. This can also be achieved by inhibition of the proinflammatory cytokine IFN-γ, which upregulates MHC-expression and, therefore, enhances the ability of APCs to activate lymphocytes. Surprisingly enough, administration of anti-IFN-γ monoclonal antibodies caused a deterioration in EAE.[176–178] This finding illustrates the complexity of the immune networks involved in the early development of an immune reaction.

Both IL-10 and TGF-β were found to suppress EAE,[179–182] whereas indomethacin (which reduces PGE-2) may enhance the disease.[183] The above treatments are apparently supposed to downregulate APCs. Recently, a new synthetic immunomodulator, linomide, was found to downregulate antigen presentation, probably through overactivation of macrophages, with a resulting increase in free radicals and PGE-2 production and auto-downregulation of APCs.[184] We have shown that linomide is one of the most potent agents in the treatment of acute and chronic-replasing EAE.[185,186]

Lymphocyte network interactions (Fig. 20.2)

Following antigen presentation be macrophages (APCs), lymphocytes (mainly of the helper CD 4-subtype) expressing the specific TCR for the antigen, differentiate further becoming either Th1 cells, producing IL-2, IL-12, TNF-α and IFN-γ (proinflammatory cytokines), or Th2 cells, which secrete IL-4, IL-6 and IL-10.[29–33,187–190] There is a 'balance' between the Th1 and Th2 subpopulations; in T-cell-mediated autoimmune diseases like MS, the lymphocytes involved in the inflammatory process are mainly of the Th1 phenotype. Therefore, a 'shift' towards the Th2 subtype[32] is

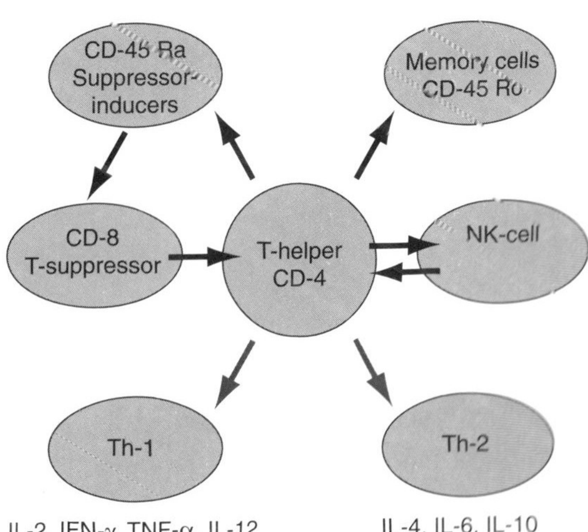

Figure 20.2 Lymphocyte network: multiple interactions between various lymphocyte subpopulations.

desirable and may lead to [illegible]tion (or at least to a relative decrease) [illegible] lympho-cytes, resulting in reduced infla[illegible] Such a shift may be achieved by oral t[illegible]n, by cytokines such as IFN-β, IL-4 and [illegible] possibly, by immunomodulating substa[illegible]and, [illegible]such as linomide. However, the acquisitio[illegible] a specific phenotype (Th1 or Th2) is [illegible]r transient and the lymphocytes status ca[illegible] be changed according to the immunological mi[illegible]u. It seems therefore, that there are no 'good' [illegible] 'bad' cells but, rather the same cell can differentiate in either direction. We believe that the Th1 to Th2 shift is a transient event that is not universally helpful in autoimmunity. Actually, such a shift may be harmful in antibody-mediated autoimmunity, as was recently shown in MOG-induced EAE,[191] whereas it might prove helpful in T-cell-mediated autoimmune diseases like MS. This shift should not be allowed to be permanent as it may be associated with increased risk of a secondary antibody-mediated autoimmunity.

CD4 lymphocytes are also functionally and phenotypically divided into two subpopulations: 'memory' cells, which—after the initial encounter with the antigen—are rapidly induced to react/proliferate following a second exposure. These cells express the CD45RO surface marker on their membranes. The second subpopulation is of the CD45RA phenotype, and consists of cells that function as 'suppressor-inducers'.[187,192–196] There is probably a cyclic relationship between CD4 subpopulations: naive CD45RA cells are converted into CD45RO memory cells upon antigen stimulation,[197–199] but without continuous antigen stimulation they lose their CD45RO expression and revert to long-lived CD45RA cells.[197–199] These CD45RO lymphocytes represent activated memory cells and they are probably identical with the CD29+ lymphocytes expressing on their surface the β-chain of the VLA-antigens (β1 integrins),[200] which is upregulated to facilitate adhesion to endothelial cells and subsequent passage to sites of inflammation. In MS and other autoimmune diseases, like rheumatoid arthritis (RA), Guillain–Barré syndrome (GBS) and SLE[114–126] the CD45RA cells are usually downregulated, especially during the active

... of the disease. In a longitudinal Phase ... hown that newly diagnosed cases study ... ve an initially higher proportion of with ... ells which, as the disease progresses, CD ... ced in number and a shift towards the ... O phenotype takes place.[126] This shift ... s to result from the conversion of resting ... s into activated memory lymphoctyes. However, since the CD45RA cells are present in lower numbers in patients with autoimmune diseases, as compared with age-matched healthy individuals, this finding may also indicate that loss of suppressor function could, at least partially, be related to the immunopathogenesis of autoimmunity in general; a low proportion of suppressor–inducer cells could permit autoreactive clones to carry out an autoimmune attack. Therefore, an increase in the CD45RA/CD45RO ratio should be an immunotherapeutic target in MS and other autoimmune diseases.

Autoreactive T cells may also be downregulated by the induction of T cells that recognize the specific T-cell receptors carried by the autoimmune lymphocytes.[112] The induction of such anti-idiotypic networks has been demonstrated in the EAE model, following T-cell vaccination or vaccination with TCRs peptides.[112,134,135,138,139] Such therapeutic approaches have been applied in patients with MS and resulted in efficient downregulation of the myelin reactive lymphocytes.[141,142,201]

Another cell population that may be involved in the delicate cell–cell interactions in this network, is composed of NK cells, which are a part of the 'natural/nonspecific immunity' (against viruses and malignant cells). NK activity is reportedly reduced in MS and other autoimmune diseases. NK cells can downregulate antigen presentation and the early phases of lymphocyte stimulation.[202] Dendritic cells, which are important APCs, can be the target of NK cells, especially after they have interacted with the antigen.[203] Recently a novel NK-cell population expressing both NK and T-cell markers was described.[204,205] These NK 1.1 cells produce large quantities of IL-4 upon activation which in turn, induces a 'shift' of T-lymphocytes towards the Th2 phenotype. Therefore, enhancement of NK-cell activity with immunodulators may also be desirable in the regulation of MS.

In a double-blind pilot trial in patients with secondary progressive MS, we showed that the new synthetic immunomodulating agent linomide inhibits the activity of the diseases (as indicated by the reduced number of active lesions in the MRI follow-up) and tends to stabilize/improve disability.[206] Preliminary immunological data indicate that linomide upregulates the NK cells and the CD45RA lymphocytes.[207] Phase III trials with this promising drug were initiated in several centres in Europe and the USA, but unfortunately, they were discontinued, following reports of myocardial toxicity (myocardial ischaemia) in some of the treated patients.

Another immunomodulating approach is to block trafficking of activated lymphocytes into the CNS by antibodies against adhesion molecules. The LFA-1,3, ICAM-1, VLA-4 adhesion molecules where shown to play an important role in the lymphocyte migration through the vessel endothelium.[20,21,23,24,26–28] Animal studies have shown that treatment of mice with antibodies against VLA-4, blocked the development of EAE.[208,209] Although experimental, such an approach, aimed at preventing the invasion of activated lymphocytes through the blood–brain barrier into the CNS parenchyma, could be applied in the treatment of MS. Intravenous immunoglobulin (IVIG) treatment also induces downregulation of ICAM-1 and LFA-1.[210]

Cytokine network

During the inflammatory process, several peptidic substances (cytokines) are excreted by the lymphocytes. These are important for inter-cell 'communication'. Some of them, such as IFN-γ, IL-2, IL-12 and TNF, are pro-inflammatory, others (IL-4, IL-6, IL-10, IFN-β and TGF-β) suppress inflammation.[29,31,33,211] Anti-TNF antibodies or soluble TNF receptors, and the cytokines IL-10 and TGF-β were shown to inhibit EAE[174,179,180,182,212,213] and may be candidates for future immunotherapeutic approaches. Surprisingly, a recent report on two patients treated with anti-TNF antibodies, not only failed to reveal any beneficial effect of this treatment, but showed that these patients deteriorated.[214]

But the most important progress in this direction has been made with the cytokine IFN-β, which effectively suppressed EAE.[215,216] IFN-β inhibits T-cell activation,[217] enhances suppressor cell activity,[218] reduces IFN-γ production and MHC-II expression[165,166] and, possibly, increases IL-10 production.[219] In two large double-blind studies performed in the USA in patients with relapsing–remitting MS, IFN-β was found to inhibit the activity of the disease.

In the first trial, recombinant IFN-β1b (Betaseron, Schering) given s.c. every other day reportedly reduced the relapse rate by 31% (0.84/year in the treated group vs. 1.27/year in the placebo group), especially at the high dose of 8 MIU, but without significantly affecting the disability status.[167] The number of exacerbation-free patients during this period was greater in the high dose protocol (8 MIU 3 times per week), compared with the placebo recipients. Several secondary outcome measures were also improved in patients receiving the high dose regimen, including a lower rate of moderate or severe exacerbations and fewer hospitalizations. An important finding in this study was the significant reduction in the MRI T2 burden of disease and a 75–80% reduction in active scans (those showing new or enlarging lesions), in patients administered the high dose.[220] This effect was long lasting even after 3–5 years of treatment.[168] The treatment was generally well tolerated, but 'flu-like' symptoms (fever, chills, myalgias and fatigue) occurred in most patients (76%), tending to decrease after the first months of treatment. Injection-site irritation was also very common (in 85% of patients), sometimes even severe, persisting for weeks after injection. About a third of the patients developed neutralizing antibodies against Betaseron, and this may be a limiting factor in long-term treatment.

In a second study, recombinant glycosylated IFN-β1a (Avonex, Biogen) at a dosage of 6 MIU i.m. once per week reduced the relapse rate from 0.90/year (placebo) to 0.61/year. The treatment also resulted in a decrease in the number and volume of Gd-DTPA-enhancing lesions in the brain MRI and, most importantly, delayed the sustained progression of disability and reduced the 1 and 2 year progression rates by about 40%.[221] The US Food and Drug Administration (FDA) has approved both Betaseron and Avonex for the treatment of ambulatory relapsing–remitting MS.

Another type of recombinant IFN-β (Rebif, Serono), almost identical with IFN-β1a, was recently made available. Rebif has shown promising effects (a reduction in the number of relapses and inhibition of MRI activity) in open phase II studies in Europe.[222,223] Recent, as yet unpublished, data from a large phase III trial with Rebif, have shown a significant beneficial effect in RR-MS patients treated with 6 or 12 million units of Rebif three times a week s.c. in all parameters tested (progression of disability, relapse rate and MRI activity). In chronic progressive MS, the only data available are the preliminary data from a European phase III trial with Betaferon, which were presented at the European Neurological Society (ENS) meeting in Nice in June 1998. According to these data treatment with Betaferon (8 million units s.c. three times a week) significantly inhibited the progression of disability and MRI activity. Studies with Avonex and Rebif in SP-MS are currently underway. It seems, therefore, that interferon beta may soon be applied for the treatment of chronic progressive MS, as well.

Treatment with high dose immunoglobulins (IVIG) produces several immunomodulatory effects: it neutralizes autoantibodies through an anti-idiotypic network and it also induces a Th1 to Th2 shift, downregulating inflammatory cytokine production.[224–226] One open-controlled study, testing the efficacy of IVIG in relapsing–remitting MS, showed that treated patients had fewer relapses.[227] However, two other studies failed to demonstrate any efficacy of this treatment in patients with relapsing–remitting or progressive MS.[228,229] MRI monitoring in the latter trial did not indicate that IVIG treatment could prevent the appearance of new lesions in the brain.[229] A pilot study examining the issue of recovery of apparently fixed, irreversible neurological deficits by IVIG treatment, showed that this modality may enhance recovery in optic neuritis patients, raising the possibility of induction of remyelination.[230–232] Recently, a placebo-controlled trial in relapsing MS patients showed a 42% reduction in the relapse rate, but no MRI data were included in the study.[233] Moreover, this trial was not completely double-blind, since the treating physician was aware of the treatment given to each participant. No controlled study with IVIG in chronic progressive MS has been reported.

CONCLUSION

Despite the extensive trials with several immunosuppressive modalities and the optimistic results with interferons and Copaxone in relapsing–remitting MS, there is no effective treatment that can substantially alter the natural course of chronic progressive MS and reverse the neurological deficits. This may be owing to the development of irreversible changes in the region of the MS plaques, i.e. axonal loss and gliosis.[234] In two studies, disability was found to correlate mainly with cerebral and spinal cord atrophy.[235,236] Therefore, future research should, in addition to immunomodulation, focus on trophic/growth factors that may promote oligodendrocyte proliferation and remyelination and nerve axonal regrowth.

REFERENCES

1. Hafler DA, Weiner HL. MS: a CNS and systemic autoimmune disease. *Immunol Today* 1989; **10 (3)**: 104–107.
2. Raine C. Biology of disease. Analysis of autoimmune demyelination; its impact upon multiple sclerosis. *Labor Invest* 1984; **50(6)**: 608–635.
3. Confavreux C, Aimard G, Devic M. Course and prognosis of multiple sclerosis assessed by the computerized data processing of 349 patients. *Brain* 1980; **103**: 281–300.
4. Runmarker B, Andersen O. Prognostic factors in a multiple sclerosis incidence cohort with twenty-five years of follow-up. *Brain* 1993; **116**: 117–134.
5. Weinshenker BG, Bass B, Rice GP et al. The natural history of multiple sclerosis: a geographically based study. I. Clinical course and disability. *Brain* 1989; **112**: 133–146.
6. Thompson AJ, Hutchinson M, Brazil J et al. A clinical and laboratory study of benign multiple sclerosis. *Q J Med* 1986; **58(225)**: 69–80.
7. Van Lambalgen R, Sanders EA, D'Amaro J. Sex distribution, age of onset and HLA profiles in two types of multiple sclerosis. A role for sex hormones and microbial infections in the development of autoimmunity? *J Neurol Sci* 1986; **76**: 13–21.
8. Comi G, Filippi M, Martinelli V et al. Brain MRI correlates of cognitive impairment in primary and secondary progressive multiple sclerosis. *J Neurol Sci* 1995; **132**: 222–227.
9. Revesz T, Kidd D, Thompson AJ et al. A comparison of the pathology of primary and secondary progressive multiple sclerosis. *Brain* 1994; **117**: 759–765.
10. Thompson AJ, Kermode AG, MacManus DG et al. Patterns of disease activity in multiple sclerosis: clinical and magnetic resonance imaging study [see comments]. *BMJ* 1990; **300**: 631–634.
11. Thompson AJ, Kermode AG, Wicks D et al. Major differences in the dynamics of primary and secondary progressive multiple sclerosis. *Ann Neurol* 1991; **29**: 53–62.
12. Miller DH. Magnetic resonance in monitoring the treatment of multiple sclerosis. *Ann Neurol* 1994; **36 (suppl)**: S91–S94.
13. Weinshenker BG. Natural history of multiple sclerosis. *Ann Neurol* 1994; **36 (suppl)**: S6–S11.
14. Sinnige LG, Teeuwissen E, Hew JM et al. Correlation between magnetic resonance imaging and clinical parameters in multiple sclerosis. *Acta Neurol Scand* 1995; **91**: 188–191.
15. Frank JA, Stone LA, Smith ME et al. Serial contrast-enhanced magnetic resonance imaging in patients with early relapsing–remitting multiple sclerosis: implications for treatment trials. *Ann Neurol* 1994; **36 (suppl)**: S86–S90.
16. Olerup O, Hillert J, Fredrikson S et al. Primary chronic progressive and relapsing/remitting multiple sclerosis: two immunogenetically distinct disease entities. *Proc Natl Acad Sci USA* 1989; **86**: 7113–7117.
17. Hillert J, Gronning M, Nyland H et al. An immunogenetic heterogeneity in multiple sclerosis. *J Neurol Neurosurg Psychiatry* 1992; **55**: 887–890.
18. Weinshenker BG. The natural history of multiple sclerosis. *Neurol Clin* 1995; **13**: 119–146.
19. Kwon OJ, Karni A, Brautbar C et al. HLA class II susceptibility to multiple sclerosis among Ashkenazi and non-Ashkenazi Jews. 1998 (in press).

20. Wilcox CE, Ward Am, Evans A et al. Endothelial cell expression of the intercellular adhesion molecule-1 (ICAM-1) in the central nervous system of guinea pigs during acute and chronic relapsing experimental allergic encephalomyelitis. *J Neuroimmunol* 1990; **30**: 43–51.
21. Dore DP, Washington R, Dragovic L. Expression of endothelial cell activation antigens in microvessels from patients with multiple sclerosis. *Adv Exp Med Biol* 1993; **331**: 243–248.
22. Sharief MK, Noori MA, Ciardi M et al. Increased levels of circulating ICAM-1 in serum and cerebrospinal fluid of patients with active multiple sclerosis. Correlation with TNF-alpha and blood–brain barrier damage. *J Neuroimmunol* 1993; **43**: 15–21.
23. Svenningsson A, Hansson GK, Andersen O et al. Adhesion molecule expression on cerebrospinal fluid T lymphocytes: evidence for common recruitment mechanisms in multiple sclerosis, aseptic meningitis, and normal controls. *Ann Neurol* 1993; **34**: 155–161.
24. Tsukada N, Miyagi K, Matsuda M et al. Increased levels of circulating intercellular adhesion molecule-1 in multiple sclerosis and human T-lymphotropic virus type I-associated myelopathy. *Ann Neurol* 1993; **33**: 646–649.
25. Tsukada N, Matsuda M, Miyagi K et al. Increased levels of intercellular adhesion molecule-1 (ICAM-1) and tumor necrosis factor receptor in the cerebrospinal fluid of patients with multiple sclerosis. *Neurology* 1993; **43**: 2679–2682.
26. Tsukada N, Matsuda M, Miyagi K et al. Adhesion of cerebral endothelial cells to lymphocytes from patients with multiple sclerosis. *Autoimmunity* 1993; **14**: 329–333.
27. Tsukada N, Matsuda M, Miyagi K et al. In vitro intercellular adhesion molecule-1 expression on brain endothelial cells in multiple sclerosis. *J Neuroimmunol* 1994; **49**: 181–187.
28. Washington R Burton J, Todd RR et al. Expression of immunologically relevant endothelial cell activation antigens on isolated central nervous system microvessels from patients with multiple sclerosis. *Ann Neurol* 1994; **35**: 89–97.
29. Bottomly K. A functional dichotomy in CD4+ T lymphocytes. *Immunol Today* 1988; **9**: 268–274.
30. Cua DJ, Hinton DR, Stohlman SA. Self-antigen-induced Th2 responses in experimental allergic encephalomyelitis (EAE)-resistant mice. Th2-mediated suppression of autoimmune disease. *J Immunol* 1995; **155**: 4052–4059.
31. Erb P, Troxler M, Fluri M et al. Functional heterogeneity of CD-4 positive T cell subsets: the correlation between effector function and lymphokine is limited. *Cell Immunol* 1991; **135**: 232–244.
32. Kuchroo VK, Das MP, Brown JA et al. B7-1 and B7-2 costimulatory molecules activate differentially the Th1/Th2 developmental pathways: application to autoimmune disease therapy. *Cell* 1995; **80**: 707–718.
33. Romagnani S. Human Th1 and Th2 subsets: doubt no more. *Immunol Today* 1991; **12**: 256–257.
34. Bernard CCA, Carnegie PR. Experimental autoimmune encephalomyelitis in mice: immunological response to mouse spinal cord and myelin basic protein. *J Immunol* 1975; **114**: 1537–1540.
35. Wisniewski HM, Keith AB. Chronic relapsing experimental allergic encephalomyelitis: an experimental model of multiple sclerosis. *Ann Neurol* 1977; **1**: 144–149.
36. Lublin FD, Maurer PH, Berry RG et al. Delayed relapsing EAE in mice. *J Immunol* 1981; **126**: 819–822.
37. Paterson PY, Day ED. Current prespectives of neuroimmunologic disease: multiple sclerosis and experimental allergic encephalomyelitis. *Clin Immunol Rev* 1981; **1**: 581–697.
38. Fritz R, Chou J, McFarlin D. Relapsing murine EAE induced by MBP. *J Immunol* 1982; **130**: 1024–1026.
39. Traugott U, Raine CS, et al. Acute EAE in the mouse. Immunopathology of the developing lesion. *Cell Immunol* 1985; **91**: 240–254.
40. Cross AH, McCarron R, McFarlin DE et al. Adoptively transferred acute and chronic relapsing autoimmune encephalomyelitis in the PL/J mouse and observations on altered pathology by intercurrent virus infection. *Lab Invest* 1987; **57**: 499–512.
41. Matsumoto Y, Fujiwara M. The immunopathology of adoptively transferred experimental allergic encephalomyelitis (EAE) in Lewis rats. Part 1. Immunohistochemical examination of developing lesions of EAE. *J Neurol Sci* 1987; **77**. 35–47.
42. Minagawa H, Takenaka A, Itoyama Y et al. Experimental allergic encephalomyelitis in the Lewis rat. A model of predictable relapse by cyclophosphamide. *J Neurol Sci* 1987; **78**: 225–235.
43. Namikawa T, Satoh J, Yamamura T et al. Recovery mechanisms from experimental allergic encephalomyelitis in rats: analyses by using encephalitogenic T cell line. *Int Arch Allergy Appl Immunol* 1987; **83**: 366–370.

44. Teuscher C, Blankenhorn EP, Hickey WF. Differential susceptibility to actively induced experimental allergic encephalomyelitis and experimental allergic orchitis among BALB/c substrains. *Cell Immunol* 1987; **110**: 294–304.
45. Tabira T. Cellular and molecular aspects of the pathomechanism and therapy of murine experimental allergic encephalomyelitis. *Crit Rev Neurobiol* 1989; **5**: 113–142.
46. Bouwer HG, Dietsch GN, Hinrichs DJ. Adoptive transfer of experimental allergic encephalomyelitis: conditions influencing memory and effector cell development. *Cell Immunol* 1990; **131**: 219–231.
47. Sobel RA, Tuohy VK, Lu ZJ et al. Acute experimental allergic encephalomyelitis in SJL/J mice induced by a synthetic peptide of myelin proteolipid protein. *J Neuropathol Exp Neurol* 1990; **49**: 468–479.
48. Cross AH, Hasim GA, Raine CS. Adoptive transfer of experimental allergic encephalomyelitis and localization of the encephalitogenic epitope in the SWR mouse. *J Neuroimmunol* 1991; **31**: 59–66.
49. Jones RE, Bourdette D, Offner H et al. The synthetic 87-99 peptide of myelin basic protein is encephalitogenic in Buffalo rats. *J Neuroimmunol* 1992; **37**: 203–212.
50. Martin R, McFarland HF. Immunological aspects of experimental allergic encephalomyelitis and multiple sclerosis. *Crit Rev Clin Lab Sci* 1995; **32**: 121–182.
51. Kupersmith MJ, Kaufman D, Paty DW et al. Megadose corticosteroids in multiple sclerosis [editorial] [see comments]. *Neurology* 1994; **44**: 1–4.
52. Miller DH, Thompson AJ, Morrissey SP et al. High dose steroids in acute relapses of multiple sclerosis: MRI evidence for a possible mechanism of therapeutic effect. *J Neurol Neurosurg Psychiatry* 1992; **55**: 450–453.
53. Barkhof F, Hommes OR, Scheltens P et al. Quantitative MRI changes in a gadolinium-DTPA enhancement after high-dose intravenous methylprednisolone in multiple sclerosis. *Neurology* 1991; **41**: 1219–1222.
54. Abbruzzese G, Gandolfo C, Loeb C. 'Bolus' methylprednisolone versus ACTH in the treatment of multiple sclerosis. *Ital J Neurol Sci* 1983; **4**: 169–172.
55. Barnes MP, Bateman DE, Cleland PG et al. Intravenous methylprednisolone for multiple sclerosis in relapse. *J Neurol Neurosurg Psychiatry* 1985; **48**: 157–159.
56. Rose AS, Kuzma JW, Kurtze JF et al. Cooperative study in the evaluation of therapy in multiple sclerosis. ACTH vs. placebo—final report. *Neurology* 1970; **20**: 1–59.
57. Thompson AJ, Kennard C, Swash M et al. Relative efficacy of intravenous methylprednisolone and ACTH in the treatment of acute relapse in MS. *Neurology* 1989; **39**: 969–971.
58. Beck RW, Cleary PA, Trobe JD et al. The Optic Neuritis Study Group. The effect of corticosteroids for acute optic neuritis on the subsequent development of multiple sclerosis. 1993; **329**: 1764–1769.
59. Beck RW, Clearly PA, Anderson MM Jr et al. The Optic Neuritis Study Group. A randomized, controlled trial of corticosteroids in the treatment of acute optic neuritis. *New Engl J Med* 1992; **326**: 581–588.
60. Cazzato G, Mesiano T, Antonello R et al. Double-blind, placebo-controlled, randomized, crossover trial of high-dose methylprednisolone in patients with chronic progressive form of multiple sclerosis. *Eur Neurol* 1995; **35**: 193–198.
61. Frequin ST, Lamers KJ, Barkhof F et al. Follow-up study of MS patients treated with high-dose intravenous methylprednisolone. *Acta Neurol Scand* 1994; **90**: 105–110.
62. Whitham RH, Bourdette DN. Treatment of multiple sclerosis with high-dose methylprednisolone pulse therapy. *Neurology* 1989; **39 (suppl 1)**: 357.
63. Lisak RP. Overview of the rationale for immunomodulating therapies in multiple sclerosis. *Neurology* 1988; **38 (suppl 2)**: 5–8.
64. Kappos L. Clinical trials of immunosuppression and immunomodulation in multiple sclerosis. *J Neuroimmunol* 1988; **20**: 261–268.
65. Kappos L, Heun R, Mertens HG. A 10-year matched-pairs study comparing azathioprine and no immunosuppression in multiple sclerosis. *Eur Arch Psychiatry Neurol Sci* 1990; **240**: 34–38.
66. Weiner HL, Hafler DA. Immunotherapy of multiple sclerosis. *Ann Neurol* 1988; **23**: 211–222.
67. Elison GW, Myers LW. A review of systemic nonspecific immunosuppressive treatment of multiple sclerosis. *Neurology* 1978; **28**: 132.
68. Rudge P. Cyclosporine and multiple sclerosis: the cons. *Neurology* 1988; **38 (suppl 2)**: 29–30.
69. Silberberg DH. Azathioprine in multiple sclerosis: the cons. *Neurology* 1988; **38 (suppl 2)**: 24–27.
70. Kappos L, Patzold U, Dommasch D et al. Cyclosporine vs azathioprine in the long-term treatment of multiple sclerosis—results of the

German multicenter study. *Ann Neurol* 1988; **23**: 56–63

71. Ellison GW, Myers LW, Mickey MR et al. Clinical experience with azathioprine: the pros. *Neurology* 1988; **38 (suppl 2)**: 20–23.
72. Goodkin DE, Bailly RC, Teetzen ML et al. The efficacy of azathioprine in relapsing–remitting multiple sclerosis. *Neurology* 1991; **41**: 20–25.
73. Steck AJ, Regli F, Ochsner F et al. Cyclosporine versus azathioprine in the treatment of multiple sclerosis: 12-month clinical and immunological evaluation. *Eur J Neurol* 1990; **30**: 224–228.
74. British and Dutch Multiple Sclerosis Azathioprine Trial Group. Double-masked trial of azathioprine in multiple sclerosis. *Lancet* 1988; **2**: 179–183.
75. Milanese C, La Mantia L, Salmaggi A et al. A double blind study on azathioprine efficacy in multiple sclerosis: final report. *J Neurol* 1993; **240**: 295–298.
76. Yudkin PL, Ellison GW, Ghezzi A et al. Overview of azathioprine treatment in multiple sclerosis. *Lancet* 1991; **338**: 1051–1055.
77. Sorensen PS, Wanscher B, Szpirt W et al. Plasma exchange combined with azathioprine in multiple sclerosis using serial gadolinium-enhanced MRI to monitor disease activity: a randomized single-masked cross-over pilot study. *Neurology* 1996; **46**: 1620–1625.
78. Hauser SL, Dawson DM, Lehrich JR. Intensive immune suppression in progressive multiple sclerosis: a randomized three arm study of high-dose intravenous cyclophosphamide, plasma exchange and ACTH. *New Engl J Med* 1983; **308**: 173.
79. Likosky WH. Experience with cyclophosphamide in multiple sclerosis: the cons. *Neurology* 1988; (in press).
80. Myers LW, Fahey JL, Moody DJ et al. Cyclophosphamide 'pulses' in chronic progressive multiple sclerosis. A preliminary clinical trial. *Arch Neurol* 1987; **44**: 829–832.
81. The Canadian Cooperative Multiple Sclerosis Study Group. The Canadian cooperative trial of cyclophosphamide and plasma exchange in progressive multiple sclerosis. *Lancet* 1991; **337**: 441–446.
82. Carter JL, Hafler DA, Dawson DM et al. Immunosuppression with high-dose i.v. cyclophosphamide and ACTH in progressive multiple sclerosis: cumulative 6-year experience in 164 patients. *Neurology* 1988; **38 (suppl 2)**: 9–14.
83. Gonsette RE, Demonty L, Delmotte P. Intensive immunosuppression with cyclophosphamide in multiple sclerosis. Follow up of 110 patients for 2–6 years. *J Neurol* 1977; **214**: 173–181.
84. Hafler DA, Orav J, Gertz R et al. Immunologic effects of cyclophosphamide/ACTH in patients with chronic progressive multiple sclerosis. *J Neuroimmunol* 1991; **32**: 149–158.
85. Weiner HL, Mackin GA, Orav EJ et al. Intermittent cyclophosphamide pulse therapy in progressive multiple sclerosis: final report of the Northeast Cooperative Multiple Sclerosis Treatment Gourp [see comments]. *Neurology* 1993; **43**: 910–918.
86. Goodkin DE, Rudick RA, VanderBrug Medendorp S et al. Low-dose (7.5 mg) oral methotrexate reduces the rate of progression in chronic progressive multiple sclerosis. *Ann Neurol* 1995; **37**: 30–40.
87. Goodkin DE, Rudick RA, VanderBrug Medendrop S et al. Low-dose oral methotrexate in chronic progressive multiple sclerosis: analyses of serial MRIs. *Neurology* 1996; **47**: 1153–1157.
88. Currier RD, Haerer AF, Meydrech EF. Low-dose oral methotrexate treatment of multiple sclerosis; a pilot study [published erratum appears in *J Neurol Neurosurg Psychiatry* 1994; **57**: 528]. *J Neurol Neurosurg Psychiatry* 1993; **56**: 1217–1218.
89. Group. TMSS. Efficacy and toxicity of cyclosporine in chronic progressive multiple sclerosis: a randomized, double-blinded, placebo-controlled clinical trial. *Ann Neurol* 1990; **27**: 591–605.
90. Zhao GJ, Li DK, Wolinsky JS et al. The MS Study Group. Clinical and magnetic resonance imaging changes correlate in a clinical trial monitoring cyclosporine therapy for multiple sclerosis. *J Neuroimaging* 1997; **7**: 1–7.
91. Beutler E, Sipe JC, Romine JS et al. The treatment of chronic progressive multiple sclerosis with cladribine. *Proc Natl Acad Sci USA* 1996; **93**: 1716–1720.
92. Sipe JC, Romine JS, Koziol JA et al. Cladribine in treatment of chronic progressive multiple sclerosis [see comments]. *Lancet* 1994; **344**: 9–13.
93. Sipe JC, Romine JS, Koziol JA et al. Cladribine improves relapsing–remitting MS: a double blind, placebo controlled study. *Neurology* 1997; **48**: A340.
94. Bastianello S, Pozzilli C, D'Andrea F et al. A controlled trial of mitoxantrone in multiple sclerosis: serial MRI evaluation at one year. *Can J Neurol Sci* 1994; **21**: 266–270.

95. Mauch E, Kornhuber HH, Krapf H et al. Treatment of multiple sclerosis with mitoxantrone. *Eur Arch Psychiatry Clin Neurosci* 1992; **242**: 96–102.
96. Krapf H, Mauch E, Fetzer U et al. Serial gadolinium-enhanced magnetic resonance imaging in patients with multiple sclerosis treated with mitoxantrone. *Neuroradiology* 1995; **37**: 113–119.
97. Noseworthy JH, Hopkins MB, Vandervoort MK et al. An open-trial evaluation of mitoxantrone in the treatment of progressive MS. *Neurology* 1993; **43**: 1401–1406.
98. Edan G, Miller D, Clanet M et al. Therapeutic effect of mitoxantrone combined with methylprednisolone in multiple sclerosis: a randomised multicentre study of active disease using MRI and clinical criteria. *J Neurol Neurosurg Psychiatry* 1997; **62**: 112–118.
99. Cook SD, Devereux C, Troiano R et al. Effect of total lymphoid irradiation (TLI) in chronic progressive multiple sclerosis. *Lancet* 1986; **8495**: 1405.
100. Comi G, Rodegher M, Colombo B et al. Low-dose total body irradiation in chronic progressive multiple sclerosis: a double blind, controlled, randomized phase II study. *Neurology* 1997; **48**: A340–A341.
101. Moreau T, Thorpe J, Miller D et al. Preliminary evidence from magnetic resonance imaging for reduction in disease activity after lymphocyte depletion in multiple sclerosis [published erratum appears in *Lancet* 1994; **344**: 486]. *Lancet* 1994; **344**: 298–301.
102. Moreau T, Coles A, Wing M et al. Transient increase in symptoms associated with cytokine release in patients with multiple sclerosis. *Brain* 1996; **119**: 225–237.
103. Weinshenker BG, Bass B, Karlik S et al. An open trial of OKT3 in patients with multiple sclerosis. *Neurology* 1991; **41**: 1047–1052.
104. Rumbach L, Racadot E, Bataillard M et al. [Open therapeutic trial of anti-T CD4 monoclonal antibody in multiple sclerosis]. *Rev Neurol (Paris)* 1994; **150**: 418–424.
105. Karussi DM, Slavin S, Lehmann D et al. Prevention of experimental autoimmune encephalomyelitis an induction of tolerance with acute immunosuppression followed by syngeneic bone marrow transplantation. *J Immunol* 1992; **148**: 1693–1698.
106. Karussis DM, Slavin S, Ben-Nun A et al. Chronic-relapsing experimental autoimmune encephalomyelitis (CR-EAE): treatment and induction of tolerance with high dose cyclophosphamide followed by syngeneic bone marrow transplantation. *J Neuroimmunol* 1992; **39**: 201–210.
107. Karussis DM, Vourka-Karussis U, Ovadia H et al. Prevention and reversal of adoptively transferred chronic-relapsing experimental autoimmune encephalomyelitis with a single high dose cytoreductive treatment followed by syngeneic bone marrow transplantation. *J Clin Invest* 1993; **92**: 765–772.
108. Slavin S, Karussis D, Weiss L et al. Immunohematopoietic reconstitution by allogeneic and autologous bone marrow grafts as a means for induction of specific unresponsiveness to donor-specific allografts and modified self in autoimmune disorders. *Transplant Proc* 1993; **25**: 1274–1275.
109. Kazis A, Kapinas K, Kimiskidis V et al. Autologous blood stem cell transplantation in the treatment of multiple sclerosis. *Eur J Neurol* 1996; **3 (suppl 3)**: 54.
110. Tindall RS, Walker JE, Ehle AL et al. Plasmapheresis in multiple sclerosis: prospective trial of pheresis and immunosuppression versus immunosuppression alone. *Neurology* 1982; **32**: 739–743.
111. Weiner HL, Dau PC, Khatri BO et al. Double-blind study of true vs. sham plasma exchange in patients treated with immunosuppression for acute attacks of multiple sclerosis. *Neurology* 1989; **39**: 1143–1149.
112. Lieder O, Reshef T, Berauud E et al. Anti-idiotypic network induced by T cell vaccination against experimental autoimmune encephalomyelitis. *Science* 1988; **239**: 181–183.
113. Cohen IR, Young DB. Autoimmunity, microbial immunity and the immunological homunculus. *Immunol Today* 1991; **12**: 105–110.
114. Bongioanni P, Fioretti C, Vanacore R et al. Lymphocyte subsets in multiple sclerosis. A study with two-colour fluorescence analysis. *J Neurol Sci* 1996; **139**: 71–77.
115. Calopa M, Bas J, Mestre M et al. T cell subsets in multiple sclerosis: a serial study. *Acta Neurol Scand* 1995; **92**: 361–368.
116. Chofflon M, Weiner HL, Morimoto C et al. Decrease of suppressor inducer (CD4+2H4+) T cells in multiple sclerosis cerebrospinal fluid. *Ann Neurol* 1989; **25**: 494–499.
117. Crucian B, Dunne P, Friedman H et al. Alterations in levels of CD28-/CD8+ suppressor cell precursor and CD45RO+/CD4+ memory T

lymphocytes in the peripheral blood of multiple sclerosis patients. *Clin Diag Lab Immunol* 1995; **2**: 249–252.

118. Eoli M, Ferrarini M, Dufour A et al. Presence of T-cell subset abnormalities in newly diagnosed cases of multiple sclerosis and relationship with short-term clinical activity. *J Neurol* 1993; **240**: 79–82.
119. Ilonen J, Surcel HM, Jagerroos H et al. T-lymphocyte subsets defined by double immunofluorescence in multiple sclerosis. *Acta Neurol Scand* 1990; **81**: 128–130.
120. Porrini AM, Gambi D, Malatesta G. Memory and naive CD4+ lymphocytes in multiple sclerosis. *J Neurol* 1992; **239**: 437–440.
121. Rose LM, Ginsberg AH, Rothstein TL et al. Selective loss of a subset of T helper cells in active multiple sclerosis. *Proc Natl Acad Sci USA* 1985; **82**: 7389–7393.
122. Rose LM, Ginsberg AH, Rothstein TL et al. Fluctuations of CD4+ T-cell subsets in remitting–relapsing multiple sclerosis. *Ann Neurol* 1988; **24**: 192–199.
123. Zaffaroni M, Rossini S, Ghezzi A et al. Decrease of CD4+CD45+ T-cells in chronic-progressive multiple sclerosis. *J Neurol* 1990; **237**: 1–4.
124. Zaffaroni M, Gallo L, Ghezzi A et al. CD4+ lymphocyte subsets in the cerebrospinal fluid of multiple sclerosis and non-inflammatory neurological diseases. *J Neurol* 1991; **238**: 209–211.
125. Khoury SJ, Guttmann CR, Orav EJ et al. Longitudinal MRI in multiple sclerosis: correlation between disability and lesion burden. *Neurology* 1994; **44**: 2120–2124.
126. Gordon C, Matthews N, Schlesinger BC et al. Active systemic lupus erythematosus is associated with the recruitment of naive/resting T cells. *Br J Rheumatol* 1996; **35**: 226–230.
127. Janeway CA. How the immune system recognizes invaders. *Scient Am* 1993; **269**: 73–79.
128. Suthanthiran M, Strom TB. Renal transplantation. *New Engl J Med* 1994; **331**: 365–376.
129. Khoury SJ, Lider O, et al. Suppression of experimental autoimmune encephalomyelitis by oral administration of myelin basic protein. III. Synergistic effect of lipopolysaccharide. *Cell Immunol* 1990; **131**: 302–310.
130. Whitacre CC, Gienapp IE, Orosz CG et al. Oral tolerance in experimental autoimmune encephalomyelitis. III. Evidence for clonal anergy. *J Immunol* 1991; **147**: 2155–2163.
131. Miller A, Zhang ZJ, Sobel RA et al. Suppression of experimental autoimmune encephalomyelitis by oral administration of myelin basic protein. VI. Suppression of adoptively transferred disease and differential effects of oral vs. intravenous tolerization. *J Neuroimmunol* 1993; **46**: 73–82.
132. Weiner HL. Double-blind pilot trial of oral tolerization with myelin antigens in multiple sclerosis. *Science* 1993; **26**: 1321–1324.
133. Sabbagh A, Miller A, Santos LM et al. Antigen-driven tissue-specific suppression following oral tolerance: orally administered myelin basic protein suppresses proteolipid protein-induced experimental autoimmune encephalomyelitis in the SJL mouse. *Eur J Immunol* 1994; **24**: 2104–2109.
134. Howell MD, Winters ST, Oless T et al. Vaccination against experimental allergic encephalomyelitis with T-cell receptor peptides. *Science* 1989; **246**: 668–670.
135. Jung S, Schluesener HJ, Tokya KV et al. Modulation of EAE by vaccination with T cell receptor peptides: V beta 8 T cell receptor peptide-specific CD4+ lymphocytes lack direct immunoregulatory activity [published erratum appears in *J Neuroimmunol* 1994; **49**: 222]. *J Neuroimmunol* 1993; **45**: 15–22.
136. Vandenbark AA, Bourdette DN, Whitham R et al. T-cell receptor peptide therapy in EAE and MS. *Clin Exp Rheumatol* 1993; **11 (suppl 8)**: S51–S53.
137. Ben-Nun A, Cohen IR. Spontaneous remission and acquired resistance to autoimmune encephalitis (EAE) are associated with suppression of T cell reactivity: suppressed EAE effector T cell as T cell lines. *J Immunol* 1982; **128**: 1450–1457.
138. Ben-Nun A, Cohen IR. Vaccination against autoimmune encephalomyelitis (EAE): attenuated autoimmune T lymphocytes confer resistance to induction of active EAE but not to EAE mediated by the intact T lymphocytes line. *Eur J Immunol* 1981; **11**: 949–952.
139. Cohen IR, Ben-Nun A, Holoshitz J et al. Vaccination against autoimmune disease with lines of autoimmune T lymphocytes. *Immunol Today* 1983; **4**: 227–230.
140. Beraud E. T cell vaccination in autoimmune diseases. *Ann NY Acad Sci* 1991; **636**: 124–134.
141. Hafler DA, Cohen I, Benjamin DS et al. T cell vaccination in multiple sclerosis: a preliminary report. *Clin Immunol Immunopathol* 1992; **62**: 307–313.
142. Zhang J, Raus J. T cell vaccination in multiple sclerosis: hopes and facts. *Acta Neurol Belg* 1994; **94**: 112–115.

143. Nicholson LB, Greer JM, Sobel RA et al. An altered peptide ligand mediates immune deviation and prevents autoimmune encephalomyelitis. *Immunity* 1995; **3**: 397–405.
144. Teitelbaum D, Webb C, Meshorer A et al. Suppression by several synthetic polypeptides of experimental allergic encephalomyelitis induced in guinea pigs and rabbits with bovine and human basic encephalitogen. *Eur J Immunol* 1973; **3**: 273–279.
145. Teitelbaum D, Milo R, Arnon R et al. Synthetic copolymer 1 inhibits human T-cell lines specific for myelin basic protein. *Proc Natl Acad Sci USA* 1992; **89**: 137–141.
146. Keith AB, Arnon R, Teitelbaum D et al. The effect of COP-1, a synthetic polypeptide on chronic-relapsing EAE in guinea pigs. *J Neurol Sci* 1979; **42**: 267–274.
147. Bornstein MB, Miller A, Slage S et al. A pilot trial of Cop 1 in exacerbating–remitting multiple sclerosis. *N Engl J Med* 1988; **317**: 408–414.
148. Bornstein MB, Miller A, Slagle S et al. Clinical experience with COP-1 in multiple sclerosis. *Neurology* 1988; **38**: 66–69.
149. Johnson KP, Brooks BR, Cohen JA et al. The Copolymer 1 Multiple Sclerosis Study Group. Copolymer 1 reduces relapse rate and improves disability in relapsing–remitting multiple sclerosis: results of a phase III multicenter, double-blind placebo-controlled trial. *Neurology* 1995; **45**: 1268–1276.
150. Whitham RH, Kotzin BL, Buenafe AC et al. Treatment of relapsing experimental autoimmune encephalomyelitis with T cell receptor peptides. *J Neurosci Res* 1993; **35**: 115–128.
151. Hiller J, Leng C, Olerup O. T-cell receptor alpha chain germline gene polymorphisms in multiple sclerosis. *Neurology* 1992; **42**: 80–84.
152. Ransohoff RM. T-cell receptor germline genes and multiple sclerosis susceptibility: an unfinished tale. *Neurology* 1992; **42**: 714–718.
153. Olive C. T cell receptor usage in autoimmune disease. *Immunol Cell Biol* 1995; **73**: 297–307.
154. Gold R, Giegerich G, Hartung HP et al. T-cell rceptor (TCR) usage in Lewis rat experimental autoimmune encephalomyelitis: TCR beta-chain-variable-region V beta 8.2-positive T cells are not essential for induction and course of disease. *Proc Natl Acad Sci USA* 1995; **92**: 5850–5854.
155. Zhang J, Raus J. Myelin basic protein-reactive T cells in multiple sclerosis: pathologic relevance and therapeutic targeting. *Cytotechnology* 1994; **16**: 181–187.
156. Karin N, Mitchell DJ, Brocke S et al. Reversal of experimental autoimmune encephalomyelitis by a soluble peptide variant of a myelin basic protein epitope: T cell receptor antagonism and reduction of interferon gamma and tumor necrosis factor alpha production. *J Exp Med* 1994; **180**: 2227–2237.
157. Bornstein MB, Miller A, Slagle S et al. A placebo-controlled, double-blind, randomized, two-center, pilot trial of Cop 1 in chronic progressive multiple sclerosis. *Neurology* 1991; **41**: 533–539.
158. De SR, Giampaolo A, Giometto B et al. The costimulatory molecule B7 is expressed on human microglia in culture and in multiple sclerosis acute lesions. *J Neuropathol Exp Neurol* 1995; **54**: 175–187.
159. Perrin PJ, Scott D, Quigley L et al. Role of B7:CD28/CTLA-4 in the induction of chronic relapsing experimental allergic encephalomyelitis. *J Immunol* 1995; **154**: 1481–1490.
160. Windhagen A, Newcombe J, Dangond F et al. Expression of costimulatory molecules B7-1 (CD80), B7-2 (CD86) and interleukin 12 cytokine in multiple sclerosis lesions. *J Exp Med* 1995; **182**: 1985–1996.
161. Jung S, Tokya K, Hartung HP. Suppression of experimental autoimmune encephalomyelitis in Lewis rats by antibodies against CD2. *Eur J Immunol* 1995; **25**: 1391–1398.
162. Archelos JJ, Jung S, Maurer M et al. Inhibition of experimental autoimmune encephalomyelitis by an antibody to the intercellular adhesion molecule ICAM-1. *Ann Neurol* 1993; **34**: 145–154.
163. Kawai K, Kobayashi Y, Shiratori M et al. Intrathecal administration of antibodies against LFA-1 and against ICAM-1 suppresses experimental allergic encephalomyelitis in rats. *Cell Immunol* 1996; **171**: 262–268.
164. Balashov EK, Smith RD, Khoury JS et al. Increased interleukin 12 production in progressive multiple sclerosis: induction by activated CD4+ T cells via CD40 ligand. *Proc Natl Acad Sci USA* 1997; **94**: 599–603.
165. Ling PD, Warren MK, Vogel SN. Antagonistic effect of interferon-β on the interferon-γ induced expression of Ia antigen in murine macrophages. *J Immunol* 1985; **135**: 1875–1863.
166. Panitch HS. Interferons in multiple sclerosis. A review of the evidence. *Drugs* 1992; **44**: 946–962.
167. Group TIMSS. Interferon beta-1b is effective in relapsing–remitting multiple sclerosis. I. Clinical

results of a multicenter, randomized, double-blind, placebo-controlled trial. *Neurology* 1993; **43**: 655–661.

168. Group TIMSS. The IFNB Multiple Sclerosis Study Group and The University of British Columbia MS/MRI Analysis Group. Interferon beta-1b in the treatment of multiple sclerosis: final outcome of the randomized controlled trial. *Neurology* 1995; **45**: 1277–1285.
169. Panitch HS, Bever C Jr. Clinical trials of interferons in multiple sclerosis. What have we learned? *J Neuroimmunol* 1993; **46**: 155–164.
170. Silberberg DH. Specific treatment of multiple sclerosis. *Clin Neurosci* 1994; **2**: 271–274.
171. Brod SA, Khan M, Kerman RH et al. Oral administration of human or murine interferon alpha suppresses relapses and modifies adoptive transfer in experimental autoimmune encephalomyelitis. *J Neuroimmunol* 1995; **58**: 61–69.
172. Wilson BA. Interferon beta for treatment of multiple sclerosis. *Medsurg Nurs* 1995; **4**: 151–153.
173. Fiorentino DF, Zlotnik A, Vieira P et al. IL 10 acts on the antigen-presenting cell to inhibit cytokine production by Th1 cells. *J Immunol* 1991; **146**: 3444–3451.
174. Racke MK, Cannella B, Albert P et al. Evidence of endogenous regulatory function of transforming growth factor-beta 1 in experimental allergic encephalomyelitis. *Int Immunol* 1992; **4**: 615–620.
175. Zicari A, Lipari M, Di Renzo L et al. Stimulation of macrophages with IFN gamma or TNF alpha shuts off the suppressive effect played by PGE2. *Int J Immunopharmacol* 1995; **17**: 779–786.
176. Voorthuis JA, Uitdehaag BM, De GC et al. Suppression of experimental allergic encephalomyelitis by intraventricular administration of interferon-gamma in Lewis rats. *Clin Exp Immunol* 1990; **81**: 183–188.
177. Duong TT, St LJ, Gilbert JJ, Finkelman FD et al. Effect of anti-inteferon-gamma and anti-interleukin-2 monoclonal antibody treatment on the development of actively and passively induced experimental allergic encephalomyelitis in the SJL/J mouse. *J Neuroimmunol* 1992; **36**: 105–115.
178. Lublin FD, Knobler RL, Kalman B et al. Monoclonal anti-gamma interferon antibodies enhance experimental allergic encephalomyelitis. *Autoimmunity* 1993; **16**: 267–274.
179. Racke MK, Dhib-Jalbut S, Cannella B et al. Prevention and treatment of chronic relapsing experimental allergic encephalomyelitis by transforming growth factor-beta 1. *J Immunol* 1991; **146**: 3012–3017.
180. Racke MK, Sriram S, Carlino J et al. Long-term treatment of chronic relapsing experimental allergic encephalomyelitis by transforming growth factor-beta 2. *J Neuroimmunol* 1993; **46**: 175–183.
181. Skias D, Reder A. IL-10 inhibits EAE. *Neurology* 1998 (in press).
182. Crisi GM, Santambrogio L, Hochwald GM et al. Staphylococcal enterotoxin B and tumor-necrosis factor-alpha-induced relapses of experimental allergic encephalomyelitis: protection by transforming growth factor-beta and interleukin-10. *Eur J Immunol* 1995; **25**: 3035–3040.
183. Ovadia H, Paterson PY. Effect of indomethacin treatment upon actively-induced and transferred experimental allergic encephalomyelitis (EAE) in Lewis rats. *Clin Exp Immunol* 1982; **49**: 386–392.
184. Lehmann D, Karussis DM, Fluresco D et al. Immunomodulation of autoimmunity by linomide inhibition of antigen presentation through downregulation of macrophage activity in a model of experimental autoimmune encephalomyelitis. *J Neuroimmunol* 1997; **74**: 102–110.
185. Karussis DM, Slavin S, Lehmann D et al. Successful treatment of chronic-relapsing experimental autoimmune encephalomyelitis with linomide (LS-2616), a synthetic immunomodulator. *Proc Natl Acad Sci USA* 1993; **90**: 6400–6404.
186. Karussis DM, Lehmann D, Slavin S et al. Inhibition of acute experimental autoimmune encephalomyelitis by the synthetic immunomodulator linomide. *Ann Neurol* 1993; **34**: 654–660.
187. Bradley LM, Duncan DD, Tonkonogy S et al. Characterization of antigen-specific CD4+ effector T cells in vivo: immunization results in a transient population of MEL-14-, CD45RB-helper cells that secrete interleukin 2 (IL-2) IL-3, IL-4 and interferon gamma. *J Exp Med* 1991; **174**: 547–559.
188. Fiorentino DF, Bond MW, Mossman TR. Two type of mouse T helper cell. IV. Th2 clones secrete a factor that inhibits cytokine production by Th1 clones. *J Exp Med* 1989; **170**: 2081–2095.
189. Goldman M, Druet P, Gleichman E. Th2 cells in systemic autoimmunity: insights from allogeneic disease and chemically-induced autoimmunity. *Immunol Today* 1991; **12**: 223–227.
190. Khoruts A, Miller SD, Jenkins MK. Neuroantigen-specific Th2 cells are inefficient suppressors of experimental autoimmune encephalomyelitis

induced by effector Th1 cells. *J Immunol* 1995; **155**: 5011–5017.

191. Genain CP, Abel K, Belmar N et al. Late complications of immune deviation therapy in a nonhuman primate. *Science* 1996; **274**: 2054–2057.
192. Sanders VM, Uhr JW, Vitetta ES. Antigen-specific memory and virgin B cells differ in their requirements for conjugation to T cells. *Cell Immunol* 1987; **104**: 419–425.
193. Sanders ME, Makgoba MW, Shaw S. Human naive and memory T cells: reinterpretation of helper-inducer and suppressor-inducer subsets. *Immunol Today* 1988; **9 (7–8)**: 195–199.
194. Jensen GS, Andrews EJ, Mant MJ et al. Transitions in CD45 isoform expression indicate continuous differentiation of a monoclonal CD5+ CD11b+ B lineage in Waldenström's macroglobulinemia. *Am J Hematol* 1991; **37**: 20–30.
195. Clement LT. Isoforms of the CD45 common leukocyte antigen family: markers for human T-cell differentiation. *J Clin Immunol* 1992; **12**: 1–10.
196. Qin Y, Van Den Noort S, Kurt J et al. Dual expression of CD45RA and CD45RO isoforms on myelin basic protein-specific CD4+ T-cell lines in multiple sclerosis. *J Clin Immunol* 1993; **13**: 152–161.
197. Rothstein DM, Sohen S, Daley JF et al. CD4+CD45RA+ and CD4+CD45RA- T cell subsets in man maintain distinct function and CD45RA expression persists on a subpopulation of CD45RA+ cells after activation with Con A. *Cell Immunol* 1990; **129**: 449–467.
198. Rothstein DM, Yamada A, Schlossman SF et al. Cyclic regulation of CD45 isoform expression in a long term human CD4+CD45RA+ T cell line. *J Immunol* 1991; **146**: 1175–1183.
199. Yamada A, Kaneyuki T, Hara A et al. CD45 isoform expression on human neonatal T cells: expression and turnover of CD45 isoforms on neonatal versus adult T cells after activation. *Cell Immunol* 1992; **142**: 114–124.
200. Pilarski LM, Yacyshyn BR, Jensen GS et al. Beta 1 integrin (CD29) expression on human postnatal T cell subsets defined by selective CD45 isoform expression. *J Immunol* 1991; **147**: 830–837.
201. Medaer R, Stinissen P, Truyen L et al. Depletion of myelin-basic-protein autoreactive T cells by T-cell vaccination: pilot trial in multiple sclerosis. *Lancet* 1995; **346**: 807–808.
202. Abruzzo LU, Rowley DA. Homeostasis of the antibody response: Immunoregulation by NK cells. *Science* 1983; **222**: 581–585.
203. Shah PD, Gilbertson SM. Rowley DA. Dendritic cells that have interacted with antigen are targets for NK cells. *J Exp Med* 1985; **162**: 625–636.
204. Yoshimoto T, Paul W. $CD4^{pos}$, $NK1.1^{pos}$ T cells promptly produce interleukin 4 in response to in vivo challenge with anti-CD3. *J Exp Med* 1994; **179**: 1285–1295.
205. Vicari AP, Zlotnik A. Mouse NK 1.1^{+} T cells: a new family of T cells. *Immunol Today* 1996; **17**: 71–76.
206. Karussis DM, Meiner Z, Lehmann D et al. Treatment of secondary progressive multiple sclerosis with the immunomodulator linomide: a pilot double-blind placebo controlled study with monthly MRI evaluation. *Neurology* 1996; **47**: 341–346.
207. Karussis D, Lehmann D, Linde A et al. Immunological evaluation of patients with secondary progressive MS treated with linomide. *Neurology* 1996; **46**: A252.
208. Yednock TA, Cannon C, Fritz LC et al. Prevention of experimental autoimmune encephalomyelitis by antibodies against alpha 4 beta 1 integrin. *Nature* 1992; **356**: 63–66.
209. Soilu-Hanninen M, Roytta M, Salmi A et al. Therapy with antibody against leukocyte integrin VLA-4 (CD49d) is effective and safe in virus-facilitated experimental allergic encephalomyelitis. *J Neuroimmunol* 1997; **72**: 95–105.
210. Dalakas MC. Immunopathogenesis of inflammatory myopathies. *Ann Neurol* 1995; **39 (suppl 1)**: S74–S86.
211. Mosman TR, Sad S. The expanding universe of T-cell subsets: Th1, Th2 and more. *Immunol Today* 1996; **17**: 138–146.
212. Samina JK, Hancock WW, Weiner HL. Oral tolerance to myelin basic protein and natural recovery from experimental autoimmune encephalomyelitis are associated with downregulation of inflammatory cytokines and differential upregulation of transforming growth factor β, interleukin 4, and prostaglandin E expression in the brain. *J Exp Med* 1992; **176**: 1355–1364.
213. Selmaj KW, Raine CS. Experimental autoimmune encephalomyelitis: immunotherapy with anti-tumor necrosis factor antibodies and soluble tumor necrosis factor receptors. *Neurology* 1995; **45(suppl 6)**: S44–S49.
214. van Oosten BW, Barkhof F, Truyen L et al. Increased MRI activity and immune activation in two multiple sclerosis patients treated with the monoclonal anti-tumor necrosis factor antibody cA2. *Neurology* 1996; **47**: 1531–1534.

215. Abreu SL. Suppression of experimental allergic encephalomyelitis by interferon. *Immunol Commun* 1982; **11**: 1–7.
216. Abreu SL. Interferon in experimental allergic encephalomyelitis (EAE): effects of exogenous interferon on the antigen-enhanced adoptive transfer of EAE. *Int Arch Allergy Appl Immunol* 1985; **76**: 302–307.
217. Rudick RA, Carpenter CS, Cookfair DL et al. In vitro and in vivo inhibition of mitogen-driven T-cell activation by recombinant interferon beta. *Neurology* 1993; **43**: 2080–2087.
218. Noronha A, Toscas A, Jensen MA. Interferon beta augments suppressor cell function in multiple sclerosis. *Ann Neurol* 1990; **27**: 207–210.
219. Porrini AM, Gambi D, Reder AT. Interferon effects on interleukin-10 secretion. Mononuclear cell response to interleukin-10 is normal in multiple sclerosis patients. *J Neuroimmunol* 1995; **61**: 27–34.
220. Paty DW, Li DK. Interferon beta-1b is effective in relapsing–remitting multiple sclerosis. II. MRI analysis results of a multicenter, randomized, double-blind, placebo-controlled trial. *Neurology* 1993; **43**: 662–667.
221. Jacobs LD, Cookfair DL, Rudick RA et al. Intramuscular interferon beta-1a for disease progression in relapsing multiple sclerosis. *Ann Neurol* 1996; **39**: 285–294.
222. Fieschi C, Pozzilli C, Koudriavtseva T et al. Human recombinant interferon beta in the treatment of relapsing–remitting multiple sclerosis: preliminary observations. *Multiple Sclerosis* 1995; **1**: S28–S31.
223. Pozzilli C, Bastianello S, Koudriavtseva T et al. Magnetic resonance imaging chages with recombinant human interferon-beta-1a: a short term study in relapsing–remitting multiple sclerosis [see comments]. *J Neurol Neurosurg Psychiatry* 1996; **61**: 251–258
224. Achiron A, Gilad R, Margalit R et al. Intravenous gammaglobulin treatment in multiple sclerosis and experimental autoimmune encephalomyelitis: delineation of usage and mode of action. *J Neurol Neurosurg Psychiatry* 1994; **57 (suppl)**: 57–61.
225. Achiron A, Cohen IR, Lider O, Melamed E. Intravenous immunoglobulin treatment in multiple sclerosis. *Isr J Med Sci* 1995; **31**: 7–9.
226. Achiron A, Barak Y, Goren M et al. Intravenous immune globulin in multiple sclerosis: clinical and neuroradiological results and implications for possible mechanisms of action. *Clin Exp Immunol* 1996; **104 (suppl 1)**: 67–70.
227. Achiron A, Pras E, Gilad R et al. Open controlled therapeutic trial of intravenous immune globulin in relapsing–remitting multiple sclerosis. *Ann Neurol* 1992; **49**: 1233–1236.
228. Cook SD, Troiano R, Rohowsky-Kochan C et al. Intravenous gamma globulin in progressive MS. *Acta Neurol Scand* 1992; **86**: 171–175.
229. Francis GS, Arnaoutelis R, Antel J. Lack of efficient of IVIG in multiple sclerosis. *Neurology* 1994; **44 (suppl 2)**: A357.
230. van Engelen BG, Hommes OR, Pinckers A et al. Improved vision after intravenous immunoglobulin in stable demyelinating optic neuritis. *Ann Neurol* 1992; **32**: 834–835.
231. Rodriguez M, Lennon VA. Immunoglobulins promote remyelination in the central nervous system. *Ann Neurol* 1990; **27**: 12–17.
232. Rodriguez M. Immunoglobulins stimulate central nervous system remyelination: electron microscopic and morphometric analysis of proliferating cells. *Lab Invest* 1991; **64**: 358–370.
233. Fazekas F, Deisenhammer F, Strausser-Fuchs S et al. Randomised placebo-controlled trial of monthly intravenous immunoglobulin therapy in relapsing–remitting multiple sclerosis. *Lancet* 1997; **349**: 589–593.
234. Lassmann H, Suchanek G, Ozawa K. Histopathology and the blood–cerebrospinal fluid barrier in multiple sclerosis. *Ann Neurol* 1994; **36 (suppl)**: S42–S46.
235. Losseff NA, Wang L, Lai HM et al. Progressive cerebral atrophy in multiple sclerosis. A serial MRI study. *Brain* 1996; **119**: 2009–2019.
236. Losseff NA, Webb SL, O'Riordan JI et al. Spinal cord atrophy and disability in multiple sclerosis. A new reproducible and sensitive MRI method with potential to monitor disease progression *Brain* 1996; **119**: 701–708.

21

Clinical results and outcome measures from the multiple sclerosis PRISMS* study

Lance D Blumhardt

INTRODUCTION

Two recent phase III, placebo-controlled, double-blind trials have demonstrated the efficacy of different forms of interferon beta (IFN-β) administered by either subcutaneous[1] or intramuscular[2] routes and at different doses, for patients with active relapsing–remitting multiple sclerosis (RRMS). Although relapses were similarly reduced in both studies, the effects on disability outcome measures were controversial and there has been considerable debate about dosage and the interpretation of the inconsistent clinical and magnetic resonance imaging (MRI) results.

The results of a randomized, double-blind, placebo-controlled study of interferon beta-1a (rIFN-β1a, Rebif®) in which high dose regimes, namely 66 and 132 μg weekly, showed significant efficacy on relapse rate, in-trial disability and MRI disease activity, and total lesion load are reviewed in this chapter.[3]

METHODS

Five hundred and sixty patients with clinically definite or laboratory supported MS of at least one year's duration, were recruited from 22 centres in nine countries. Each patient was required to have had at least two documented relapses or attacks[3] in the 2 years before the study as an indicator of recent disease activity. Disability levels at the time of enrolment had to be within the range of 0–5.0 on the Kurtzke expanded disability status scale (EDSS).[4] Patients who had any prior treatment with cyclophosphamide, systemic IFNs, lymphoid irradiation, or any other immunomodulatory or immunosuppressive therapies in the 12 months before the trial were excluded. The study was approved by hospital ethical committees and all patients gave informed consent.

Patients were randomized to IFN-β1a (Rebif®, Ares-Serono), 22 μg, 44 μg or placebo, administered three times weekly by subcutaneous injection. Scheduled neurological assessments were carried out by a neurologist 'blinded' to the treatment category on the first study day and thereafter at 3-monthly intervals and within 48 h of an MRI scan. All injection sites were covered during these evaluations to avoid unblinding due to local skin reactions. Wherever possible, additional examinations were carried out on patients experiencing relapses. The neurological rating scales used in the study included the EDSS,[4] Scripps neurological rating scale[5] (for assessment of relapse severity) and the ambulation index.[6]

*PRISMS; Prevention of Relapses and Disability by interferon beta 1a, subcutaneously in multiple sclerosis

The general medical care of patients, including management of adverse events was carried out by an independent 'treating' neurologist. Relapses could be treated with a 3-day course of intravenous methylprednisolone (1 g daily), and influenza-like side-effects were treated with paracetamol.

All patients had twice-yearly proton density (PD/T_2-weighted) MRI. In addition, 205 patients had monthly PD/T_2 and T_1 gadolinium-enhanced MRI at the start and for the first 9 months of the study, and 39 had monthly MRI throughout the whole 24 months.

Throughout the trial all patients had haematological and biochemical monitoring at 3-monthly intervals (fortnightly for the first 2 months). Assays for IFN-β neutralizing antibodies (NABs) were carried out every 6 months.

The primary outcome measure was the number of relapses during the 24-month study period. Secondary outcome measures included: the time to the first and second relapses; the proportion of patients who remained free of attacks at the end of the trial; patients whose disability progressed (as defined by a sustained increase of 1.0 EDSS point, confirmed on two occasions 3 months apart); the number of hospitalizations and steroid courses given for relapses; and the disease activity and total lesion load on PD/T_2 MRI.

RESULTS

Five hundred and sixty patients were randomized into the three treatment groups (Table 21.1). The mean age (34.9 years), female to male ratio (2.2) and disability levels (2.5) were characteristic of patients with RRMS, relatively early in the disease course. There were no significant demographic differences between the three treatment arms at study entry (Table 21.1). Pre-study relapse rates were higher than average at 1.5 relapses per annum.

At the end of the study period complete data sets were available on 533 patients (95.2%) and the inclusion of follow-up data for those who withdrew from treatment during the study allowed an intention-to-treat analysis for 98% of the total cohort (1094 out of a possible maximum of 1120 patient-years of data was available for final analysis).

Table 21.1. Baseline characteristics of patients by treatment group.

	All	Placebo	rIFN-β1a 22 μg	rIFN-β1a 44 μg
n	560	187	189	184
Mean (SD) age (years)	34.9 (7.5)	34.7 (7.5)	34.8 (7.0)	35.2 (7.9)
M:F (%)	31:69	25:75	33:67	34:66
Mean (SD) disease duration (years)	7.2 (5.8)	6.1 (4.8)	7.7 (6.1)	7.8 (6.3)
Mean (SD) baseline EDSS	2.5 (1.2)	2.4 (1.2)	2.5 (1.2)	2.5 (1.3)
Mean (SD) baseline SNRS	84.6 (12.2)	85.7 (11.8)	83.8 (12.2)	84.2 (12.6)

EDSS = expanded disability status scale.[4]
SNRS = Scripps neurologic rating scale.[5]

Conventional analysis

Primary outcome measure

The mean number of relapses per patient over the 2 years of the study was reduced to 1.82 (Rebif 22 μg) and 1.73 (Rebif 44 μg), compared with 2.56 for the placebo group ($p \leqslant 0.0002$), a percentage reduction of 29% and 32% (Figure 21.1), respectively.

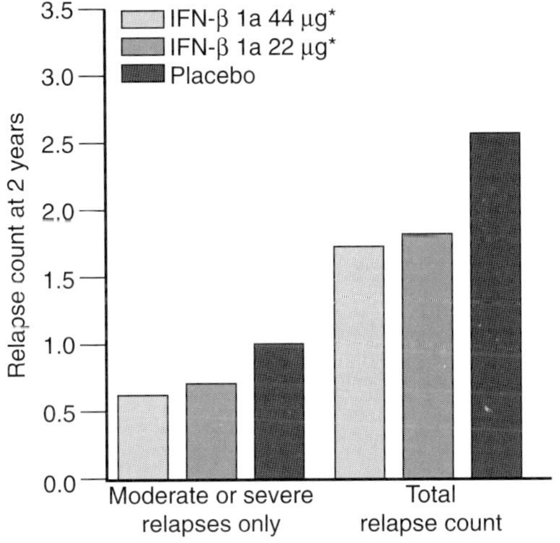

Figure 21.1 Mean number of total and moderate or severe relapses by treatment group.

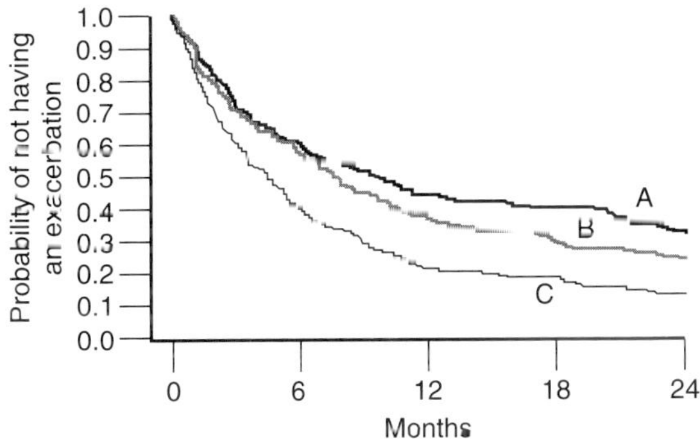

Figure 21.2 Kaplan–Meier plots of probability of not having a first exacerbation during the trial by treatment group. A, IFN-β 1a 44 μg; B, IFN-β 1a 22 μg; C, placebo.

Other outcome measures

The mean number of moderate and severe relapses was reduced from 0.99 in the placebo group to 0.71 ($p < 0.005$) and 0.62 ($p < 0.001$) in the 22 μg and 44 μg treatment groups, a percentage reduction of 28% and 37% (Figure 21.1), respectively.

There was a significant increase in the proportion of patients who were relapse-free during the trial period, from 14.6% in the placebo group to 24.6% ($p = 0.01$) and 32.1% ($p < 0.0001$) in the low and high dose arms, respectively.

The median time to the first relapse was prolonged from 4.5 months in the placebo group to 7.6 months by 22 μg ($p < 0.001$) and to 9.6 months by 44 μg ($p < 0.0001$) (Figure 21.2). Similarly, the median time to the second relapse was increased from 15 months (placebo) to 23.4 months by the 22 μg treatment and to more than 24 months by the 44 μg treatment (both $p < 0.01$).

Patients given placebo had a mean of 1.39 steroid courses during the trial compared with 0.97 ($p < 0.05$) for the 22 μg dose and 0.75 ($p < 0.001$) for the 44 μg dose of Rebif. The mean number of hospitalizations was reduced from 0.48 in the placebo arm to 0.38 (not significant) in the 22 μg treatment arm and 0.25 in the 44 μg treatment arm ($p < 0.05$).

The mean change in EDSS (baseline to end of study change) declined by 0.48 points in the placebo group compared to 0.23 points ($p < 0.05$) and 0.24 points ($p < 0.05$) in the 22 μg and 44 μg Rebif treatment groups, respectively.

Sixty-nine of the 180 (38%) patients in the placebo group had confirmed progression in disability (1.0 point sustained change in EDSS) in a Q1 (i.e. median time to progression for first 25% of patients reaching this endpoint) of 11.8 months (Figure 21.3). This was significantly more than the 54/182 (30%) of the 22 μg treated patients who progressed in a Q1 of 18.2 months ($p < 0.05$) and the 48/179 (27%) who progressed in a Q1 of 21 months ($p < 0.05$).

In the placebo group, 13% of patients worsened on the ambulation index (by two

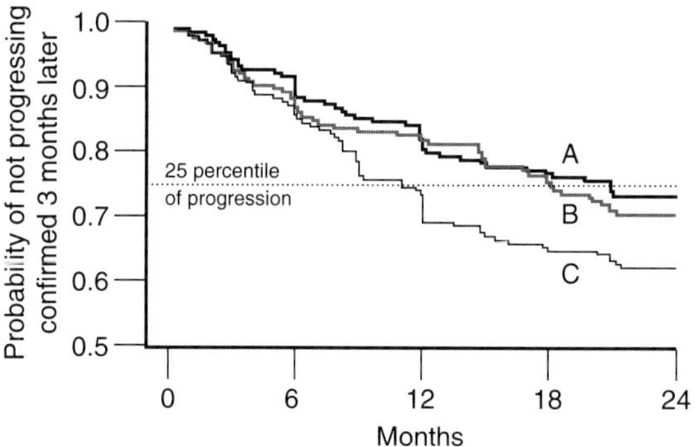

Figure 21.3 Kaplan–Meier plots of probability of not progressing by 1.0 EDDS point (confirmed at 3 months) during the trial according to treatment group. A, IFN-β 1a 44 μg; B, IFN-β 1a 22 μg; C, placebo.

steps confirmed at 3 months) compared with 12% of patients treated with rIFN-β1a 22 μg (not significant) and 7% given the 44 μg dose ($p < 0.05$).

Analysis by summary measure statistic

The area under time–disability curves (EDSS, SNRS) adjusted for baseline (entry score) was calculated for each patient using the trapezoidal rule (Figure 21.4).[7] The median area under the curve (AUC) for the EDSS showed a reduction from 0.479 EDSS-years in the placebo group to 0.051 EDSS-years in the patients on IFN-β1a 22 μg ($p = 0.0142$) and 0.056 EDSS years in the patients on IFN-β1a 44 μg ($p = 0.0084$) (Figure 21.5).

For the SNRS, the median AUC for the placebo group was –1.678 SNRS-years compared with –0.249 SNRS-years in the 22 μg group ($p = 0.1307$) and +0.166 in the 44 μg group ($p = 0.0450$).

Analysis by 'global score'

Using a multiple rank sum test as proposed by O'Brien,[8] we constructed an overall assessment

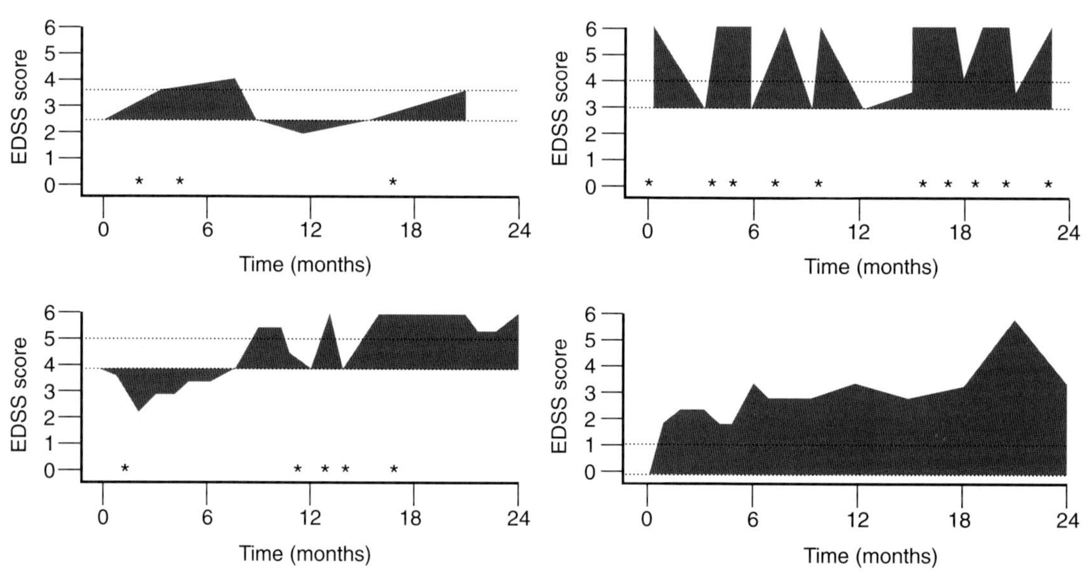

Figure 21.4 Area under the EDSS–time plots (normalized to baseline entry scores) for four individual patients in the trial. *Y* axis = EDSS scores (for both scheduled and unscheduled visits).[3]

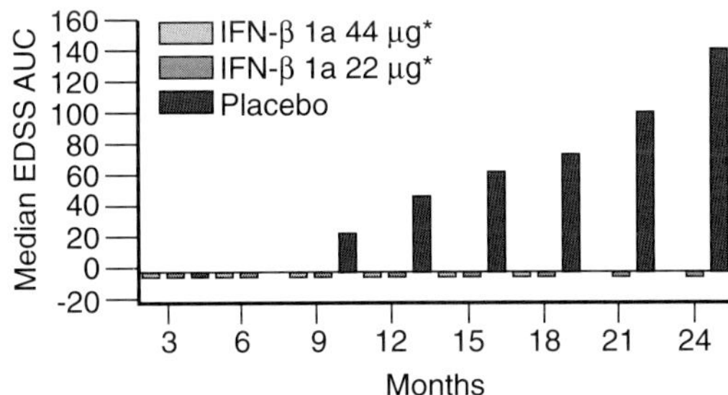

Figure 21.5 Accumulated median scores (normalized to baseline) for AUC of the EDSS–time plots by group.

of the efficacy of rIFN-β1a. This multiple procedure takes into account five endpoints: exacerbation count, the time to first confirmed progression on the EDSS, percentage change of the burden of disease from baseline to 24 months, the mean number of PD/T_2 active lesions, and the AUC of the EDSS–time plots. This method gave a probability of 74% of responding better when treated with Rebif on 44 μg versus placebo (for 4.24 of the five endpoints) ($p < 0.0001$), of 68% of responding better given a 22 μg dose versus placebo (for 4.04 of the five endpoints) ($p < 0.001$) and, of 57% of responding better given a 44 μg dose versus 22 μg (for 3.77 of the five endpoints) ($p = 0.0248$).

Safety and tolerability

IFN-β1a was well tolerated and only 4% of patients dropped out of the study during the 2 year period because of adverse events. Influenza-like side-effects were prevalent in the first 3 months of the study but tended to become less important with time, and overall there was little difference between the groups. Injection site reactions (redness and swelling) were significantly more common in the rIFN-β1a-treated groups than in the placebo-treated patients, although there was no difference between high and low dose arms. The mostly mild and asymptomatic reductions in white cells, granulocytes and lymphocytes were significantly more common in rIFN-β1a-treated patients. Most side-effects were less common in the second year of the trial. Two patients on high dose rIFN-β1a had to withdraw from treatment owing to marked asymptomatic increases in liver transaminases.

Depression occurred in 21% of patients given 22 μg rIFN-β1a and in 24% of patients given 44 μg rIFN-β1a, compared with 28% of patients taking placebo. Three patients in each group reported suicidal ideation or suicide attempts and one placebo-treated patient committed suicide during the study. There were no significant inter-group differences for the 267 English-speaking patients who underwent periodic assessment using the Beck's hopelessness scale, Centre for Epidemiological Studies depression mood scale and the general health questionnaire.

The proportions of patients with NABS in a titre of 20 nU/ml or greater were 23.8% and 12.5% in the two treated groups (low and high dose, respectively) at 24 months. In each case the lower incidence of NABs in the high dose group attained significance ($p < 0.05$).

DISCUSSION

We aimed to evaluate the effects of rIFN-β1a on the prevention of relapses and disability in patients with relapsing–remitting multiple sclerosis (RRMs). The phase III, placebo-controlled, double-blind PRISMS study was the largest and most complete study of RRMS carried out to date, with complete data available on 95% of the patients at 2 years. It demonstrated significant benefits of treatment for all major outcome measures, with consistent trends in favour of the high dose. Both low and high dose treatments resulted in a significant reduction in the number and severity of attacks, an increased proportion of patients who remained exacerbation-free, and an increased time to first and second exacerbations. In addition, there was a significant reduction of hospitalizations and the need for steroids. A significant dose-dependent reduction was seen in the number of active lesions and the proportion of active scans on MRI.

Both doses significantly delayed progression of disability on a conventional outcome measure (1.0 EDSS point deterioration sustained at 3 months). As disability experienced by patients with RRMS is predominantly transient, an assessment of the overall in-trial disability can be obtained by using an additional statistical tool that is more appropriate to the fluctuating levels of disability in this disease population and therefore more clinically meaningful. The AUC of a disability–time plot (using data from any suitable clinical rating scale) summarizes all the disability experienced by a patient during a trial, including both the fixed disability that either persists after attacks or results from secondary progression, and the transient disability owing to exacerbations that subsequently resolve. In addition, because it uses all available data from both scheduled and unscheduled visits, it is likely to be more sensitive than conventional outcome measure statistics. It also has the advantage that it takes into account any further deterioration or improvements (erroneous treatment failures) that may occur after a rigid 3-month endpoint has been achieved. Applying the AUC method to all available EDSS data showed there was a more than eight-fold difference in the median EDSS disability experienced by patients given placebo compared with those given 44 μg of rIFN-β1a, a result which was highly significant. Expressed in a different way, patients given placebo experienced a median increase in disability of 1.0 EDSS-year during the trial compared with only 0.28 EDSS-year in those treated with rIFN-β1a 44 μg.

For the SNRS, patients given placebo deteriorated by 3.4 SNRS-years during the trial compared with an improvement of 0.33 SNRS-years in the 44 μg or rIFN-β-treated group.

CONCLUSION

Treatment with rIFN-β1a subcutaneously three times weekly significantly benefits patients with active RRMS with respect to relapse rate, on-trial disability reduction, and MRI outcome measures. Long-term follow up of patients treated with rIFN-β1a is now required to see how these clear short-term benefits translate into long-term reductions of chronic disability.

REFERENCES

1. The IFNB Multiple Sclerosis Study Group. Interferon beta-1b is effective in relapsing–remitting multiple sclerosis. I. Clinical results of a multicentre, randomized, double-blind, placebo-controlled trial. *Neurology* 1993; **43**: 655–661.
2. Jacobs LD, Cookfair DL, Rudick RA et al. and the Multiple Sclerosis Collaborative Research Group (MSCRG). Intramuscular interferon beta-1a for disease progression in relapsing multiple sclerosis. *Ann Neurol* 1996; **39**: 285–294.
3. PRISMS (Prevention of Relapses and Disability by Interferon beta-1a Subcutaneously in Multiple Sclerosis) Study Group. Randomized double-blind placebo-controlled study IFN-β1a in relapsing–remitting multiple sclerosis. *Lancet* 1998; **352**: 1498–1504.
4. Poser CM, Paty DW, Scheinberg L et al. New diagnostic criteria for multiple sclerosis: guidelines for research protocols. *Ann Neurol* 1983; **13**: 227–231.
5. Kurtzke JF. Rating neurologic impairment in multiple sclerosis: an expanded disability status scale (EDSS). *Neurology* 1983; **33**: 1444–1452.
6. Sipe JC, Knobler RL, Braheny SL et al. A neurologic rating scale (NRS) for use in multiple sclerosis. *Neurology* 1984; **34**: 1368–1372.
7. Hauser SL, Dawson DM, Lehrich JR et al. Intensive immunosuppression in progressive multiple sclerosis. A randomized, three-arm study of high-dose intravenous cyclophosphamide, plasma exchange, and ACTH. *N Engl J Med* 1983; **308**: 173–180.
8. Liu C, Li Wan Po A, Blumhardt LD. 'Summary measure' statistic for assessing outcome of treatment trials in relapsing and remitting multiple sclerosis. *J Neurol Neurosurg Psychiatry* 1998; **64**: 726–729.
9. O'Brien PC. Procedures for comparing samples with multiple endpoints. *Biometrics* 1984; **40**: 1079–1087.

22

Magnetic resonance techniques for monitoring multiple sclerosis pathology in clinical trials

Donald W Paty and David KB Li

INTRODUCTION

Magnetic resonance (MR) techniques have helped considerably in the definition and understanding of multiple sclerosis (MS) lesions in both the diagnosis and the natural history of the evolution of pathology. More recently MR techniques have been used to monitor clinical trials. The ability to define clearly the lesions in the brain has resulted in many studies directed toward the goal of being precise about the type of pathology as it evolves. In addition, the quantitation of pathology and the extent of active pathology are being defined.[1] There is also evidence that the pathological process differs between the various clinical categories of MS such as primary progressive, secondary progressive and benign disease. The pathological process in MS is quite dramatically active. Systematic studies have shown that brain activity is 5–10 times more frequent than clinical activity.[2] The location of the lesion probably determines whether a correlation between MRI findings and neurological symptoms is or is not precise. The primary use of magnetic resonance imaging (MRI) in MS is in diagnosis, and the reason that MRI is so useful is that it shows many asymptomatic lesions. We cannot, however, have the situation in both ways, i.e. show many asymptomatic lesions in diagnosis, and have a high degree of correlation between clinical and MRI findings for clinical trials.

MRI AS A MEASURE OF PATHOLOGY IN VIVO

In the early 1980s systematic studies of unenhanced MRI scans in natural history studies showed that in frequently sampled patients, new lesions could appear and old lesions could enlarge.[3] Eventually these 'active lesions' became smaller in size. These morphological phenomena were subsequently aided by gadolinium-enhanced imaging,[2] which has shown even greater degrees of disease activity.

In the evolution of new lesions in MS, the first stage is the apparent breakdown of the blood–brain barrier (BBB).[4] Breakdown in the BBB can be preceded by subtle changes detectable by magnetic transfer imaging.[5] Gadolinium enhancement can detect the disruption in the BBB. Gadolinium enhancement is usually followed by the appearance of the lesion, which is identifiable on a proton density or T_2-weighted scan, and can be seen to enlarge over time. Eventually after some stabilization, this same lesion is usually reactivated with subsequent enhancement, enlargement, and shrinkage to a stable state.[6]

Most of these lesions become permanent over time, probably because they are fully demyelinated. Newer techniques such as magnetization transfer imaging,[7] T_2 relaxation analysis,[8] and MR spectroscopy[9] may be able to identify specific degrees of pathology that have occurred during the evolution of a lesion. In addition, MR spectroscopy may be able to identify the active phase of demyelination by detecting the appearance of neutral fat.[10]

The final irreversible damage in the MS lesion is axonal loss.[11] Axonal integrity can be measured as the *N*-acetyl aspartate (NAA) peak on MR spectroscopy.[9] Spectroscopy and other new MR techniques will eventually be able to identify specific pathologies as they evolve, and these techniques can then be applied to the adjudication of new treatments in clinical trials.

Table 22.1. Disease activity measures in MS.

(A) Acute dynamic phase monitoring:		
1. Clinical:	Relapse counts	
	Severity of relapses	
	Hospitalizations for relapses	
2. MRI:	Activity analysis in frequent scans	
	New lesions—counts, duration	
	Enlarging lesions—counts, duration	
	Stable lesions	
	Enhancing lesions—counts, area involved	
(B) Chronic dynamic phase monitoring:		
1. Clinical:	Impairment scales	
	Disability scales	
	Ambulation scales	
	These measures should be confirmed at 3–6 months to eliminate the effect of relapses	
2. MRI:	Quantitative measures of extent of disease T_1 unenhanced, PD/T_2 (BOD or LL)	

MRI = Magnetic resonance imaging; BOD = burden of disease; LL = lesion load.

PATHOLOGICAL CORRELATION WITH MRI

There have been several studies of pathological correlation that show a good individual correlation between single lesions seen on pathology and single lesions seen on MRI.[12] In addition, biopsy studies have shown a very good correlation between gadolinium enhancement and inflammatory lesions.[13]

More recently, unenhanced T_1 black holes seemed to correlate very well with both disability and axonal loss.[14]

As experience increases, other aspects of MRI should also be examined for their contribution to the identification of specific pathologies.

THE USE OF MRI IN ADJUDICATING CLINICAL TRIALS

The concept of MRI in monitoring clinical trials includes, as does clinical monitoring, the use of acute phase and chronic phase monitoring techniques (see Table 22.1). Acute clinical activity is manifested as clinical relapses. The dynamic MRI activity seen by frequent scanning is the MRI correlate to acute clinical activity. New lesions, as they appear, should have correlates in clinical measures, if our clinical measures are sensitive enough. However, some of the clinical manifestations of MRI lesions may be very subtle or non-existent.

Chronic phase monitoring for clinical outcomes is usually dependent upon the use of impairment or disability scales. Since the disease is so dynamic, impairment scales must usually be confirmed as a sustained change not thought to be owing to the effect of clinical relapses. A quantitative measure of the extent of the lesions on proton density or the T_2-weighted scans is the MR equivalent for a chronic measure. The total extent of proton density MRI abnormality, however, includes both acute inflammatory, chronic demyelinating and axonal pathology. Chronic active inflammatory lesions are very hard to differentiate. Eventually new MR methods should allow one to specifically distinguish between these pathologies.

Currently clinical trials are generally divided into phase I, (primarily safety trials), phase II (early trials at one site or a small number of sites in order to get a hint of efficacy), and phase III (multicentre trials that are randomized, placebo or otherwise controlled, that are designed to show proof of efficacy using a number of different parallel outcome measures). At present the primary outcome measures in definitive trials are the clinical measures of disease activity and chronicity. MRI serves as a secondary outcome measure in those trials. As the correlation between MRI changes and the evolving pathology of the disease becomes more and more widely recognized, however, there is a possibility that MRI could reach a position parallel to clinical activity as a co-primary measure of outcome.

Phase II studies can use MRI as a primary outcome measure in order to get a hint of efficacy.[15] The design of such studies is usually parallel groups of treated and placebo patients looking for signs of activity such as enhancing lesions, new lesions, and enlarging lesions. An alternative approach is to use repeated pretreatment baseline scans (at least once a month for 3 months) to give a reasonable idea of baseline (untreated) MRI activity rates. Patients can then be randomized to treated or untreated limbs in order to make comparisons between the untreated and treated periods.

Table 22.1 lists the disease activity measures used in MS clinical trials (see A2 for definitions of the MRI activity measures). Also, note the examples in Figures 22.1–22.3 of new, enlarging, and enhancing lesions.

Since stable lesions can enhance and enlarging lesions can develop out of previously stable ones, it is important to use multiple methods to identify activity so that evidence of activity that involves new lesions, enlarging lesions, and/or enhancing ones is not counted twice.

Chronic phase monitoring by MRI is shown in Table 22.1, B2. Basically the area involved, slice by slice, is measured by determining the border. An estimate of the volume of lesions can be calculated by multiplying the area in square millimetres by the slice thickness to get cubic millimetres (see Figures 22.4 and 22.5). The border of the lesions can be determined by manual tracing, contour tracing, threshold techniques, and fully automated methods. In our laboratory we use the manual tracing method because of its reliability, sensitivity to change, and efficient use of manpower.[13]

The quantitative measures are referred to as the burden of disease (BOD) or the lesion load (LL) in various publications. Quantitative measures can also be used in the unenhanced or enhanced T_1 scan by tracing out the area of the hypointensity (black holes) (see Figure 22.2), or hyperintensity (see Figure 22.3, enhancing lesions).

USE OF MRI AS A MEASURE OF PATHOLOGY IN VIVO

In the past few years we have seen very exciting changes in the application of MR techniques to understand MS. MR techniques are now generally acknowledged to reveal the evolving pathology of the disease.[16] Some, but not all, lesions detected by MRI are reflected in clinical changes. Clinical signs and symptoms in MS are an indirect reflection of the pathology. These signs and symptoms usually depend upon the location and intensity of pathological activity in lesions that develop in 'eloquent' tracts of the nervous system. There are large areas within the nervous system that deal with emotional and cognitive function that are not measured very well on the neurological examination. It is

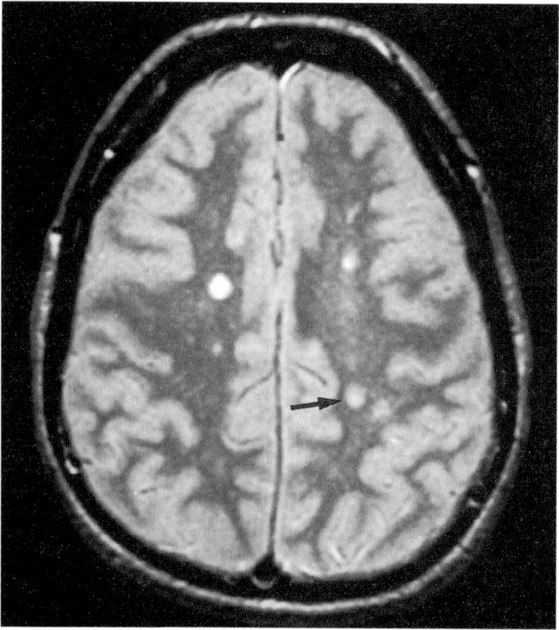

Figure 22.1 A typical axial proton density MRI above the level of the ventricles showing multiple white spots (lesions) in the white matter typical of MS. The arrow indicates a new lesion that had not been present previously.

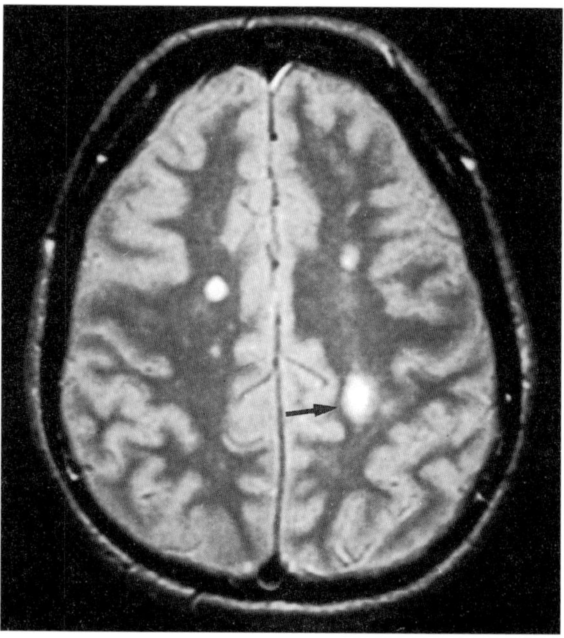

Figure 22.2 A proton density scan at the same level and tilt as Figure 22.1, taken 1 month later. The arrow indicates where the new lesion seen in Figure 22.1 has enlarged. Note that the four or five additional lesions were stable from scan to scan.

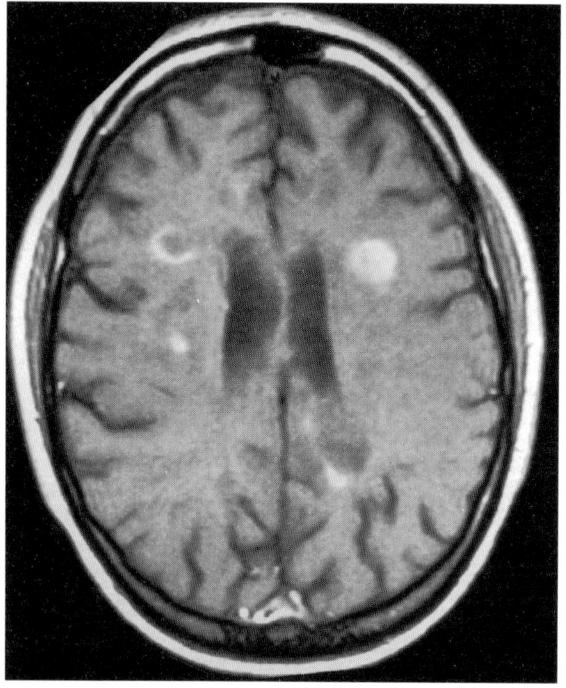

activity in these less expressive areas of the brain that are captured equally as well by MRI as are the more eloquent areas.

Currently the use of MR techniques in clinical trials has provided a unique and objective measure of the evolution of pathology. Such applications were not possible 15 years ago and are a major advance in the understanding of the pathology of MS and the effects of treatment.[17]

Figure 22.3 A T_1 post-gadolinium scan showing several enhancing lesions. Note the crescent shape of several of the lesions. The lesion in the left occipital area consists of a dark area ('black hole') and a small crescent enhancing area.

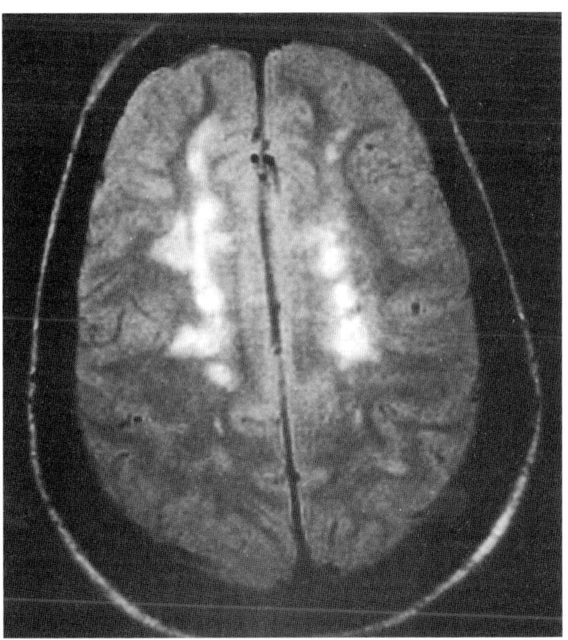

Figure 22.4 A proton density scan of a patient with moderately advanced MS (white areas).

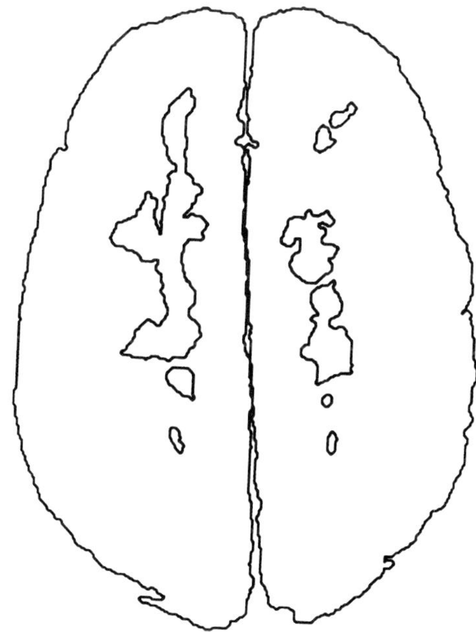

Figure 22.5 A traced outline of the lesions seen in Figure 22.4 that can be used for calculation of the burden of disease or lesion load.

REFERENCES

1. Paty DW, McFarland A. Magnetic resonance techniques to monitor the long term evolution of multiple sclerosis pathology and to monitor definitive clinical trials. *J Neurol Neurosurg Psychiatry* 1998; **64**: S47–51.
2. Miller DH, Rudge P, Johnson G et al. Serial gadolinium enhanced magnetic resonance imaging in multiple sclerosis. *Brain* 1988; **111**: 927–939.
3. Paty DW. Magnetic resonance imaging in the assessment of disease activity in multiple sclerosis. *Can J Neurol Sci* 1988; **15**: 266–272.
4. Thorpe JW, Kidd D, Moseley IF et al. Serial gadolinium-enhanced MRI of the brain and spinal cord in early relapsing–remitting multiple sclerosis. *Neurology* 1996; **46**: 373–378.
5. Comi G, Rocca MA, Rovaris M et al. Magnetization transfer changes in the normal-appearing white matter precede the appearance of enhancing lesions in patients with multiple sclerosis. *Neurology* 1998; **50**: A191.
6. Koopmans RA, Li DKB, Oger JJF et al. The lesion of multiple sclerosis: imaging of acute and chronic stages. *Neurology* 1989; **39**: 959–963.
7. Van Walderveen MA, Scheltens P, Barkof F et al. Histopathologic correlates of hypointense lesions on T1-weighted SE MR images in multiple sclerosis. *J Neurol* 1996; **243**: S18.
8. MacKay A, Whittall KP, Adler J et al. *In vivo* visualization of myelin water in brain by magnetic resonance. *Magn Res Med* 1994; **31**: 673–677.
9. Arnold DL, Matthews PM, Francis GS et al. Proton MR spectroscopic imaging (SI) for metabolic characterization of the brain plaques of demyelinating disease. *Neurology* 1991; **41(suppl 1)**: 144.
10. Wolinsky, JS, Naryana PA, Fenstermacher MJ. Proton magnetic resonance spectroscopy in multiple sclerosis. *Neurology* 1990; **40**: 1764–1769.
11. Trapp BD, Peterson J, Ransohoff RM et al. Axonal transection in the lesions of multiple sclerosis. *N Engl J Med* 1998; **338**: 278.
12. Stewart WA, Hall LD, Berry K et al. Correlation between NMR scan and brain slice: data in multiple sclerosis. *Lancet* 1984; **2**: 412.

13. Katz D, Taubenberger JK, Canella B et al. Correlation between magnetic resonance imaging findings and lesion development in chronic, active multiple sclerosis. *Ann Neurol* 1993; **34**: 661–669
14. Dousset V, Grossman RI, Ramer KN et al. Experimental allergic encephalomyelitis and multiple sclerosis, lesion characterization with magnetization transfer imaging. *Radiology* 1992; **182**: 483–491. (Erratum *Radiology* 1992; **183**: 878.)
15. Miller DH, Albert PS, Barkhof F et al. Guidelines for the use of magnetic resonance in monitoring the treatment of multiple sclerosis. *Ann Neurol* 1996; **39**: 6–16.
16. McDonald WI. The pathological and clinical dynamics of multiple sclerosis. *J Neuropathol Exp Neurol* 1994; **53**: 338–343.
17. PRISMS (Prevention of Relapses and Disability by Interferon beta-1a Subcutaneously in Multiple Sclerosis) Study Group. Randomized double-blind, placebo-controlled study of interferon-β1a in relapse–remitting multiple sclerosis. *Lancet* 1998; **352**: 1498–1504.

23

Combination therapy in multiple sclerosis*

Michel Clanet

INTRODUCTION

The new therapies licensed for relapsing–remitting multiple sclerosis (MS) offer to patients the first opportunity in the effort to cure the disease. However, as for other major complex autoimmune diseases, these therapies only produce a partial beneficial effect, which can be increased either by the development of new therapeutic procedures or by the use of combination therapies. Two main goals are followed in combination therapies: reduction of toxicity and improvement of efficacy. Cancer therapy, treatment of the haematological diseases or AIDS are examples in which these strategies have been successfully performed.

As shown in AIDS, combination therapy can be either concordant or discordant. A concordant therapy targets the same disease stage or aspect of the disease process: this is the case when the use of two agents enhance significantly the inhibition of HIV reverse transcriptase. A discordant therapy target different stages or different aspects of the disease process: in AIDS, this is the case when inhibitors of both reverse transcriptase and viral protease are used.[1]

Combination therapies must be tolerable over the long term. Agents that are well tolerated alone may not be tolerated in combination. This statement must be taken in account in clinical trials as the lack of tolerability can decrease the power of the study because of an unwanted number of drop outs.

In AIDS the clinical evaluation of treatments follows a well-defined strategy: comparison of monotherapies with placebo, comparisons of monotherapies with each other, paired combinations with monotherapies, then paired combinations with each other, and so on for tripled combinations. This means that the number of patients in these trials raises a new problem because the importance of the cohorts necessary to detect a moderate difference in efficacy between the different arms. However, in many chronic complex diseases the strategy of combination therapy is the main development in the improvement of therapeutic research.

RATIONALE FOR COMBINATION THERAPY IN MS

The new compounds used in relapsing–remitting MS act as disease modulators without a complete curative, action. The different main trials performed with interferon beta 1a (IFN β1a), beta 1b (IFN-β1b) or copolymer 1 showed a global 35% decrease in the relapse rate of

*This work highlights some key points presented at the 1st meeting of the Task Force on Combination Therapy, organized by the National Multiple Sclerosis Society. The final conclusions of the Task Force on Combination Therapy are yet to be published.

treated patients compared to placebo.[2–4] Their action is targeted at different aspects of the immune inflammatory process which is involved in the development of MS lesions. As toxicity is not a principal issue, combination therapy should improve the control of the disease process. Some combinations are suggested by biological synergistic actions in vitro such as interferon and copolymer 1 which enhance the suppressive effect of T cells (see later).

However, many discrepancies exist in the literature about the in vivo effects of these complex modulating agents. In two different experimental trials interleukin IL-10 shows either a beneficial or a deleterious effect in the treatment of experimental autoimmune encephalitis (EAE).[5,6] The combination of IFN-β1b and copolymer 1 has been reported to have additive effects on the immune response to myelin basic protein (MBP).[7] However, in a mouse model of EAE, oral IFN-α and copolymer 1 should have paradoxical effects with an increase of the disease process (J. Wolinsky, personal communication). These observations mean that the design of any combination therapy trial in humans must include a safety trial before the efficacy trial.

It is highly probable that the new therapeutical agents for relapsing–remitting (RR) MS will be evaluated in trials with combination therapies. Although most neurologists consider that the use of placebo in trials is justified, the feasibility of such trials in the northern countries is highly unlikely. So, as in the therapy of epilepsy, combination treatments will become the gold standard for the evaluation of new drugs at this stage of the disease.

WHICH COMBINATION TO TRY?

Combination therapy can involve three types of compounds: drugs currently licensed for MS indications, drugs licensed in other indications and unavailable drugs still in development.

Among the first category the first combination which can be suggested is copolymer 1 and IFN-β. As previously shown this combination was found to have an additive effect on the immune response to MBP.[7] Copolymer 1 exerts two main actions on the immune system: it inhibits epitope binding (as well MBP as proteolipid protein (PLP) or myelin oligodendrocyte glycoprotein (MOG)) with the class II molecules and induces the production of T-suppressor cells specific for MBP.[8] Knowledge about the mechanisms by which interferon beta affects MS is still limited but they include: downregulation of activation markers on activated immune competent cells, inhibition of the proliferation of T lymphocytes, amplification of the Th2 cytokines responses, enhancement of the suppressive cell function, diminution of the capacity of T lymphocytes to traverse the blood–brain barrier.[9] In the combined in vitro experiments, copolymer 1 and IFN-β1b had additive effects either on the suppression of the proliferation of MBP-specific T-cell lines or on the synthesis of the proinflammatory cytokines IL-2 and IFN-γ by MBP-specific lines. These in vitro data cannot be easily extrapolated in vivo. Different complex behaviours can be observed in experimental disease in animals as has been shown with many immune modifiers tested as potential therapeutical agents: as an example, cyclophosphamide used before the induction of EAE worsens the disease, whereas introduced after sensitization it improves the outcome dramatically. Some preliminary data could suggest an unwaited enhancing effect of the combination of copolymer 1 acetate and oral IFN-γ on EAE severity in mice (Wolinski, personal communication).

Among the other licensed drugs, the combination of long-term high doses of methylprednisolone and IFN-β can be proposed. The optic neuritis study suggested that pulse methylprednisolone could have a salutary effect on the disease course.[10] Although this issue remains controversial, this combination therapy could be of interest in a future trial.

Mitoxantrone, azathioprine and acyclovir are three drugs which are licensed in other indications than MS but at least the first two are used in many countries as a treatment for MS. Mitoxantrone, a very potent immunosuppressive agent, was confirmed as a candidate for the treatment of MS in the first trials.[11] In a highly selected group of MS patients with a very active disease, this drug was effective in improving both clinical and MRI indices of activity over a 6 months.[12] The cardiotoxicity of the drug is a limiting factor for prolonged use. A combination sequential therapy of mitoxantrone as an induction drug and IFN-β as a maintenance therapy in patients with very active MS would logically follow the preceding trial. The aim of this study, which is in under investigation, will be to evaluate the clinical efficacy of the combination of these two drugs over a long time (3–5 years) in patients with active RRMS at an early stage of their disease and with a moderate disability.

Azathioprine (AZA) was the first and most widely used immunosuppressant drug in MS, but without a careful evaluation. A recent meta-analysis of most of the published trials with AZA suggested a moderate therapeutical effect by decreasing the relapse rate and a marginal effect on disability progression.[13] Despite the lack of experimental data that confirms the additive effects of the two drugs, it is highly probable that a combination of AZA and IFN-β should have synergistic effects and should decrease anti-IFN antibodies production. Erazimus is an European program designed to test this combination (C Confavreux, personal communication). A safety trial preceding the efficacy trial is in progress.

Two subtypes of HHV6 herpes viruses should play a pathogenic role in MS.[14] This is the rationale for designing preliminary trials of MS with acyclic nucleoside derivative like acyclovir, antiherpes virus drugs, either isolated or in combination with IFN-β.

Many emerging therapies for MS will be used in combination therapies. Animal studies have demonstrated that IFN-β and oral myelin have synergistic effects when given together in animal models.[15] However, the recent report of the absence of any beneficial effect of oral administration of daily capsules of bovine myelin in a large phase III trial in RRMS patients means such a study is unlikely. The retinoids superfamily, such as vitamin A or vitamin D, are substances which exert antiproliferative, immunomodulatory and anti-inflammatory actions.[16] A pilot study is in progress in MS patients. Rolipram and pentoxifylline are two drugs which have an inhibiting effect on the tumor necrosis factor (TNF-α) production. Pentoxifylline has been used in combination therapy with IFN-β1b in a pilot trial.[17] These are some of many potential candidates to be proposed as disease modifiers in addition to the recognized therapies. In the long term, it is probable that a discordant form of combination therapy will be the association of disease modifiers and therapeutical strategies targeting the repair of damaged white matter.

WHICH DESIGN FOR COMBINATION THERAPIES TRIALS?

It is probable that the philosophy behind the regulations for acceptance of fixed combinations trials by health authorities would drive any consideration of combination therapy delivered in a nonfixed combination approach.[18] In the case of effectiveness of combinations therapy studies with licensed drugs, these agents might be used in combination therapy in some countries since neurologists can independently prescribe them. However, most of the time, an official approval is needed for this new use, or at least for marketing and advertising of these combinations.

In fixed combination trials, this driving philosophy is that each component must make a contribution to the therapeutical effects and the dosage of each component is safe and effective for a significant population of patients. With two drugs A and B, it means that the major concern of a trial is to demonstrate that a combination of A + B is more efficient than the therapeutical effect of A or B alone. This 'full factorial design' may or may not require a placebo arm.

It is probable that these rules will be applied to combination therapies in MS: a trial in RR patients must prove that a combination of drugs represents an improvement over monotherapy and that each component is playing a role in the ultimate outcome. Only a full factorial design can provide this level of certainty.

Because of economical, logistic and practical reasons, some less rigorous designs would be considered as compromises. However they will be less pertinent and there will be greater regulatory hurdles. An example can be a combination sequential study in which the goal of the trial is the demonstration of the superiority of A, then B more than A alone or B alone with the use of a placebo.

SAMPLE SIZE AND POWER OF THE STUDY

The magnitude of the anticipated effect and the definition of the main outcome will determine sample size. A general rule is that sample size requirements increase in combination therapies compared to monotherapy tested versus placebo, and in inverse relation with the magnitude of effect. In most cases the magnitude of this effect is not anticipated, so the larger estimates must be used. The practical rule coming from these considerations is to maximize the major criteria of the trial such as strengthening the entry criteria, using a pertinent outcome easy to measure, and selecting the best statistical tests for the analysis.

AN EXAMPLE OF STUDY DESIGN

Whatever the drugs used in combination, the full phase III trial in relapsing MS—either RR and relapsing progressive, or RR patients only—must be preceded by a short-term safety trial. This safety trial can be followed in sequence with an efficacy study if appropriate. This study should be phased as following. A + PBO will be followed with the addition of B. In the best design half the patients would have the sequence A + PBO > A + B, and half B + PBO > B + A.

The primary outcome should be MS activity measurement on MRI number of active scans, number of new, enlarging or reappearing lesions on T2-weighted fast spin-echo and number and volume gadolinium (Gd)-enhancing lesions on T1-weighted MRI.[19] Sample size and power calculations will be calculated from extrapolations of MRI activity studies in previous trials. There is an agreement to consider that a change between the subgroups will be significant beyond 50%, that is to demonstrate more than global equivalence of monotherapy versus combination therapy.

The other safety assessments are of primary importance and must be followed each week for 4 weeks, then monthly during the trial. These parameters will depend on the drugs used. With injected drugs intramuscular (i.m.) or subcutaneously the rhythm of injections for the local tolerance should not be a problem. Neurological assessment with a composite scale (expanded disability status scale (EDSS), ambulation measurement, nine hole peg test (NHPT), neuropsychological function) will be a secondary outcome measurement.[20]

Study duration should be a 'run-in' phase of 2 or 3 months and combination therapy for 6 months. The short run-in phase is sufficient for establishing a baseline value to demonstrate the safety of the combination, not the efficacy.

The efficacy study theoretically include three arms, i.e. A versus B versus A + B with a clinically composite primary outcome. The sample size will be calculated from extrapolations of the safety study and the major pivotal studies with monotherapy. The minimum duration will be 2 years.

ACKNOWLEDGEMENTS

This article was written after the 1st meeting of the 'Task Force on Combination Therapy' organized by the National Multiple Sclerosis Society. The author would l;ike to acknowledge F. Lublin (Chairman) and S. Reingold for their invitation to the group.

REFERENCES

1. Proceedings of the MS Forum. Modern Management Workshop. *Design and Interpretation of Clinical Trials in MS. Clinical Trials with Multiple Agents*. PPS Europe, 1996; 24–27.
2. IFNB MS Study Group and the University of British Columbia MS/MRI Analysis Group. Interferon beta 1b in the treatment of MS: final outcome of the randomized controlled trials. *Neurology* 1995; **45**: 1277–1285.
3. Jacobs LD, Cookfair DL, Rudick RA et al. Intramuscular interferon beta 1a for disease progression in relapsing MS. *Ann Neurol* 1996; **39**: 285–294.

4. Johnson KP, Brooks BR, Cohen JA et al. Copolymer 1 reduces relapse rate and improves disability in RR MS. *Neurology* 1995; **45**: 1268–1276.
5. Rott O, Fleischer B, Cash E. IL 10 prevents EAE in rats. *Eur J Immunol* 1994; **24**: 1434–1440.
6. Canella B, Gao YL, Brosnan C et al. IL 10 fails to abrogate EAE. *J Neurosci Res* 1996; **45**: 735–746.
7. Milo R, Panitch H. Additive effects of copolymer 1 and interferon beta 1b on the immune response to MBP. *J Neuroimmunol* 1995; **61**: 185–193.
8. Lobel E, Riven-Kreitman R, Amselen A et al. Copolymer 1. *Drugs Future* 1996; **21**: 131–134.
9. Hartung HP. Targets for the therapeutic action of interferon beta in MS. *Ann Neurol* 1996; **40**: 825–826.
10. Beck RW. Strategies to delay the onset of clinically definite MS in patients with monosymptomatic presentations of optic neuritis, brainstem syndromes or myelopathy. In: Goodkin DE, Rudick RE, eds. *Multiple Sclerosis Advances in Clinical Trial Design, Treatment and Future Perspectives*. New York: Springer-Verlag, 1996; 201–223.
11. Gonsette RE, Demonty L. Immunosuppression with mitoxantrone in MS; a pilot study for 2 years in 22 patients. *Neurology* 1990; **40 (suppl 1)**: 261 [abstract].
12. Edan G, Miller D, Clanet M et al. Therapeutic effect of mitoxantrone combined with methylprednisolone in MS. *J Neurol Neurosurg Psychiatry* 1997; **62**: 889–894.
13. Yudkin PL, Ellison GW, Ghezzi A et al. Overview of azathioprine treatment in MS. *Lancet* 1991; **338**: 1051–1055.
14. Challoner PB, Smith KT, Parker JD et al. Plaque associated expression of human herpes virus 6 in MS. *Proc Natl Acad Sci* 1995; **92**: 7440–7444.
15. Al-Sabbagh A, Nelson P, Weiner H. Beta interferon enhances oral tolerance to MBP and PLP in EAE. *Neurology* 1994; **44 (suppl 2)**: A242.
16. Mehta K, McQueen T, Tucker S et al. Inhibition by all trans retinoic acid of TNF and NO production by peritoneal macrophages. *J Leukoc Biol* 1994; **55**: 336–342.
17. Rieckmann P, Weber F, Günther A et al. Pentoxifylline, a phosphodiesterase inhibitor, induces immune deviation in patients with MS. *J Neuroimmunol* 1995; **60**: 9–15.
18. Fonichel RR, Lipicky RL. Combination products as first line pharmacotherapy. *Arch Intern Med* 1994; **154**: 1429–1430.
19. Miller DH, Albert PS, Barkhof F et al. Guidelines for the use of MRI in monitoring the treatment of MS. *Ann Neurol* 1996; **39**: 6–16.
20. Rudick R, Antel J, Confavreux C et al. Recommendations from the National MS Society clinical assessment task force. *Ann Neurol* 1997; **42**: 379–382.

24

Evidence of early axonal damage in multiple sclerosis lesions and its implications for therapeutic intervention

Daniel C Anthony, Margaret M Esiri and V Hugh Perry

INTRODUCTION

Axonal loss occurs in MS lesions and is thought likely to be responsible for the permanent disability characterizing the later chronic progressive stage of the disease. This raises two key issues central to the pathogenesis of MS that are often ignored. First, at what stage in the pathogenesis of MS does the damage to axons occur? And, secondly, why should there be any axon loss at all in what is thought to be principally an axon-sparing demyelinating disease? Concerning the timing of axon loss, there are two possibilities: it could happen either at the time of myelin damage, or later on as a consequence of myelin damage. From a position of understanding about the timing of axon damage, we can begin to investigate the question of why. Clearly, in order to develop therapeutics that might prevent axon loss, these problems need to be addressed. In this chapter, we shall discuss the difficulties associated with the detection of axon damage and review evidence for the presence of early axonal loss in MS lesions. In addition, a mechanism that may lead to axon damage will be described, and, lastly, the implications of early axonal loss for therapy will be considered.

DETECTING AXON LOSS

Perhaps the principal reason for the problem in accepting axonal loss has been the difficulty in detecting it in post-mortem tissue specimens. In the laboratory, axon loss in experimental models can be assessed by a variety of means. Using electron microscopy it is possible to visualize the whole spectrum of axon sizes and quantify axon loss. This approach is not practical in post-mortem MS tissue; not only does it require stringent fixation techniques, but the considerable variation in axon density in different fibre tracts, and differences between individuals, will confound assessment. The presence of oedema and leucocytes within the tissue will also influence axon density estimates. A qualitative approach to the detection of axonal degeneration is to take advantage of the higher affinity of degenerating axoplasm for binding silver, relative to normal axoplasm. Herein lies the basis of the Nauta,[1] Fink–Heimer,[2] and related silver stains.[3,4] These methods and their various modifications over the years have not only proved capricious, but again require well-defined fixation of the tissue. While their application in the neurohistology laboratory may become routine, they are still laborious and they are not useful for the analysis of post-mortem tissue.

Thus, the neuropathologist has to rely on methods that are relatively robust and less sensitive to artefact of tissue fixation. The silver stains that reveal the cytoskeleton of the axon are the methods of choice, although immunocytochemistry for neurofilament triplet may replace these methods. Indeed, it has been demonstrated that the Bodian silver stain does, in fact, stain the 200 kDa neurofilament.[5] However, the detection of axon loss by comparison of the number of axons in normal-appearing white matter with the number of axons remaining in MS lesions employing neurofilament stains is not without problems. Firstly, neither the silver stains nor the immunocytochemical methods reveal more than a subpopulation of axons—namely, the largest. Precisely what percentage of the myelinated fibres are visualized has not to our knowledge been examined. Secondly, it has become increasingly apparent that neuronal numbers and thus axon numbers are highly variable in the human population.[6] Thus, comparison of axon numbers, or densities, between patients and controls requires a large group to be examined.

Methods that reveal the neurofilaments do, in principle, provide an opportunity to visualize axons that have been severed and the degenerating distal segment. The proximal end of a severed axon appears as a small swelling or 'retraction bulb' on the end[7] and the distal segment will, for a short time, appear as a fragmenting process. These two histological profiles are, however, also sensitive to fixation artefact.

Thus, there is a clear need for a method that would detect axon damage in post-mortem tissue. Such a method would preferably detect the damaged axon rather than axon absence, since the positive signal would reveal the number of damaged axons, and the method would need to have the potential to detect axons of all sizes and in all parts of the central nervous system. Finally, the method would have to be sufficiently robust not to be easily influenced by post-mortem fixation artefact.

EVIDENCE FOR EARLY AXONAL LOSS IN MS

A recently described new technique for investigating axon damage depends for its ability on the immunoreactivity of amyloid precursor protein (APP).[8] The method has been shown to be more sensitive than silver stains for detecting damaged axons. Indeed, by employing this new technique it was concluded that silver staining markedly underestimated the frequency of axon damage in the traumatized human brain.[9] Diffuse axon damage[10] is associated with the traumatic head injury that may arise from rapid acceleration or deceleration of the head. In the injured axons axoplasmic flow is interrupted, and APP or APP-containing organelles build up at the sites of injury.[11] Within these axons, the presence of APP—which normally is transported in an anterograde direction[12] and cannot be detected by standard immunocytochemistry on formalin-fixed paraffin embedded sections[8]—can be readily seen. Thus, the presence of APP immunoreactivity is thought to represent the arrest of axon transport and the development of an end-bulb at the proximal end of the severed axons (Fig. 24.1). APP is not unique in its ability to reveal axon damage in this way; synaptosome-associated protein of 25kDa (SNAP-25), chromogranin A and cathepsin D also mark injured axons, although they are not as sensitive or specific as APP.[8] Recently, we used the APP immunoreactivity method to investigate whether axon damage occurs in acute MS lesions.[13]

The results of our APP staining showed that the expression of APP in MS lesions is associated with acute MS lesions and the active border of less acute lesions (Fig. 24.2). There was little, if any, APP expression in the chronic lesions. This was an unexpected finding, and suggests that axonal damage—like demyelination—is closely associated with active inflammation. When the macrophage distribution in the MS lesions was compared to the distribution of APP immunoreactive particles there was a striking similarity (Fig. 24.3). If axon loss were to develop progressively during the course of the disease, then we would have expected to find some immunoreactivity in the chronic lesions. Indeed, our own

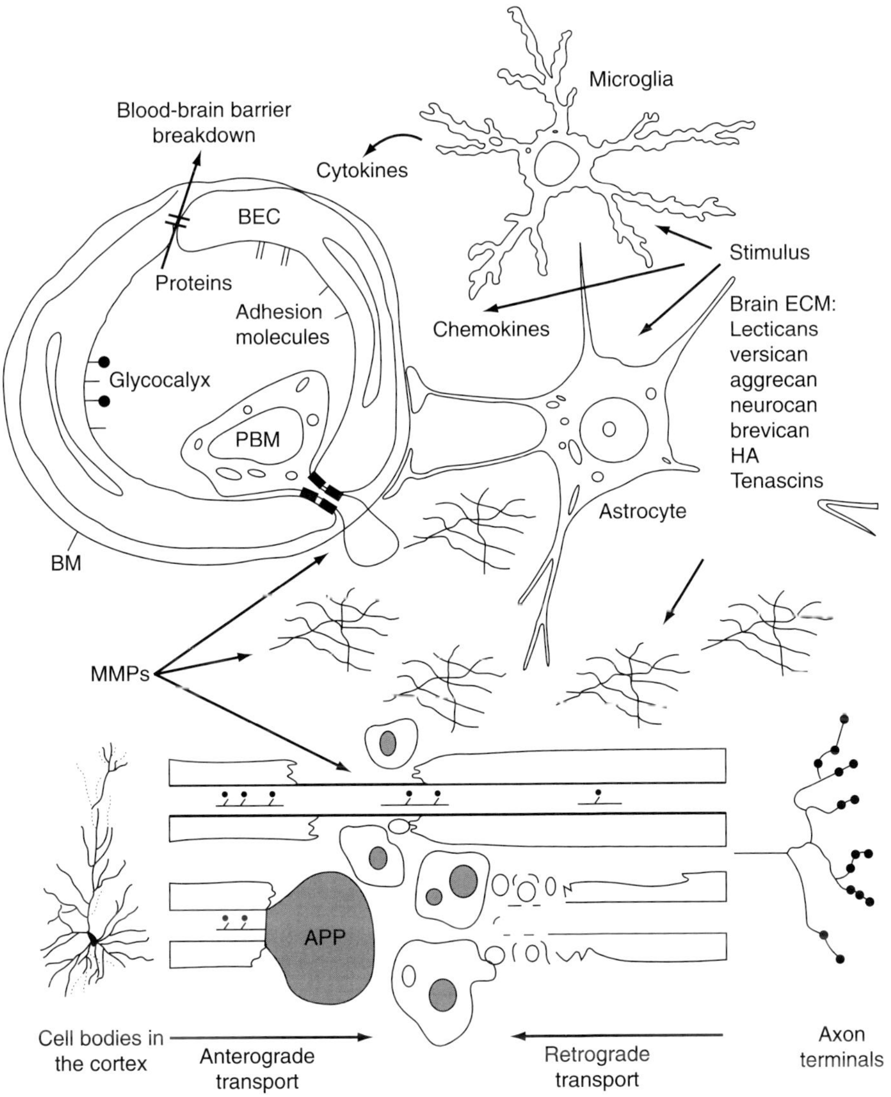

Figure 24.1
Bystander damage in the CNS. Peripheral blood monocytes (PBM) and other leucocytes are recruited to active MS lesions in response to inflammatory stimuli. The recruitment of leucocytes is associated with blood–brain barrier breakdown and oedema. Matrix metalloproteinases, required by leucocytes to cross basement membrane (BM), may be released into the CNS parenchyma in active MS lesions, causing destruction of the matrix, damage to myelin and possibly to axons as well. APP containing structures, with a morphology similar to the end bulbs generated in experimental axotomy, are present within regions of active inflammatory MS lesions.

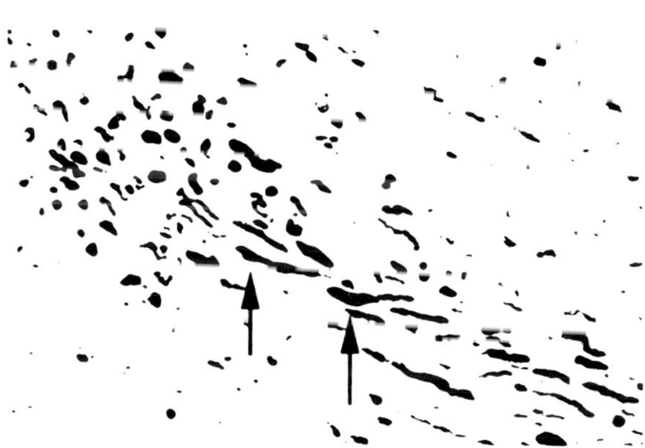

Figure 24.2 APP immunoreactivity in an acute multiple sclerosis lesion. Staining with the LN27 monoclonal antibody (ant-APP) shows many APP positive axons (arrows) inside the lesion.

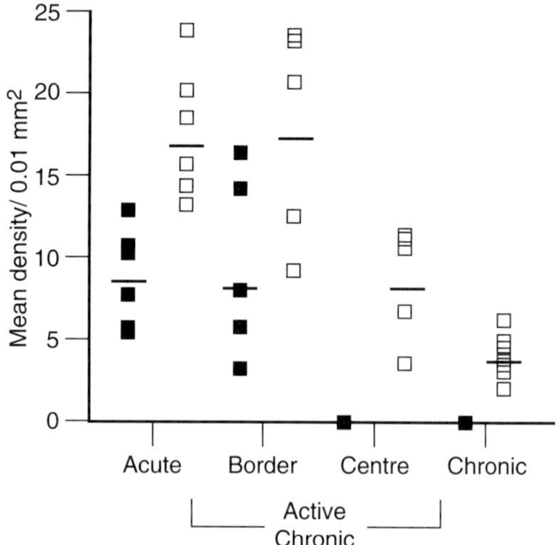

Figure 24.3 Scatter plots showing the mean density of APP-positive axons (■) and macrophages (□) in all the lesions studied by Ferguson et al.[13] Note that the presence of APP immunoreactivity is associated with the presence of active inflammation in MS lesions, as evidenced by the increased number of macrophages.

observations of APP staining following the transection of fibre tracts in the rodent brain indicate that APP immunoreactivity can persist for up to 3 months (T Woolley, unpublished observations) and for at least 1 month in rodents that have been subject to a traumatic brain injury.[14] It is not clear whether, in these long-term experiments, the presence of APP staining represents different axons at different stages of degeneration or the persistence of the same APP-positive end-bulbs. In either case, the absence of APP staining in the chronic lesions is all the more remarkable, as it indicates that axon damage must be occurring at a very low level, if at all, in these plaques. In a chronic lesion, conduction, and thus function, along axons eventually recovers after a period of demyelination, by the upregulation and redistribution of ion channels.[15] Thus, within a noninflammatory quiescent lesion with only a portion of the axon demyelinated, perhaps we shouldn't be so surprised that there appears to be no overt axonal damage.

While the presence of APP undoubtedly represents a perturbation of axoplasmic flow in the MS lesions, it is unclear what percentage of the APP-positive axons are irreversibly damaged and what percentage are likely to recover. Much of the staining has the appearance of the swollen end-bulbs that are associated with axotomy as described by Cajal.[7] Most of the other studies in human tissue that have employed the APP technique are of conditions which are known to be associated with axotomy, such as stroke[16,17] and head injury,[9] and the staining had a similar appearance to that seen in the MS lesions. Thus, it would seem likely that among all the APP-stained axons in the acute MS lesions a substantial proportion of them are likely to be irreversibly damaged.

Another important issue that surrounds the use of the APP technique concerns the amount of time APP remains immunoreactive after injury. As mentioned above, we know that the APP staining remains present in a lesion long after axotomy. Thus, the presence of APP in a lesion does not necessarily represent an absolute measure of the amount of axon damage that is taking place at any one time. Clearly, it would be useful to have markers which could identify 'sick' axons or acutely damaged axons.

However, there is other evidence that damage to axons occurs early in the pathogenesis of MS. This comes from our studies examining axon loss in the post-mortem spinal cords of individuals that suffered from MS, from magnetic resonance imaging (MRI)/magnetic resonance spectroscopy (MRS) studies, and from studies examining brain atrophy. These will be discussed in turn.

Recently, we found that significant axon loss is present even in those individuals with recently-diagnosed MS.[18] In this study, the lateral white matter columns of spinal cord from 11 males without spinal cord disease and 23 males with neuropathologically confirmed MS were subject to computational image analysis. Overall, the MS sufferers were found to have significant lateral column atrophy and significantly fewer fibres in the corticospinal tracts than the controls. Surprisingly, these findings were not related to the length of history, the patient's age, weakness, or the clinical type of MS. Spinal cord atrophy has also been identified, using MRI, in MS patients with secondary progressive and, to a lesser extent, benign MS.[19]

The application of MRI and MRS to the study of MS has also provided evidence of axon loss in MS.[20,21] The earliest detectable event in the development of a new lesion is an increase in permeability of the blood–brain barrier, associated with inflammation and demyelination. Both of these processes contribute to conduction block and functional loss. During remission, oedema resolves and conduction is restored, often to the point where it is hard to detect any increase in permanent disability. However, MRS of cerebellar white matter in a group of MS patients with cerebellar deficits showed a highly significant reduction in the concentration of *N*-acetylaspartate (a neuronal marker) compared with an MS group with minimal or no signs of cerebellar involvement, and with healthy controls.[20] Furthermore, the MS group with severe cerebellar signs also had significant cerebellar atrophy as determined by MRI studies. Marked atrophy of the spinal cord in MS patients has also been demonstrated in MRI studies,[19] where the degree of disability was inversely correlated with both the cross-sectional area and the transverse diameter of the cord. These results support the hypothesis that axonal loss is important in the development of persistent clinical disability in MS. In their report, Tourbah et al. also observe a reduction in the *N*-acetylaspartate signal in the normal-appearing white matter of MS patients, suggesting a more generalized atrophy in the brains of MS patients.[21]

Interestingly, in a recent report investigating the extent of axon damage in Guillain–Barré syndrome, which is often described as the peripheral equivalent of MS, Sobue et al. report that in 7 out of 15 autopsy cases there was significant axon loss associated with the pathology.[22] Indeed, in 5 of the 15 cases there was little segmental demyelination. Like MS, Guillain–Barré syndrome was also classically considered to be a predominantly demyelinating disease.

BYSTANDER DAMAGE IN MS

If we accept that the APP staining represents irreversible damage to some axons, the next question is: what factors are responsible for mediating damage to axons in MS? Since the primary target in MS is likely to be a component of the central nervous system (CNS) other than the axon, a constituent of myelin for example, then the damage suffered by axons is likely to be mediated by a 'bystander' phenomenon. The interaction of tissue macrophages with T cells and/or other resident cells in the CNS leads to the release of many proinflammatory cytokines, complement, eicosanoids, oxygen radicals and proteolytic enzymes, all of which may be involved to a greater or lesser extent in axon loss. However, as direct mediators of destructive events in inflammatory lesions the proteolytic enzymes present themselves as rational targets for intervention. Indeed, the matrix metalloproteinases (MMPs), which as a family of enzymes are able to degrade all of the components of the extracellular matrix,[23] have turned out to be promising therapeutic targets. The MMPs are endopeptidases that contain Zn^{2+} at the active site and are Ca^{2+}-dependent. The production of MMPs is tightly regulated at the various levels of synthesis, secretion and activation. The presence of cytokines within inflamed tissue, such as an MS lesion, induces enzyme expression.[24] The active forms of metalloproteinases may be inactivated by forming a complex with tissue inhibitors of metalloproteinases (TIMPs) or with α_2-macroglobulin.[25,26] It has been useful to subdivide the MMPs into four subclasses based on sequence homology and on substrate specificity: collagenases, gelatinases, stromelysins, and the membrane-type matrix metalloproteinases (MT-MMPS).

A potential role for the involvement of MMPs in CNS inflammatory disease is suggested by their ability to degrade myelin basic protein (MBP) to release immunogenic fragments,[27] by their elevation in the cerebrospinal fluid of patients with MS,[28] by the ability of specific inhibitors of MMPs to reduce the severity of disease in experimental neuroinflammatory disease,[29-31] and by their ability to disrupt the blood–brain barrier following direct of purified enzyme into the brain parenchyma[32] (Fig. 24.1).

Most studies have also found undetectable or very low level expression of these enzymes in normal brain.[33–35] The extracellular matrix of the brain is comprised predominantly of lecticans, which contain a lectin domain and a hyaluronic acid binding domain, and two extracellular matrix components—tenascins and hyaluronic acid—to which the lecticans bind.[36] Many of the lecticans are known to be substrates of the MMPs. Thus, the low level of expression of some of the MMPs may be reflecting turnover of the brain extracellular matrix as part of normal 'housekeeping' processes.

MMPs are expressed in inflammatory lesions in the CNS, and their pattern of expression is highly dependent on the nature and chronicity of the lesion. When MS lesions at various stages of disease were examined for the presence of MMPs, expression was most marked within regions of active inflammation, with a spatial distribution similar to that of the APP stain.[35] MMP staining was most intense in the acute lesions and the active borders, and least intense in the chronic lesions. Within the lesions, elevated MMP expression was most often associated with leucocytes cuffed around vessels. The recruitment of leucocytes to brain parenchyma requires that leucocytes cross the specialized brain endothelium and the basement membrane, which is rich in type-IV collagen, laminin and fibronectin.[37] Those MMPs present in acute MS lesions—gelatinase-A, gelatinase-B and matrilysin—are all capable of degrading basement membrane and may, therefore, aid in leucocyte diapedesis.[38] Leucocyte recruitment to the brain parenchyma is often associated with blood–brain barrier breakdown; the excessive production of MMP may give rise to such breakdown. Studies by Rosenberg and co-workers have shown that intracerebral injection of purified gelatinase-A will damage the blood–brain barrier.[39]

It is well established that demyelination is a feature of traumatic spinal cord injury, which may be a consequence of the influx of inflammatory cells and the release of proteases and cytokines in a nonspecific 'bystander' phenomenon.[40] We have recently described a model in which heat-killed bacillus Calmette–Guérin (BCG), sequestered behind the blood–brain barrier, can be targeted by a delayed-type hypersensitivity (DTH) response after subcutaneous injection of BCG[41] to produce 'bystander' damage. The lesions are characterized by macrophage and lymphocyte infiltration, breakdown of the blood–brain barrier and tissue damage including myelin loss and damage to axons—all the hallmarks of an MS lesion. We have previously shown that development of these lesions may be inhibited by the administration of an MMP inhibitor (BB-1101).[30] It would seem, therefore, that the MMPs may be some of the principal mediators of 'bystander' damage. Indeed the injection of MMP-9 into the CNS parenchyma was associated with loss of MBP immunoreactivity around the injection site, loss of Nissl staining, and recruitment of leucocytes (DC Anthony, unpublished). Thus, in these simple experiments we have demonstrated that the release of a protease from leucocytes present in the CNS parenchyma can give rise to undirected bystander demyelination and possibly to axon damage as well.

IMPLICATIONS FOR THERAPY

The expression of the MMPs within MS lesions, and their ability to degrade myelin and kill neurones, places them firmly in the list of potential targets for the development of therapies. Evidence that the modulation of MMP activity can be of benefit in experimental demyelinating neuroinflammatory disease comes from studies on experimental autoimmune encephalomyelitis (EAE) and in bystander tissue damage in a CNS DTH lesion. Selective inhibition of MMP activity results in a reduction in the clinical score of animals with EAE[29] and significantly reduces the volume of the DTH lesions.[30] In a model of cerebral oedema, following intra-cerebroventricular administration of TNF-α, increased vessel permeability was inhibited by a synthetic hydroxymate-based metalloproteinase inhibitor.[42] Clearly, whether or not MMPs turn out to be important mediators of axon damage in MS, it will be those measures taken to prevent axon damage that will be most likely to reduce the level of permanent disability. Two recent findings—our observation that damage to axons occurs in the inflammatory lesions and evidence from MRI spectroscopy, which suggests that the MS plaque is a more destructive lesion than was previously thought—indicate that earlier intervention may be essential to delay the disabling aspects of MS. If axonal loss occurs as part of the same process that brings about demyelination, rather than by a temporally separate process, then those steps taken to reduce the number of relapses may also improve the long-term survival of neurons. Finally, note that while the overt manifestations of MS are clear indications for therapy, there is often a more insidious cognitive decline, which is observed in >50% of MS patients—probably reflecting cumulative axon loss in the brain. Early intervention and axon-sparing therapy is, therefore, also likely to benefit these patients.

REFERENCES

1. Nauta WJH, Gygax PA. Silver impregnation of degenerating axons in the central nervous system: a modified technique. *Stain Technol* 1954; **29**: 91–93.
2. Fink RP, Heimer L. Two methods for the selective silver impregnation of degenerating axons and their synaptic endings in the central nervous system. *Brain Res* 1967; **4**: 369–374.
3. De Olmos JS, Beltramino CA, Olmos De Lorenzo SD. Use of an amino-cupric-silver technique for the detection of early and semiacute neuronal degeneration caused by neurotoxicants, hypoxia, and physical trauma. *Neurotoxicol Teratol* 1994; **16**: 545–561.
4. Gallyas F, Wolf JR, Bottcher H et al. A reliable and sensitive method to localize terminal degeneration and lysosomes in the central nervous system. *Stain Technol* 1980; **55**: 299–306.
5. Autiliogambetti L, Crane R, Gambetti P. Binding of bodian silver and monoclonal-antibodies to defined regions of human neurofilament subunits—bodian silver reacts with a highly charged unique domain of neurofilaments. *J Neurochem* 1986; **46**: 366–370.
6. Curcio CA, Allen KA. Topography of ganglion-cells in human retina. *J Comp Neurol* 1990; **300**: 5–25.
7. Cajal R. Degeneration and regeneration of the white matter. In: May RM, ed. *Degeneration and Regeneration of the Nervous System*, vol. 2. New York: Hafner Publishing, 1959: 484–516.
8. Sherriff FE, Bridges LR, Gentleman SM et al. Markers of axonal injury in post-mortem human brain. *Acta Neuropathol* 1994; **88**: 433–439.
9. Gentleman SM, Roberts GW, Gennarelli TA et al. Axonal injury—a universal consequence of fatal closed-head injury. *Acta Neuropathol* 1995; **89**: 537–543.
10. Maxwell WL, Povlishock JT, Graham DL. A mechanistic analysis of nondisruptive axonal injury: a review. *J Neurotrauma* 1997; **14**: 419–440.
11. Povlishock JT. Traumatically induced axonal injury—pathogenesis and pathobiological implications. *Brain Pathol* 1992; **2**: 1–12.
12. Koo EH, Sisodia SS, Archer DR et al. Precursor of amyloid protein in Alzheimer-disease undergoes fast anterograde axonal-transport. *Proc Natl Acad Sci USA* 1990; **87**: 1561–1565.
13. Ferguson B, Matyszak MK, Esiri MM et al. Axonal damage in acute multiple sclerosis lesions. *Brain* 1997; **120**: 393–399.
14. Bramlett HM, Kraydieh S, Green EJ et al. Temporal and regional patterns of axonal damage following traumatic brain injury: a beta-amyloid precursor protein immunocytochemical study in rats. *J Neuropath Exp Neurol* 1997; **56**: 1132–1141.
15. Bostock H, Sears TA. The internodal axon membrane—electrical excitability and continuous conduction in segmental demyelination. *J Physiol* 1978, **280**: 273–301.
16. Cochran E, Bacci B, Chen Y et al. Amyloid precursor protein and ubiquitin immunoreactivity in dystrophic axons is not unique to Alzheimer's-disease. *Am J Pathol* 1991, **139**: 485–489.
17. Yam PS, Takasago T, Dewar D et al. Amyloid precursor protein accumulates in white matter at the margin of a focal ischaemic lesion. *Brain Res* 1997; **760**: 150–157.
18. Prince C, Esiri MM. A quantitative study of axonal loss in the spinal cord in multiple sclerosis. *Neuropathol Appl Neurobiol* 1997; **23**: 432 [abstract].

19. Filippe M, Campi A, Colombo B et al. A spinal-cord MRI study of benign and secondary progressive multiple-sclerosis. *J Neurol* 1996; **243**: 502–505.
20. Davie CA, Barker GJ, Webb S et al. Persistent deficit in multiple-sclerosis and autosomal-dominant cerebellar-ataxia is associated with axon loss. *Brain* 1995; **118**: 1583–1592.
21. Tourbah A, Stievenart JL, Ibazizen MT et al. In-vivo localized NMR proton spectroscopy of normal appearing white-matter in patients with multiple-sclerosis. *J Neuroradiol* 1996; **23**: 49–55.
22. Sobue G, Li M, Terao S et al. Axonal pathology in Japanese Guillain–Barré syndrome: a study of 15 autopsied cases. *Neurology* 1997; **48**: 1694–1700.
23. Murphy G, Reynolds J. Extracellular matrix degradation. In: Royce P, Steinmann B, eds. *Connective Tissue and its Heritable Disorders*. New York: Wiley-Liss, 1993: 287–316.
24. Fabunmi RP, Baker AH, Murray EJ et al. Divergent regulation by growth-factors and cytokines of 95-kDa and 72-kDa gelatinases and tissue inhibitors of metalloproteinase-1, metalloproteinase-2 and metalloproteinase-3 in rabbit aortic smooth-muscle cells. *Biochem J* 1996; **315**: 335–342.
25. Cawston TE, Galloway WA, Mercer E et al. Purification of rabbit bone inhibitor of collagenase. *Biochem J* 1981; **195**: 159–165.
26. Ward RV, Hembry RM, Reynolds JJ et al. The purification of tissue inhibitor of metalloproteinases-2 from its 72 kDa progelatinase complex. Demonstration of the biochemical similarities of tissue inhibitor of metalloproteinases-2 and tissue of metalloproteinases-1. *Biochem J* 1991; **278**: 179–87.
27. Chandler S, Coates R, Gearing A et al. Matrix metalloproteinases degrade myelin basic-protein. *Neurosci Lett* 1995; **201**: 223–226.
28. Gijbels K, Masure S, Carton H et al. Gelatinase in the cerebrospinal fluid of patients with multiple sclerosis and other inflammatory neurological disorders. *J Neuroimmunol* 1992; **41**: 29–34.
29. Gijbels K, Galardy RE, Steinman L. Reversal of experimental autoimmune encephalomyelitis with a hydroxymate inhibitor of matrix metalloproteases. *J Clin Invest* 1994; **94**: 2177–2182.
30. Matyszak M, Perry V. Delayed-type hypersensitivity lesions in the central nervous system are prevented by inhibitors of matrix metalloproteinases. *J Neuroimmunol* 1996; **69**: 141–149.
31. Clements JM, Cossins JA, Wells GMA et al. Matrix metalloproteinase expression during experimental autoimmune encephalomyelitis and effects of a combined matrix metalloproteinase and tumor necrosis factor-alpha inhibitor. *J Neuroimmunol* 1997; **74**: 85–94.
32. Rosenberg GA. Matrix metalloproteinases in brain injury. *J Neurotrauma* 1995; **12**: 833–842.
33. Sawaya RE, Yamamoto M, Gokaslan ZL et al. Expression and localization of 72 kDa type IV collagenase (MMP-2) in human malignant gliomas in vivo. *Clin Exp Metastasis* 1996; **14**: 35–42.
34. Rao JS, Yamamoto M, Mohaman S et al. Expression and localization of 92 kDa type IV collagenase/gelatinase B (MMP-9) in human gliomas. *Clin Exp Metastasis* 1996; **14**: 12–18.
35. Anthony DC, Ferguson B, Matyzak MK et al. Differential matrix metalloproteinase expression in cases of multiple sclerosis and stroke. *Neuropathol Appl Neurobiol* 1997; **23**: 406–415.
36. Ruoslahti E. Brain extracellular-matrix. *Glycobiology* 1996; **6**: 489–492.
37. Nag S. Immunohistochemical localization of extracellular matrix proteins in cerebral vessels in chronic hypertension. *J Neuropathol Exp Neurol* 1996; **55**: 381–388.
38. Murphy G, Cockett MI, Ward RV et al. Matrix metalloproteinase degradation of elastin, type IV collagen and proteoglycan. A quantitative comparison of the activities of 95 kDa and 72 kDa gelatinases, stromelysins-1 and -2 and punctated metalloproteinase (PUMP). *Biochem J* 1991; **277**: 277–279.
39. Rosenberg GA, Kornfeld M, Estrada E et al. TIMP-2 reduces proteolytic opening of blood–brain barrier by type IV collagenase. *Brain Res* 1992; **576**: 203–207.
40. Blight AR. Delayed demyelination and macrophage invasion: a candidate for secondary cell damage in spinal cord injury. *CNS Trauma* 1985; **2**: 299–315.
41. Matyszak MK, Perry VH. Demyelination in the central nervous system following a delayed-type hypersensitivity response to bacillus Calmette–Guérin. *Neuroscience* 1995; **64**: 967–977.
42. Rosenberg GA, Estrada EY, Dencoff JE et al. Tumor necrosis factor-alpha-induced gelatinase-B causes delayed opening of the blood–brain-barrier—an expanded therapeutic window. *Brain Res* 1995; **703**: 151–155.

25

Long-term management and rehabilitation in multiple sclerosis

Jürg Kesselring

INTRODUCTION

There are many conference reports on multiple sclerosis (MS) but only rarely is rehabilitation and long-term management the subject of such volumes. Knowledge about pathogenesis of MS has deepened considerably over the recent past and new medical treatments have opened new ways of patient management in MS. A new area in MS therapy began when interferon-β-1b (IFN-β1b) was approved by the FDA in April 1993 confronting MS researchers and clinicians alike with new economical and political dimensions. Diagnosis of MS may have become less difficult than in earlier years and some drugs are available that have been proven in good clinical trials to be of some benefit for some patients in some phases of their disease, but the astute clinician has by no means been rendered superfluous since the long-term management of MS patients has remained the same great challenge as ever.[1]

But how may rehabilitation contribute to the long-term management of MS?

PRINCIPLES OF NEUROLOGICAL REHABILITATION

Rehabilitation has been defined as 'an active process by which those disabled by injury or disease achieve a full recovery or when a full recovery is not possible realise their optimal physical, mental and social potential and are integrated into their most appropriate environment'. Rehabilitation does differ from many medical specialties in that it is an active process of education and enablement. It is focused on the proper management of disability and the minimization of handicap. Often rather simple measures such as prone lying and standing which help to maintain a full range of movements of the joints make the difference between independence and dependence. It is less focused on the problems of diagnosis and impairment. The necessity of daily standing does not depend on the underlying cause nor does the management of contractures.

Thus, neurological rehabilitation is a speciality that requires both skills and training in neurology and training in the complementary skills of the rehabilitation physician. It is a process that requires an understanding and knowledge of the value and importance of other therapies and nursing and of the problems of disability and caring for someone with a disabling condition, as well as an empathetic approach.

MS appears to be a particularly important clinical entity well suited for implementing the International Classification of Impairment, Disability and Handicap (ICIDH).[2,3] This classification system should provide a common language based on new thinking. The ICIDH sets a framework for gaining information about the long-term consequences of diseases such as MS.[4] This information is relevant for care and includes the lowering of natural and social barriers; it makes the description of life circumstances possible. On the level of institutions and of the community it facilitates the determination of personal and financial resources and needs.

A disease sets the stage for an inevitable decision between loss or gain, and in this sense it is always also a chance. The decision does not depend on the disease itself but on what we make out of it. If one thinks to depend only on the disease itself, the decision is already taken—for loss.

Some service values should underpin any neurological rehabilitation service:

- *choice* as to where to live and how to maintain independence without over-protection—or the risk of unnecessary hazards—including help in learning how to choose
- *consultation* with disabled people and their families on services as they are planned
- *information* clearly presented and readily available to the most severely disabled consumers
- *participation* in the life of local and national communities in respect to both responsibilities and benefits
- *recognition* that long-term disability is not synonymous with illness and that the medical model of care is inappropriate in most cases
- *autonomy*, that is, freedom to make decision regarding that way of life best suited to an individual disabled person's circumstances.

The underlying principle is therefore that disabled people, and their carers, should be intrinsically involved in the rehabilitation process. It is a process that should be carried out by or with disabled people and not for disabled people.

WHY HAVE A NEUROLOGICAL REHABILITATION SERVICE?

There are significant benefits from a dedicated neurological rehabilitation service:

(a) *Functional benefit.* There is now considerable evidence that the rehabilitation process does produce real functional benefit and improved outcomes for disabled people.[5,6]
(b) *Reduction of unnecessary complications.* Many problems with disability are caused by unnecessary complications.[7] Poorly managed spasticity can result in contractures and thus unnecessary further restrictions on mobility or use of arms.[8] Pressure sores are nearly always preventable but if allowed to develop can cause pain, infection, increasing disability and often require expensive hospital admission and surgery. A neurological rehabilitation team can assure that proper attention is paid to nutrition and the assessment and management of swallowing disorders. Many behavioural disorders, anxiety, depression and other emotional problems often accompany physical disability and are amenable to appropriate intervention.
(c) *Coordination and use of resources.* A neurological rehabilitation team can provide a better coordinated service for the disabled person and family. This should lead to a better use of limited resources and prevention of duplication of assessment and treatment.
(d) *Reduction of crisis admission to hospital.* A properly planned goal-orientated rehabilitation service should offer long-term support to the disabled person and carer to prevent inappropriate crisis or other residential admission.
(e) *Lessened handicap.* Maximum improvements in independence and quality of life should lead to better changes of employment. Social and leisure opportunities should be increased and overall rehabilitation will maximize the chances of the disabled person leading a full and active life and making a significant contribution to the local community.

(f) *Cost effective.* An efficient rehabilitation process—because of shorter assessment time and less duplication as well as more accurate needs assessment—should result in an improved effectiveness of service provision and, in the long term, lead to cost savings.
(g) *Education and teaching.* A neurological rehabilitation team should act as a focus for education and teaching of medical, nursing and therapy colleagues. Such improvement of knowledge will further ease the problems that disabled people face when in contact with health services.
(h) *Research.* There is a considerable need for research in many aspects of neurological rehabilitation, particularly applied research into the best method of service delivery and reduction of disability. A coordinated neurological rehabilitation team should act as a base for such research projects.
(i) *Point of contact.* There is a complicated array of services necessary for the disabled person. Often there is poor coordination between different departments, and a neurological rehabilitation team can act as a point of contact for information and advice for the disabled person and family and ease the path through health and social systems.

We recommend that every person with a neurological disability should have access to support and advice from a physician expert in neurological rehabilitation. The numbers of such experts in any country will clearly depend on the design and scope of rehabilitation and neurological facilities and services. However, as a general rule most countries with an established network of such physicians find that one physician per 100 000 population is sufficient to provide reasonably quick and efficient access to such individuals within the disabled population.

In some countries the physicians will have a neurological background and training while in other countries rehabilitation services are provided from the separate specialty of rehabilitation or physical medicine. The dual training in both fields is important, and medical authorities should support and promote a comprehensive programme of training in neurology and rehabilitation medicine. It is important for neurologists to have a period of exposure and training in rehabilitation medicine or for rehabilitation physicians to have a period of exposure and training programmes may be difficult to fund or establish. Organizations such as ECTRIMS and RIMS, ACTRIMS and the Consortium of MS Centers could become the platforms to promote cross-national training programmes and move towards international standards for such training programmes.

Every neurologically disabled person should have access to a full multidisciplinary team trained in the management of neurological disabilities. The composition of such a team will clearly vary from country to country. We think that the team should be led by a physician for various reasons and we consider the minimum discipline requirements for a comprehensive team are:

- physiotherapy
- occupational therapy
- access to speech and language therapy
- access to clinical neuropsychology
- nursing—I know from experience that the nurses play a cardinal role in the team
- occasional and intermittent access to other relevant disciplines such as dietetics, social work and to other medical disciplines including orthopaedics, urology and plastic surgery may be required.

Teamwork means pulling on the same rope—and in the same direction! A rehabilitation team implies multidisciplinary or interdisciplinary working and is a client-centred goal-setting process. There are different methods of leading a team; requirements are clear indications that allow individually and private initiative. Such methods also imply a blurring of strict professional boundaries, with proper team coordination to avoid unnecessary duplication and overlap of scarce resources. In contrast to the overorganized and hyperindividualized structures which have been commonplace in our societies and which lead to isolation, in rehabilitation centres a setting which facilitates communication must be installed. The first and most crucial step in this process is *assessment*.

The quality or appropriateness of rehabilitation can only be as good as the assessment on which it is based.[9] In MS, where there is frequently a wide range of problems many of which interact in a complex fashion, it can often be a challenging and difficult process. It can be formative, i.e. an ongoing process to target and develop appropriate interventions.[10] It can also be summative, i.e. an expert analysis and statement of current problems and needs at a point in time. The assessment team needs to gather all relevant information leading up to the assessment from their own disciplines and beyond, and work together to identify appropriate areas of input. The initial assessment will identify areas in which there is potential for a change which will be of benefit to the person with MS (*goal setting*). It should allow the team to define the extent of change possible, i.e. the long-term goal and the length of time required to achieve it. The long-term goal needs to be broken down into small measurable steps which are seen to be important to the person with MS, not simply areas regarded as being important by the therapist or physician. In any rehabilitation process it is essential to measure the effect of the process in relation to outcome, the basis of evidence-based clinical decision making. It can be addressed from two distinct perspectives:

(1) the success of the rehabilitation process in relation to goal achievement
(2) the effect of the rehabilitation process on the person with MS.

The first, although difficult, may be measured using integrated care pathways,[11] while the evaluation of the effect of the rehabilitation process on the patient requires the use of outcome measures in the context of audit or clinical trials.[5,6] When measuring outcome in MS, four levels should be considered: physiological parameters such as MRI, clinical endpoints such as relapse rate, aspects of health status such as disability and handicap, and health-related quality of life. A scientifically sound scale used to measure outcome must be reliable (free from random error), valid (measures what it intends to measure), and responsive (capable of measuring clinically significant changes even if that change is small).[9] In a stratified, randomized, waitlist controlled study to evaluate the effectiveness of short-term (25 days) multidisciplinary inpatient rehabilitation in MS, at the end of 6 weeks the treatment group showed significantly improved levels of disability and handicap compared to those in the waitlist control group,[5] and this effect was carried over 6 months after discharge.[6] These studies underline the conviction that inpatient rehabilitation should not be seen in isolation and must be part of a continuum of care involving inpatient, outpatient and community services.

MEDICAL SYMPTOMATIC TREATMENT[8]

Spasticity

For the clinician confronted with a patient with MS, it is of particular importance to determine signs of spasticity. This complex clinical syndrome consists of muscle hypertonia and exaggerated tendon reflexes (including clonus). Clinically, spasticity is characterized by weakness, slowness in building up to maximal power of muscle activity and relaxing again, and clumsiness of voluntary movements. This usually results from a lack of coordination of synergistic muscles or failure of inhibition of antagonists. Thereby, the range of functional voluntary movements may be reduced to a few stereotyped patterns. Spasticity is largely responsible for the disability of affected individuals and it is often amenable to efficient treatment. In MS, the legs are usually more markedly affected by spasticity than the arms.[7] Extensor spasticity of the legs, particularly of the quadriceps, might be considered for muscular weakness. The 'clasp-knife' response, however, which is only known in extensor muscles may annihilate this apparent functional gain. Part of the clinical impression of a progressive course in MS may therefore be owing to inadequate management of spasticity[7] that leads to such structural changes of muscles with subsequent functional impairment.

Treatment

Treatment of spasticity should be considered only after careful assessment of the patient's functional status to clearly identify treatment goals and to evaluate the potential risks and likely benefits of various therapeutic interventions.[12]

Clinical observations suggest that spasticity in MS may be triggered or aggravated by many conditions, noxious or potentially painful afferent activity,[12,13] including urinary tract infections, faecal impaction, contractures, ingrowing toenails, skin ulcerations and increased sensory stimuli from ill-fitting, orthotic appliances, catheter bags or even tight clothing or footwear. These conditions should routinely be looked for and, when present, appropriately managed. Correct positioning is most important for preventing limbs becoming fixed in the position imposed by the pattern of spasticity. 'The use of a well-structured physiotherapy programme is certainly the most effective way of retraining motor functions in patients with upper motorneuron lesions and of reducing spasticity.'[14] Since there is little scientific evidence that any particular technique is more efficacious than another for the promotion of functional gait or for the management of spasticity,[13,14] it is difficult to evaluate the role of dynamic physiotherapy in the overall management of spasticity. One fundamental aim of physiotherapy in the management of MS is adaptation of muscle tone according to behavioural demands. Normal tone has to be high enough to provide optimal stabilization against gravity and low enough to allow for selective movements in all their graduations. This harmonious interplay of muscle activity is governed by the principle of reciprocal inhibition of agonists and antagonists. According to the Bobath concept,[15] abnormal postural tone and spasticity can be positively influenced by facilitation of the movements of certain key points of postural control. By producing reflex inhibiting patterns, normal movement sequences are facilitated. This learning process set apace by special treatment must be supported and enhanced by carry-over of the relevant exercise programme into the activities of daily life. With the help of ongoing assessment of the patient's abilities, the therapeutic aims are continuously adjusted to the special requirements of the individual situation. All different physiotherapeutic methods in MS aim at prevention and treatment of muscle contractures, allowing as full range of movements of joints as possible, reduction of muscle hypertonia, training of posture and automatically performed movements with the induction of voluntarily initiated and controlled complex movements, and learning and training of coordinated movements by the involvement of tactile, vestibular, auditory and visual cues.[13] In one of the first randomized controlled trials on physiotherapy in MS it was demonstrated that a 15-week aerobic training programme may lead to statistically significant improvements in the short term (up to 10 weeks) in aerobic capacity, isometric strength, body composition, blood lipid levels, depression, anger and fatigue in comparison to a nonexercise group.[16] Physiotherapy may lead to a significant reduction in mobility-related distress in MS patients as measured by the patient visual analogue scale even though this is not reflected in significant changes in objective disability or mobility scores.[17]

Several drugs are available which effectively reduce increased muscle tone and painful muscle spasms in a variety of clinical disorders, including MS. Before introducing drug treatment for reducing spasticity, it should be considered, however, that a relatively rigid or spastic limb may be useful for walking or transferring for an individual with muscle weakness, and that inappropriate alleviation of spasticity in such circumstances can lead to a functional reduction in mobility and independence. Since, like all clinical manifestations of MS, spasticity tends to change over time it is important to re-evaluate antispastic treatment at intervals. As a rule, the use of only one substance at a time is recommended, although combinations of drugs with different mechanisms of action may eventually be tried. Because relief of muscle spasms and muscle hypertonia may be achieved only at the cost of reduced muscle power, and because all antispastic drugs may induce side-effects, doses should be kept to a minimum, especially immobile patients.[13]

Tizanidine acts by stimulation of alpha-2 adrenergic receptors in the spinal cord. In controlled trials the effective dose of tizanidine for reducing spasticity ranged from 12 to 36 mg (average 18 mg). All basic symptoms associated with spasticity, e.g. increased muscle tone, muscle spasms and clonus, improved to a similar extent (60–80% responders).[18] A useful improvement of the clinical applicability of tizanidine is the introduction of 'constant-release' forms of 6 mg and 12 mg tablets. The most frequent side-effects are tiredness, drowsiness and dry mouth.

Baclofen is an agonist of gamma-aminobutyric acid (GABA)-B receptors, acting mainly at the terminals of primary afferent fibres in the spinal cord. Baclofen as oral medication is given in doses starting at 10 mg and increased stepwise until the desired benefit is achieved or side-effects (such as drowsiness, fatigue and muscle weakness) become unacceptable. On average, 40–80 mg/day are given in three doses. Abrupt discontinuation may result in withdrawal symptoms such as hallucinations and seizures.

In very severe spasticity, as may occur in longstanding MS, baclofen may be given intrathecally via a subcutaneously placed infusion pump. This may be indicated for facilitating nursing and for alleviating painful muscle spasms and automatic movements of the legs.

Dantrolene has a peripheral target of action and exerts its antispastic effect within the muscle itself. Because of this different site of action it may be used in combination with one of the above-mentioned antispastics of first choice. Side-effects include drowsiness, weakness and fatigue and can be minimized by starting dose at 25 mg and slowly increasing to a maximum of 400 mg over several weeks. Hepatotoxicity, depending on dosage and duration of treatment often limits the use of dantrolene. In spite of their excellent antispastic effect, benzodiazepines have only limited usefulness as single agents to treat spasticity of MS patients because of their serious side-effects, such as drowsiness, tolerance and dependency.

Treatment with botulinum toxin A is usually a safe procedure and has an established role in various movement disorders. Its usefulness in the treatment of spasticity, however, is only recently being investigated. In a double-blind, placebo-controlled, cross-over study[19] on non-ambulatory patients with longstanding MS, local injection of botulinum toxin into severely spastic hip adductors was shown to make peroneal hygiene, urethral catheterization, sitting and positioning in bed much easier. This benefit lasted an average of 3 months.

ATAXIA

Ataxia is a lack of reduction in coordination. Ataxia is a common symptom in MS occurring in 85% of patients at some stage in the course of their condition. It may be aggravated by weakness, spasticity and reduced sensory and visual input. Classification of ataxic tremor is still at a relatively early stage in development.

Management

Three broad approaches may be taken for management:

(a) practical management, which is fundamental and aimed at addressing disability and handicap
(b) drug treatment, which is limited and often not well tolerated
(c) surgical intervention, which is often discouraged in MS and includes thalamotomy and thalamic stimulation.

Occupational therapy plays a key role in teaching practical compensatory strategies, for example stabilizing body parts during activities, reviewing posture and seating, which may allow improved control over ataxic limbs, providing advice on adaptations to the home environment,[20] and teaching carers easier ways of tackling the problem. The physiotherapist aims to improve proximal stability, thereby improving motor control. Other therapeutic manoeuvres have included using weights[21] which have not proved very successful though the results are somewhat better if a computer-controlled damping device is incorporated.

Medical treatment

Isoniazid (with pyridoxine) up to 1200 mg/day in divided doses has been shown to be of some, albeit limited, value in tremor in MS. It is usually introduced gradually over 2 weeks. Isoniazid is not always well tolerated and causes gastrointestinal disturbance including diarrhoea. Other medications which have been tried with limited success in small studies include carbamazepine.

Surgical treatment

Thalamotomy of the ventral intermediate nucleus (VIM) has been shown to be beneficial in alleviating tremor in MS. The results in relation to cerebellar tremor have been variable. These patients had generally lost all upper limb function and following thalamic stimulation were able to carry out simple tasks such as grasping an object; six patients were able to feed themselves. So significant change was seen in the EDSS and only one patient developed a transient motor deficit. Thalamic stimulation has an important role in the management of cerebellar tremor in MS with clear advantages over thalamotomy.[22] The tremor, especially its proximal component, was improved in 70% of patients not surprisingly. The greatest functional improvement was observed in those patients whose disability related to tremor (marked improvement in 80% of cases). The effect on truncal ataxia and gait is not known as most of the patients studied were severely disabled. It would of course be preferable that patients had unilateral tremor and were in a position to make the most of the functional benefit acquired from the procedure.

FATIGUE

Fatigue is reputed to be the most common symptom in MS, affecting over 85% of patients,[23] and it is certainly one of the most disabling from the patient's perspective. Fatigue poses a great challenge for clinicians, researchers and the MS population, particularly because of difficulty in defining the entity, understanding the underlying mechanisms, measuring its impact and alleviating it. MS fatigue is defined as an overwhelming sense of tiredness, lack of energy, or feeling of exhaustion. It is far in excess of what might be expected for the associated level of activity and can be distinguished from 'normal' tiredness experienced by everyone.[24] It should be distinguished from depression, which will usually be associated with symptoms such as lack of self esteem, despair or feelings of hopelessness, though these two entities may co-exist and may aggravate each other.[25] Various mechanisms contribute to the global symptom: a poor sleep pattern, which can result from other MS symptoms such as nocturia, pain and spasticity, and the increased effort, both physical and mental, required for mobility because of weakness, spasticity and ataxia. An immunological effect is supported by the known capacity of cytokines to produce fatigue and myalgia, and abnormalities of the hypothalamic pituitary axis, including impaired response to stress, may contribute. Fatigue in MS has also been associated with impaired motor function. Fatigue impacts on all activities of the person with MS, both task related (disability) and social (handicap). Identifying fatigue as a relevant and disabling symptom is the first and most important step, to be followed by education and support. Patients benefit directly when their symptoms are recognized as genuine, and it is equally important for family and carers to understand the nature of the problem.

Medication

Several medications have been shown to be partly effective in the management of fatigue: amantadine, pemoline and 4-aminopyridine.[26–28]

Addressing the issue of fatigue is particularly relevant in the rehabilitation setting, and there is evidence to suggest that failure to allow for its impact on the patient with MS will lead to less than satisfactory goal achievement.[11]

PAIN

Pain in MS is present in one-third to one-half of cases and may be considered by up to one-third of patients to be the most disturbing symptom. The frequency of occurrence of pain is not related to the degree of disability: it is more frequent in older people, when disease onset has occurred at a late age, in those with chronic progressive disease and when there is spastic paresis and disturbances of coordination. It can be classified as follows.

(a) pain due to the disease process itself, e.g. trigeminal neuralgia and painful chronic spasms
(b) shooting spasms of the extremities, particularly marked flexor spasticity of the legs
(c) pain due to disability and its associated problems.

In most cases the last type of pain can be prevented by adequate physiotherapy and comprehensive rehabilitation: 60% of wheelchair patients complain of neck pain and the comfort of those sitting in wheelchairs is not always considered carefully enough. In chronic MS, painful osteoporosis may be due to inactivity or to irresponsible long-term prescription of steroid therapy.[7]

SERVICES

The most efficient outcomes will be obtained by a two-tier system of neurological service delivery. Individuals should have access to regional specialist expertise, particularly for the management of the most complex and severe disabilities. Regional neurological rehabilitation centres are required to provide access to specialist experts familiar with the management of complex and severe disabilities. Taking disability seriously may have repercussions on our understanding of disease mechanisms. There is new experimental evidence that mechanical factors are important in lesion development.

Regional centres should also act as a focus for education, training and research, and should be linked to university teaching centres. They must be staffed by adequate numbers of physicians trained in neurological rehabilitation with the support and cooperation of specialized therapists and nurses. The numbers of such regional centres in each country will depend on available resources, geography and the general organization of the health system, and the services delivered will vary depending on available staff and resources.

Standards of education and training in neurological rehabilitation are generally inadequate. There are very few coordinated training programmes for physicians, therapists and nurses in this field. Regional centres should act as a focus for education and training programmes within their own country and be part of an international network such as RIMS which should focus its activities on setting standards concerning symptomatic treatment, long-term management, assessment and on the integration of rehabilitation into academic teaching. The move towards standardization of training is to be encouraged. Regional centres should also act as a focus for education and training of other health professional colleagues. Many problems for disabled people arise when they have contact with other health services who have minimal understanding of the problems of disability.

Training programmes for disabled people and carers in the proper management of disability are also important, both for the development of self esteem and to make best use of scarce resources. This is an important task for local and regional centres.

There is inadequate evidence on which to base proper rehabilitation decisions regarding the best method of service delivery, the best type of intervention and the best means of management of various disabilities. All regional centres should therefore develop research programmes, and universities should become more active in the establishment of academic centres for rehabilitation. Governments should invest more health research money into this important field of neurorehabilitation. Research into rehabilitation and neurological disability will not only produce benefits for the disabled people and their carers but also in the long term should produce benefits for the national economy.

LOCAL AND COMMUNITY

However, most disability can be managed at a local community level and most disabled people will not need access to regional services. Thus, we strongly encourage the development of more locally orientated neurological disability teams. They may be based in local hospitals for the sake of convenience. But we firmly encourage such teams to develop community outreach into local clinics, health centres or into the individual's home. Because we are aware that the economic situation in many European countries will not allow the development of teams that are staffed only by qualified therapists or doctors, we encourage serious consideration of the community-based rehabilitation (CBR) model developed by the World Health Organization. This model allows local communities to deliver their own support mechanisms for disabled people, often with a locally trained worker supervised by qualified staff, but providing basic rehabilitation, treatment and advice within their own community.

Although this chapter is mainly focused on health rehabilitation, I am fully aware that the needs for disabled people go beyond the boundaries of health. Local disability teams have to work together with other relevant local services, particularly social services, housing and employment agencies. This would enable a more comprehensive disability service to be provided for all disabled people.

INTERNATIONAL COOPERATION

Neurological rehabilitation is insufficiently developed across Europe and indeed across the world as a whole. There is much to be gained by international cooperation with regard to sharing of models of good practice, and education and research initiatives. International cooperation in these developing fields is vital and the cooperation of European and global bodies such as ECTRIMS, ACTRIMS, RIMS, the consortium, IFMSS and the European Platform of MS societies must be strengthened to develop international clinical, education or research initiatives.

REFERENCES

1. Bauer HJ, Kesselring J. *Medizinische Rehabilitation und Nachsorge bei Multipler Sklerose.* Stuttgart, New York: Gustav Fischer, 1995.
2. World Health Organization. *International Classification of Impairments, Disabilities, and Handicaps. A Manual of Classification Relating to the Consequences of Disease.* Geneva: WHO, 1980.
3. Thompson AJ. Rehabilitation of progressive neurological disorders: a worthwhile challenge. *Curr Opin Neurol* 1996; **9(6)**: 437–440.
4. Badley EM. An introduction to the concepts and classifications of the international classification of impairments, disabilities and handicaps. *Disability Rehab* 1993; **4**: 161–178.
5. Freeman JA, Langdon DW, Hobart JC et al. Long-term effects of neurorehabilitation in multiple sclerosis: a longitudinal study. *J Neurol Neurosurg Psychiatry* 1997; **65**: 694.
6. Freeman JA, Langdon DW, Hobart JC et al. The impact of inpatient rehabilitation on progressive multiple sclerosis. *Ann Neurol* 1997; **42**: 236–244.
7. Kesselring J, ed. *Multiple Sclerosis*. Cambridge: Cambridge University Press, 1997.
8. Kesselring J, Thompson AJ. Management of spasticity, fatigue and ataxia in multiple sclerosis. In: Miller DH, ed. *Multiple Sclerosis, Baillière's Clinical Neurology*, 1998 (in press).
9. Thompson AJ. Neurorehabilitation in MS. *Schweiz Arch Neurol Psychiatry* 1997; **148 (suppl 197)**: 182–186.
10. Ward C, McIntosh S. The rehabilitation process: a neurological perspective. In: Greenwood R, Barnes MP, McMillan TM et al., eds. *Neurological Rehabilitation*. Singapore: Churchill Livingstone, 1993; 13–27
11. Rossiter D, Edmonson A, al-Shahi R, Thompson AJ. Integrated care pathways in MS rehabilitation: completing the audit cycle. *Mult Scler* 1998; **4**: 85–89.
12. Bakheit AMO. Management of muscle spasticity. *Crit Rev Phys Med Rehab* 1996; **8 (3)**: 235–252.
13. Dietz V, Young RR. The syndrome of spastic paresis. In: Brandt T, Dichgans J, eds. *Neurological Disorders: Course and Treatment*. London: Academic Press, 1996; 861–871.

14. Hömberg V. Rehabilitation in spastic syndromes—nonpharmacological treatment. In: Emre M, Benecke R, eds. *Spasticity. The Current Status of Research and Treatment.* Parthenon, London, 1989; 97–114.
15. Mertin J, Paeth B. Physiotherapy and multiple sclerosis—application of the Bobath concept. *MS Management* 1994; **1**: 10–13.
16. Petajan JH, Gappmaier E, White AT et al. Impact of aerobic training on fitness and quality of life in multiple sclerosis. *Ann Neurol* 1996; **39**: 432–441.
17. Fuller KJ, Dawson K, Wiles CM. Physiotherapy in chronic multiple sclerosis: a controlled trial. *Clin Rehab* 1996; **10**: 195–204.
18. Emre M. Review of clinical trials with tizanidine (Sirdalud®) in spasticity. In: Emre M, Benecke R, eds. *Spasticity. The Current Status of Research and Treatment.* Parthenon, London, 1989; 153–184.
19. Snow BJ, Tsui JKC, Bhatt MH et al. Treatment of spasticity with botulinum toxin: a double-blind study. *Ann Neurol* 1990; **28**: 512–515.
20. Britell CW. Soup through a straw: tremor in MS. *MS Q Rep* 1997; **16(1)**.
21. Michaelis J. Mechanical methods of controlling ataxia. *Baillière's Clin Neurol* 1993; **2**: 121–139.
22. Nguyen J, Feve A, Keravel Y. Is electrostimulation preferable to surgery for upper limb ataxia? *Curr Opin Neurol* 1996; **9 (6)**: 445–450.
23. Vercoulen JH, Hommes OR, Swanink CM et al. The measurement of fatigue in patients with multiple sclerosis. A multidimensional comparison with patients with chronic fatigue syndrome and healthy subjects. *Arch Neurol* 1996; **53 (7)**: 642–649.
24. Krupp LB, Pollina DA. Measurement and management of fatigue in progressive neurological disorders. *Curr Op Neurol* 1996; **9**: 456–460.
25. Schwartz CE, Coulthard Morris L, Zeng Q. Psychosocial correlates of fatigue in multiple sclerosis. *Arch Phys Med Rehab* 1996; **77 (2)**: 165–171.
26. The Canadian MS Research Group. A randomized controlled trial of amantadine in fatigue associated with multiple sclerosis. *Can J Neurol Sci* 1987; **14 (3)**: 273–278.
27. Krupp LB, Coyle PK, Dosiher C et al. Fatigue therapy in multiple sclerosis: results of a double-blind, randomized, parallel trials of zanatadine, penioline and placebo. *Neurology* 1995; **45**: 1956–1961.
28. van Diemen HAM, Polman CH, von Dangen JMMM et al. The effects of 4-amino pyridine on clinical signs in multiple sclerosis: a randomized, placebo-controlled, double-blind crossover study. *Ann Neurol* 1992; **32**: 123–130.

26

Raising issues in multiple sclerosis: Part I

Rana Karabudak and Anthony T Reder

INTRODUCTION

In October 1997 Istanbul played host to the 13th ECTRIMS meeting at which over 1000 delegates attended. During 3 days a packed program of plenary lectures, symposia, platform and poster presentations was held; 55 platform and 280 poster presentations allowed for discussion of new data. The plenary papers are presented in the earlier chapters of this book. In this chapter we attempt to provide a concise summary of ECTRIMS '97. The elements presented in this overview highlight some of the key platform and poster presentations and discussions. Additionally emerging data coming from AAN and ENS 1997 meetings are included in related topics.

Two different and exceptional techniques—the introduction of MRI and its increasing application, and the production and proven efficacy of recombinant proteins in multiple sclerosis—have revolutionized our understanding and management of MS. Not surprisingly most of the presentations at the 13th ECTRIMS meeting dealt with these two areas: neuroimaging and immunomodulating therapies in MS.

Neuroimaging with its proven and potential power was in the centre of many studies dealing with the diagnosis, natural history, clinical correlations, pathology, evaluation of clinical trials and therapy in MS. We focus from this point of view in the first part. The main focus of the second part is on the neuroimmunology of MS. Important issues raised at the meeting are included below.

NEUROIMAGING AND METHODOLOGY

There is an ongoing search to refine and enhance magnetic resonance imaging (MRI) techniques so that the pathological specificity of MRI and our understanding the dynamics of MS can be increased. Another important aim of this search is to use MRI in the most effective way to monitor the treatment effects of potentially active therapies. Several studies have shown that the use of a triple dose (TD) of gadolinium (Gd)-DTPA markedly increased the sensitivity of enhanced MRI for detecting active lesions. MRI obtained after the injection of a TD of gadolinium detects 70% more enhancing lesions than that of a standard dose.[1–3]

Filippi and colleagues[4] compared the unenhanced and enhanced MRI techniques in detecting new lesions. Their comparison indicated that conventional spin echo (CSE) could be substituted by fast liquid-attenuated inversion recovery (FLAIR) when monitoring short-term disease activity. Gd-enhanced MRI remained the most sensitive method to detect 'active' lesions in MS.

The temporal relationship between Gd enhancement and the breakdown of the blood–brain barrier (BBB) has been recently addressed at the AAN 97 Boston Meeting. According to the current hypothesis BBB breakdown is believed to occur earlier than morphological changes. Dr Li and the UBC MS/MR Group have reported that in most lesions enhancement occurred at the same time or before the morphological changes (new, enlarging or recurrent lesions).[5]

The Queen Square NMR group[6] has shown that lesion volume gain increased 34% with the three-dimensional fast FLAIR (3D-fFLAIR) technique when compared to CSE images. High resolution 3D MRI (magnetisation-prepared rapid acquisition gradient echo—MP RAGE) increased the ability to detect the hypointense lesion load, and significantly correlated with the expanded disability status scale (EDSS) scores.[7] The median volume of hypointense lesions increased from 1190 mm^3 on 5 mm^3 MP RAGE, to 1733 mm^3 on 3 mm^3, and to 1862 mm^3 on 1 mm^3 MP RAGE. The hypointense lesion volumes measured on three scans significantly correlated with the EDSS score ($r = 0.58$, $p = 0.02$). MP RAGE sequence technique may improve clinical and MRI correlations compared to conventional T2 (where $r = 0.37$ or less).

Serial brain MRI is widely used in pilot studies of new agents to monitor treatment efficacy. For secondary progressive MS patients separate sample size calculations are not available. Tubridy et al.[8] addressed this issue at the AAN 97. They showed that with a single baseline scan, demonstration of a 70% reduction in a newly active lesion required 2 × 30 relapsing–remitting (RR) and 2 × 50 secondary progressive (SP) patients. An extra baseline scan 1 month before treatment reduced sample sizes to 2 × 20 for RR and to 2 × 30 for SP MS patients (2 arm trials).[8]

Magnetization transfer imaging (MTI) and magnetic resonance spectroscopy (MRS) provide new dimensions to MR imaging. MTI, which obtains T1-weighted spin-echo images with a magnetization transfer pulse, provides in vivo information about the pathological nature of the MS lesions. A comparison study of the short-term evolution of the magnetization transfer ratios of MS lesions (enhancing after the injection of a standard or a TD of Gd-DTPA) implied that the amount of tissue damage occurring within lesions seen only with the TD injection might be less severe than that of standard dose.[9]

MRS may provide a better appreciation of the role of axonal degeneration in MS lesion evolution. However, it is not easy to make comparisons of the results because of different methodology and techniques used in different centres at present.

Spinal cord MRI

Imaging of the spinal cord is difficult and time consuming. New techniques have been applied to improve spinal cord imaging, including cardiac gating and large field of view receiver coils. Additionally, post-mortem MRI investigations have revealed supplementary data. The preliminary results of an ongoing study on multiparameter MRI characteristics of the spinal cord with a high resolution 7 Tesla spectrometer was presented by the Queen Square Group.[10] In addition to T1 and T2 measurements, apparent diffusion coefficient (ADC) and MTR were also calculated. Areas of demyelination were characterized by reduced MTR and increased T1, T2 and ADC. Among these parameters the correspondence between T2 and the histology was less straightforward. Lyclama and colleagues,[11] of the Dutch MS MR Research group, carried out another high-resolution post-mortem study. They imaged formalin-fixed cervical cord specimens from 15 MS patients at 4.7 Tesla; 1-mm slice thickness and contiguous axial proton-density were used. No abnormalities were seen with the three control specimens. All MS specimens were associated with heterogeneous pathological changes. In the lateral and dorsal white matter columns of eight cases, there were focal areas of increased signal intensity which corresponded to the presence of foam cells and demyelination. In two cases the spinal cord was diffusely involved. The results suggest that high field strength MR imaging is sensitive and that it reflects the histopathology of MS. In another study, the same group pointed out that in early phases of MS a high proportion of patients showed focal spinal cord lesions. However diffuse abnormalities might also be found in the early cases and might not necessarily indicate late MS pathology.[12]

NATURAL HISTORY OF MULTIPLE SCLEROSIS

As clinical measures are often not the most objective assessment of MS, various MRI parameters are currently used to monitor the natural history of the disease. Serial imaging studies have provided some important information on the natural history of MS:

(a) Disease activity, as detected by MRI, is visible at 6–20 times the clinical relapse rate.[13–16]
(b) In untreated patients the extent of abnormality increases on average at a rate of 10% per patient per year.[17,18]

    Lesion activity and change of burden of disease (BOD) are currently used to measure lesion changes. Recently at AAN 97, Zhao and colleagues,[19] as part of a beta interferon (IFN-β) trial, presented a 5-year follow-up of their 115 placebo patients' data. In untreated patients, the mean percentage change in BOD was a 28% increase per patient per year. The change in BOD significantly correlated with the change in EDSS.
(c) Most active lesions seen on MRI are clinically silent. However many lesions re-occur in the same place, and these areas of reactivation are associated with large areas of residual damage.[20]

A small study of seven patients, followed by monthly MRI for 1 year, evaluated the natural history of hypointense lesions. Pre- and post-gadolinium T1-weighted images were obtained and 100 enhancing lesions were identified as baseline activity; 79% of them appeared hypointense on corresponding unenhanced T1 SE images. Of these acute lesions 27% stayed hypointense; 73% became isointense during the first 5 months. However 19% of these isointense lesions became hypointense after 2–3 months in the second follow-up period. Of the baseline isointense group 10% changed into hypointense status during follow-up.[21] It has been already suggested that the increasing lesion hypointensity might correspond to significant breakdown in the macromolecular structure of myelin.[22]

Some clinical MS subtypes have MRI correlates. Benign MS patients may have extensive MRI abnormalities though few of their lesions are symptomatic. They also seem to have less MRI-evident disease activity over time. Secondary progressive MS patients are prone to show a large and confluent lesions on MRI. Many of them enhance though this correlates poorly with their clinical symptoms. Primary progressive patients tend to have relatively few and less dynamic MRI lesions to explain their clinical disability. Nevertheless, this classification of subtypes does not complete the whole clinical spectrum in MS. A large number of 'variants' from clinically isolated monophasic demyelinating syndromes (optic neuritis, transverse myelitis), to ADEM and Balo's disease generally is included in this picture.

The long-term prognostic ability of MRI for recognizing the patients at risk of developing MS was evaluated in a 10-year follow-up study; 83% of patients with clinically isolated syndromes with abnormal MRI scans at presentation, converted to MS.[23]

A long-term follow-up of ADEM patients was presented at the ENS97;[24] 12 patients with a mean age of 29 years were followed-up for a mean duration of 5.6 years—none had a recurrence. Like other examples in the literature this study indicated that most ADEM cases have a favourable and a monophasic course.

In Balo's disease, MRI clearly shows a concentric pattern of alternating myelinated and unmyelinated bands so that ante-mortem diagnosis is possible. Based on the clinical and the MRI follow-up of the patients detected with MRI, the disease may not have a fulminant course.[25]

MS particularly affects young women in their child bearing years. Results of the PRIMS study were presented at the ECTRIMS '97. A total of 254 patients and 269 pregnancies were followed for 12 months after delivery. The mean annual relapse rate decreased from 0.73 relapses/year to

0.54 during the first two trimesters and to 0.22 in the last trimester. However the 3-month post-partum period saw a significant deleterious effect—the relapse rate rose to 1.23 relapses/year during the 3 months post-partum. Breastfeeding and epidural anaesthesia were safe.[26]

Another prospective study dealing with the paraclinical profile and prognosis of optic neuritis was presented,[27] in which 116 patients were evaluated: 55% of them had three or more high signal lesions and 35% had normal MRI. In 72% of the patients, immunoglobulin G (IgG) oligoclonal bands (OB) were positive. The presence of OB, plus three or more MS-like MRI lesions were strongly associated with the conversion to MS: 50% of the optic neuritis patients with three or more MRI lesions plus OB developed MS in 1 year.

The 5-year risk and the prognostic factors for the development of clinically definite MS (CDMS) following optic neuritis has also been investigated by the Optic Neuritis Study Group; data were published in November 1997. Because of the patient enrolment criteria, large sample size and a high follow-up rate (88%) the 5-year prospective study provides compelling results; 388 patients were followed from the onset of an acute episode of optic neuritis. The 5-year risk of development of CDMS was 30%. Brain MRI with three or more lesions was a strong predictor of CDMS (51%). Even with a normal MRI the 5-year risk of development of CDMS was still 16%. Additionally, certain clinical features of optic neuritis such as lack of pain, presence of mild visual loss, and absence of prior neurological symptoms and history of optic neuritis in the fellow eye were associated with a low risk of developing CDMS. However comparing data on this issue is not easy, since the size and the duration of the studies differ.[28]

There is no single paraclinical test that is diagnostic for MS. In young adults many conditions may mimic a multifocal central nervous system syndrome running a multiphasic course. This year at the AAN Meeting in Boston and at the ENS Meeting at Rhodes, Karussis and colleagues drew our attention to primary antiphospholipid antibody syndrome possibly mimicking MS both clinically and radiologically. They described 16 patients with optic neuropathy and myelopathy. All of the patients had high titres of anticardiolipin antibodies (mean levels were almost seven times above normal values). As the management of each of the diseases is different they recommended that probable MS cases should be checked for the presence of these antibodies.[29] A divergent report on this issue was that of Cordoliani and colleagues. They studied the levels of antiphospholipid antibodies in 66 MS patients but could not find any significant increase.[30]

Kozić and colleagues concentrated on the MRI side of the differential diagnosis. They applied spin-echo inversion recovery (IR), and fFLAIR to test the reliability of the techniques in differentiating between demyelinating and ischaemic lesions. Ischaemic lesions were hyperintense on T2 fFLAIR and were iso- or hyperintense on proton fFLAIR, whereas demyelinating lesions appeared still hyperintense on proton fFLAIR.

T2 fFLAIR was less reliable for detecting posterior fossa lesions but, in detecting cortical and subcortical MS lesions, was superior to fast spin-echo (FSE)[31] which allows the generation of T2-weighted images with similar contrast to conventional spin echo in far less time.

EVALUATION OF MS USING MRI

A multicentre European study of 191 patients with primary progressive and transitional MS (progressive disability with a single relapse at the onset or during the course of the disease) confirmed some previous findings. Primary progressive patients were older and had later disease onset. Additionally, no significant differences were found in the disease duration, disability and MRI T2 and T1 'black hole' load between the two groups. The transitional MS patients had significantly higher lesion load in the spinal cord.[32]

As part of a MAGNIMS project the cognitive functions of 55 patients with primary progressive MS and 20 with transitional MS were presented at the 13th ECTRIMS Meeting by Thompson and colleagues.[33] The short repeatable battery, the

VESPAR, the MADRS and a measure of depression and reasoning were evaluated in a controlled manner. Patients performed poorly on tests of memory, attention, and spatial reasoning; however, no significant differences were scored between the two groups.

A 3-year longitudinal cohort study evaluated the clinical features and the disease course of primary progressive MS (PPMS) patients. PPMS typically began as a noncompressive cord disease in the fifth and the sixth decade, was more common in women and the mean time for bilateral assistance and loss of independent living were 15.9 and 27.7 years, respectively. There were no gender differences in rate of progression.[34]

Wang and colleagues[35] compared MRI lesion distribution between RR and secondary progressive MS (SPMS). Compared to 502 RR patients, 108 SPMS patients had a higher percentage of confluent cerebral (5.3% vs. 4.3%, $p < 0.025$), brainstem (78% vs. 64% $p < 0.025$) and cerebellar lesions (4.8% vs. 3.5% $p < 0.005$), and greater number of periventricular lesions (11.9% vs. 10.4%, $p < 0.001$). From this data it can be concluded that differences occur in the distribution of MS lesions in RRMS and SPMS patients.

In parallel to the clinical studies, trials have been conducted to determine the MRI changes and the relevant pathology. According to current hypothesis, BBB breakdown is believed to occur earlier than the morphological changes. Dr Li and the UBC MS/MR Group[5] as part of a IFN-β trial, evaluated 93 patients for morphological changes in active lesions before the breakdown of the BBB. In most lesions enhancement occurred on the same scan (86.6%) as morphological change that is defined either by new, enlarging or recurrent lesions in proton-density T2-weighted scans (PD/T2W).

Chronic MS lesions have been evaluated by proton magnetic resonance spectroscopy[1] (HMRS) and magnetization transfer technique (MT) in 18 MS patients. Davie and colleagues[36] observed a significant correlation between the reduction in absolute concentration of *N*-acetylaspartate (NAA) and the reduction in the MT value (myelin disruption) in the same chronic lesions. They proposed that axonal loss and demyelination might occur together in the chronic lesions of MS.

At the 7th ENS Meeting a study on the histopathology of these chronic hypointense, so-called 'black holes' was presented.[37] Postmortem unfixed whole brains from five MS patients were obtained and scanned (T1,T2) within 24 hours after death. The degree of hypointensity correlated with the degree of matrix destruction/widening of extracellular space. The hypointense lesions might be the MRI equivalent of severe tissue destruction, and axonal loss and might serve as a marker of persistent deficit.

MRI AND CLINICAL TRIALS

One of the most controversial issues is the relationship between MRI dynamics and clinical disease activity. In search of a clear picture in this area, MRI has been used in monitoring both acute and chronic phase and evaluation of the natural history of MS. The results of the fourth and the largest, double-blind randomized controlled study on IFN-β (IFN-β1a; Rebif-Serono) were presented at the 13th ECTRIMS Meeting by Drs Paty and Li of the University of British Columbia.[38] Compared with placebo, IFN-β1a had a highly significant impact at both 6 MIU (33% after 1 year and 29% after 2 years) and 12 MIU (37% after 1 year and 32% after 2 years) doses. Over the 2-year follow-up the placebo group showed a progressive median increase in BOD of 10.9% while the 6 MIU group showed a median decrease of –1.2% and the 12 MIU group –3.8% ($p < 0.0001$).

Association between MRI changes and neutralizing antibodies (NAb) to IFN β was also addressed at the 13th ECTRIMS Meeting. Calabresi and colleagues[39] presented data from 33 patients with serial MRIs and serum samples taken before and after the initiation of IFN-β1b 12 out of 33 patients became NAb+; however not all of them had a return of Gd+ MRI lesions. Furthermore, over time seven of the NAb+ MS patients had a complete resolution of titres to undetectable, and had a sustained MRI response to therapy. Currently the relationship between

NAb and MRI is not clear, and factors such as amount of pre-existing disease activity on MRI, titre of NAb, dose of IFN, and other immune and clinical variables may determine whether NAb are important in a given patient.

There is an emerging consensus that treating MS early is beneficial. This view has been crystallized over recent years by MRI studies.[40–42] National Institutes of Health (NIH) MRI studies were reviewed at AAN 97. They evaluated the natural history data on MRI lesion frequency in a cohort of 75 RRMS patients who were relatively early in their MS course. Nearly 80% of the patients had evidence of activity on at least one of the 3-monthly MRIs. The mean lesion frequency was 1.7 per month. Thus, even during the early RR phase, MS can be a progressive disease, and initiating therapy early might be of importance for limiting the accumulation of disability.[42]

NIH MRI studies showed an extensive amount of fluctuating activity in T2-weighted lesion load. Some of the fluctuations were related to Gd enhancement. However, some T2 changes appeared to be independent of Gd enhancement, suggesting that once the lesion is established it might be able to progress independently of BBB breakdown.[42] One implication is that therapy should be directed at multiple components of the disease process.

REFERENCES

1. Filippi M, Yousry T, Campi A et al. Comparison of triple dose versus standard dose gadolinium-DTPA for detection of MRI enhancing lesions in patients with MS. *Neurology* 1996; **46**: 379–384.
2. Filippi M, Capra R, Campi A et al. Triple dose gadolinium-DTPA and delayed MRI in patients with benign multiple sclerosis. *J Neurol Neurosurg Psychiatry* 1996; **60**: 526–530.
3. Filippi M, Campi A, Martinelli V et al. Comparison of triple dose versus standard dose gadolinium-DTPA for detection of MRI enhancing lesions in patients with primary progressive multiple sclerosis. *J Neurol Neurosurg Psychiatry* 1995; **59**: 540–544.
4. Filippi M, Rovaris M, Bastianello S et al. A comparison of the sensitivity of monthly unenhanced and enhanced MRI techniques in detecting new multiple sclerosis lesions. *Multiple Sclerosis* 1997; **3**: 333.
5. Li DKB, Zhao GJ, Koopmans RA et al. Can morphological changes in MRI active lesions occur prior to their blood–brain barrier breakdown in MS? *Neurology* 1997; **48 (suppl 2)**: A311.
6. Tubridy N, Barker GJ, MacManus DG et al. Fast FLAIR: a new sequence which increases the detectable cerebral lesion load in multiple sclerosis. *Multiple Sclerosis* 1997; **3**: 334.
7. Rovaris M, Filippi M, Rocca MA et al. High resolution 3D MRI increases hypointense lesion load detection in multiple sclerosis. *Neurology* 1997; **48 (suppl 2)**: A361.
8. Tubridy N, Ader H, Barkhof F et al. Sample size calculations for MRI outcome pilot trials in MS: relapsing–remitting versus secondary progressive subgroups. *Neurology* 1997; **48 (suppl 2)**: A175.
9. Filippi M, Rocca M, Rovaris M et al. A comparison of the short-term evolution of the magnetisation transfer ratios of MS lesions enhancing after the injection of a standard or a triple dose of gadolinium-DTPA. *Multiple Sclerosis* 1997; **3**: 334.
10. Mottershead JP, Clemence M, Thornton JS et al. Multi-parameter NMR imaging of the spinal cord post-mortem in MS. *Multiple Sclerosis* 1997; **3**: 264.
11. Lyclama GJ, Nikolay K, Barkhof F et al. Post-mortem MR appearance of the spinal cord in MS high field strength. *Multiple Sclerosis* 1997; **3**: 264.
12. Lyclama GJ, Uitdehaag BMJ, Barkhof F et al. MR imaging appearance of spinal cord in early MS: occurrence of diffuse abnormalities. *Multiple Sclerosis* 1997; **3**: 298.
13. Isaac C, Li DKB, Garten M et al. Multiple sclerosis: a serial study using MRI in relapsing patients. *Neurology* 1988; **38**: 1511–1515.
14. Willoughby EW, Growchowsky E, Li DK et al. Serial magnetic resonance scanning in multiple sclerosis: a second prospective study in relapsing patients. *Ann Neurol* 1989; **25**: 43–49.
15. Koopmans RA, Li DKB, Oger JJF et al. Chronic multiple sclerosis: serial magnetic resonance brain imaging over six months. *J Neurol Neurosurg Psychiatry* 1989; **51**: 1126–1133.
16. Paty DW. MRI in the assessment of disease activity in MS. *Can J Neurol Sci* 1988; **15**: 266–272.
17. Paty DW. Trial measures in MS: the use of magnetic resonance imaging in the evaluation of clinical trials. *Neurology* 1988; **38**: 82–83.

18. Zhao GJ, Redekop WK, Li DKB et al. Clinical and magnetic resonance imaging changes correlate in a clinical trial monitoring cyclosporine therapy for MS. *J Neuroimaging* 1997; **7**: 1–7.
19. Zhao GJ, Li DKB, Koopmans RA, Bedell L et al. Correlation of clinical status with MS lesion changes in untreated patients: a 5-year study by yearly MRI. *Neurology* 1997; **48**: A361.
20. Koopmans RA, Li DKB, Oger JJF et al. The lesion of multiple sclerosis: imaging of acute and chronic stages. *Neurology* 1989; **39**: 959–963.
21. Waesberghe JHTM, Walderveen MAA, Scheltens P et al. Natural history of hypointense lesions in MS. *J Neurology* 1997; **244**: S87.
22. Loevner LA, Grossman RI, McGowan JC et al. Characterisation of multiple sclerosis plaques with T1-weighted MR and quantitative magnetisation transfer. *Am J Neuroradiol* 1995; **16**: 1463–1479.
23. Sailer M, O'Riordan J, Kingsley DPE et al. Long term predictive value of quantitative brain MRI in patients presenting with a clinically isolated syndrome suggestive of demyelination. *J Neurology* 1997; **244**: S38.
24. O'Riordan J, Thompson AJ, McManus DG et al. The long term prognosis of acute disseminated encephalomyelitis. *J Neurology* 1997; **244**: S10.
25. Karabudak R, Bolay H, Selekler K. Clinical and neuroimaging features of Balo's concentric sclerosis. *Multiple Sclerosis* 1997; **3**: 290.
26. Hutchinson M, Hours M, Cortinovis-Tournaire P et al. and the PRESTIMUS Group. PRESTIMUS: predictive estimates in multiple sclerosis: a European multicenter prospective study. *Multiple Sclerosis* 1997; **3**: 266.
27. Söderström M, Jin Y, Hillert J et al. Optic neuritis in Stockholm, Sweden 1990–1995: paraclinical profile and its prognosis for MS. *Multiple Sclerosis* 1997; **3**: 267.
28. Optic Neuritis Study Group. The five year risk of MS after optic neuritis: experience of the optic neuritis treatment trial. *Neurology* 1997; **49**: 1404–1413.
29. Karussis D, Ashkenazi A, Leker R et al. Primary antiphospholipid syndrome mimicking clinically and radiologically MS. *Neurology* 1997; **48 (suppl 2)**: A425.
30. Cordoliani MA, Pasturel UM, Rerat K et al. Lack of association between MS and antiphospholipid antibodies. *J Neurol* 1997; **244**, S76.
31. Kozić D, Vucurevic G, Eric M et al. Application of fast FLAIR and spin echo IR in differentiation between MS and ischaemic lesions. *Neurology* 1997; **48 (suppl 2)**: A310.
32. Stevenson V, Thompson AJ, Miller DH et al. Primary progressive and transitional multiple sclerosis: a cross sectional clinical, MRI and neuropsychological study. *Multiple Sclerosis* 1997; **3**: 264.
33. Camp SJ, Langdon DW, Stevenson VL et al. Cognitive function in primary progressive MS: a controlled study with MR correlates. *Multiple Sclerosis* 1997; **3**: 302.
34. Andersson PB, Waubant E, Gee L et al. Primary progressive MS (PPMS): clinical characteristics and progression of disability. *Neurology* 1997; **48 (suppl 2)**: A423.
35. Wang X, Zhao G, Li DKB et al. Comparison of MRI lesion distribution between relapsing–remitting and secondary progressive MS. *Neurology* 1997; **48 (suppl 2)**: A311.
36. Davie CA, Barker GJ, Thompson AJ et al. Does axonal loss and demyelination occur in the same lesions in MS? *Multiple Sclerosis* 1997; **3**: 264.
37. Walderveen MAA, Scheltens P, Waesberghe JHTM et al. Hypointense lesions on T1-weighted MR images correlate with axonal loss in MS. *J Neurol* 1997; **244**: S84.
38. Paty DW and the PRIMS Study Group. Interferon beta 1a (Rebif®) in the treatment of relapsing–remitting multiple sclerosis: the MRI results of a large multicentre study. *Multiple Sclerosis* 1997; **3**: 269.
39. Calabresi PA, Frank JA, Maloni HW et al. Association between neutralising antibodies to interferon beta and contrast enhancing lesions in MS patients. *Neurology* 1997; **48 (suppl 2)**: A80.
40. Paty DW, Li DKB, UBC MS/MRI Study Group and the IFNB MS Group. Interferon beta-1b is effective in RRMS. II. MRI analysis results of a multicenter, randomised, double blind, placebo controlled trial. *Neurology* 1993; **43**: 662–667.
41. Stone LA, Frank JA, Albert PS et al. The effect of IFN-β on blood–brain barrier disruptions demonstrated by contrast-enhanced MRI in RRMS. *Ann Neurol* 1995; **37**: 611–619.
42. McFarland HF, Stone LA, Calabresi PA et al. MRI studies of multiple sclerosis: implications for the natural history of the disease and for monitoring effectiveness of experimental therapies. *Multiple Sclerosis* 1996; **2**: 198–206.

Raising issues in multiple sclerosis: Part II

Anthony T Reder and Rana Karabudak

EPIDEMIOLOGY

MS has been linked to many environmental factors. Several new ideas appeared at ECTRIMS and other recent meetings.

ENVIRONMENT

There is an epidemiological link between intake of smoked sausage and development of MS.[1] The mechanism is unclear but suggests that free radicals and other toxins could affect development of MS. Anti-oxidants are potential therapy for stroke and degenerative neurological disease, but have largely been overlooked for treatment of inflammatory lesions in MS.

VIRAL AND BACTERIAL EFFECTS ON MS AND MS EXACERBATIONS

Virus and bacteria—cross-reactions with myelin antigens and cytokine stimulation

Some infections induce interleukin (IL)-12, which in turn increases IFN-γ secretion[2]—probably deleterious in MS. T cells from experimental autoimmune encephalitis (EAE)-resistant B10.S mice have defective IFN-γ production. High levels of IL-12 can reverse this EAE resistance. Superantigens, SEA and SEB, also induce IL-12 and enhance EAE severity.[3] Bacterial infections are three times more common in patients with exacerbations than in patients without exacerbations.[4] These studies suggest that infections can enhance autoimmune disease and MS, and interruption of the IL-12 pathway is a potential target for MS treatment.

Vaccinations

Recombinant hepatitis B vaccination was linked to 51 cases of central demyelinating syndromes in 10 000 000 vaccinated subjects over 7 years, an incidence of 0.51/100 000 over 7 years.[5] The yearly incidence of MS in France is approximately 2.5/100 000, so 7 years × 2.5/100 000 yields 17.5/100 000 expected cases of MS. This suggests there was no increased incidence in the vaccinated subjects.

Viruses

HHV-6 is the latest virus suspect. Many viruses have been linked to MS, but none convincingly. An entire session at ACTRIMS was devoted to HHV-6. HHV-6 causes focal encephalitis and febrile seizures in children.[6] In HIV infection, myelin pallor correlates with numbers of HHV-6^{+} brain cells. Some cases of subacute HHV-6 leukoencephalitis could be misdiagnosed as MS. For instance, rapidly progressive demyelination in three young (16-, 18-, 24-year-old) patients was caused by HHV-6B.[7] In support of a link to MS, high levels of HHV-6 DNA are present in brain tissues of some patients with MS, as are high titres of serum and cerebrospinal fluid (CSF) anti-HHV-6 antibodies.[8] Reactivation of HHV-6 by inflammation was deemed unlikely because subacute sclerosing panencephalitis (SSPE), progressive multifocal leukoencephalopathy (PML), post-infectious encephalomyelitis, and progressive rubella panencephalitis brains were negative for HHV-6. There is evidence against the HHV-6 hypothesis, however. Almost all children are exposed to HHV-6 by age three, and almost all adults are HHV-6 positive. Moreover, there is no meaningful correlation between the location of HHV-6 staining and MS lesion activity.[9] Multiple viruses including HHV-6, however, could potentially affect immune reactions in the CNS.

Antiviral drugs are possible therapies—either for treatment of a primary viral cause of MS (unproven), or because one out of three virus infections triggers attacks of MS. Of interest, acyclovir tends to lower the exacerbation rate in RRMS (34%, $p = 0.083$),[10] and warrants further investigation.

GENETICS

Recent genomic searches in England, Canada and the USA found HLA-DR2 was the strongest candidate (*Nature Genetics* 1993; **13**). Several other genes are also likely to be involved.

HLA-DR2 is common in Northern Europeans with MS, but this connection is not universal. There is a low frequency of DR2 in Turkish MS patients (0%), but high DQ2 and DR14 (6) (odds ratios of 11 and 3, respectively).[11] DR4 is associated with MS in Sardinia.[12] In Japan, Western forms of MS are still linked to DR2.[13] However, most Japanese MS is more often similar to Devic's disease (eye and spinal cord involvement), and is not linked to DR2. There may be different immunologic routes to the development of MS in different populations. Genetic searches of MS populations where HLA-DR2 is uncommon could lead to other important genes.

SOME MEDICAL PROBLEMS

Osteoporosis in MS is from reduced weight bearing at the hip, secondary to loss of ambulation and excess bone resorption.[14] Glucocorticoid treatment was not a risk factor for osteoporosis. Nonfatiguing exercise should be encouraged.

The diagnosis of MS is not always simple. In young adults, many conditions may mimic a multifocal central nervous system syndrome with a multiphasic course. Primary antiphospholipid syndrome may mimic MS, clinically and on MRI. Twenty Israeli patients (13 women, 7 men) with MS-like symptoms had high titres of anticardiolipin antibodies (mean = 42.2 GPL units (IgG-phospholipid); normal = up to 8);[15] 9 of 20 had headaches; 7 of 16 with typical 'MS' changes on MRI had a slowly progressing myelopathy and 4 had optic neuropathy. Since a number of other autoantibodies are increased in MS serum, it is unclear whether these patients truly had MS or had multiple infarcts without pathological confirmation. Only 4 of 20 had CSF oligoclonal bands, pointing out the importance of CSF studies in the diagnosis of MS. In contrast, others find no association between MS and antiphospholipid antibodies.[16] As management is different, some cases of probable MS should be checked for the presence of these antibodies.

CLINICAL ASPECTS OF MS

Menses and MS

Half (43%) of women with MS reported worsening of symptoms right before menses (Day –3 to onset).[17] The proportion of relapses starting in the premenstrual period was also higher. The mechanism is unknown.

Visual memory

The higher the total lesion load, the more visual memory decreased.[18] There was no specific region responsible, but only frontal areas were tested; 'normal-appearing white matter' could be involved too. Proton-density load correlated better with cognitive changes than clinical examination did. Since most of the visual pathways are posterior, even better correlation would be expected with posterior pathways.

One other group found decreased visual memory in MS. Also, working memory performance was more easily disrupted by interference tasks carried out during memory consolidation.[19]

IFN-β1b causes improvement in Stroop 3 and verbal dichotomy tests.[20] (The Stroop measures frontal lobe function and is dependent on adequate vision.) IFN-β1b improves visual memory, possibly because the visual pathways have to go around the ventricle twice—both times through white matter.[21] Balanced white matter function should be reflected in improved vision.

HOW IS THE IMMUNE SYSTEM ACTIVATED IN MS?

An unknown peripheral event can cause immune activation in the blood first, before the onset of inflammation in the brain. The underlying trigger that causes these immune abnormalities is a mystery.

IFN-γ-induced calcium influx in MS lymphocytes precedes clinical attacks and MRI changes by 2–4 weeks.[22,23] In active MS, there is increased serum IgM against αB-crystallin, a glial component.[24] The presence of immunoglobulin M (IgM) recognizing this protein suggests this is a new humoral response. (But, if this IgM is a new response each time there is a flare, why is it repeated over and over?) The antibody response in MS was greatest in serum. In CSF, patients with Guillain–Barré had higher responses than MS patients. This again suggests a peripheral immune response precedes the CNS lesions in MS.

Epstein–Barr virus (EBV)-transformed B cells also express αB-crystallin, a heat shock family protein which is associated with CNS myelin.[25] (Cytokines and multiple other viruses also induce αB-crystallin, and there is increased αB-crystallin in MS glia.[26]) Th1 lines proliferate in response to EBV-transformed B cells, suggesting that virus induction of αB-crystallin could be one element driving a Th1 response in MS.

Natural killer (NK) cell function shows periodic 10-week fluctuations.[27] MS attacks and MRI activity are preceded by a drop in NK cytolytic function. The set point in MS patients is high—average NK function is highest in patients likely to have attacks, so the relative fall in NK function during exacerbations is greatest in this subset. (IFN-β had no effect on NK function.)

Activation of immune cells in MS by myelin antigens

Class II MHC-restricted responses by peripheral blood mononuclear cells (PBMNC) against myelin oligodendrocyte glycoprotein (MOG) were decreased in MS (28%) compared to controls (57%).[28] Similar differences were seen in response to myelin basic protein (MBP) (0 vs. 7%) and PLP (7 vs. 17%). Reduced responses to myelin antigens in MS do not fit some current thinking.

Costimulation

B7-1 and B7-2 (CD80 and CD86) are costimulatory molecules which provide a necessary second signal for immune activation. T-cell receptor (TCR) stimulation alone causes anergy, but TCR plus B7 stimulation results in proliferation and cytokine secretion.

B7-2 is present on CSF immune cells in optic neuritis and viral meningitis, but appears less frequently in MS.[29] It is expressed on monocytes more than B cells, but not on CSF T cells. However, others find more B7-1^{+} B cells in MS CSF.[30] B7-1 staining is strong on CSF cells in viral meningitis and cells within MS plaques, but only weakly on MS CSF cells. Technical difficulties with flow cytometry of cells with low antigen expression, or variation between B7-1 and B7-2, may explain the differences. The signals which downregulate B7 expression or which induce B7^{low} cells to die or migrate out of MS plaques are unknown. Possibly related, exogenous IFN-β reversed IFN-γ-induced B7-1 and B7-2 expression on mouse microglia in vitro.[31]

TCRγδ T-cell lines recognize heat shock proteins (HSP), and appear to recognize HSP better in the absence of antigen-presenting cells

(APCs).[32] Proliferative responses to HSP are roughly twice as high in MS as in normal γδ T-cell lines. This response suggests B7 and MHC class II molecules are expressed on these T-cell lines, allowing them to function as APCs. Monocytes—not needed as APC—might secrete inhibitory cytokines (PGE and IL-10 are likely suspects). This raises a question: if monocytes are not necessary for activation of γδ T cells, which other cells function as APCs in the immune response in MS?

Cytokines

IL-15 is a proinflammatory cytokine which stimulates T-cell proliferation and IFN-γ and TNF-α secretion. There are increased IL-15$^+$ cells in MS, but not in myasthenia gravis, based on in situ hybridization of MNC and CSF cells.[33] IL-15$^+$ cells are more frequent in CSF than in blood, suggesting a role for IL-15 in MS inflammation.

Cytokine mRNA and protein

Multiple ECTRIMS presentations agreed with prior papers by Rieckmann et al.[34] and Byskosh and Reder[35] showing that levels of cytokines in blood cells change with disease activity and after IFN therapy. There were a few discrepancies, however. Some of the disagreement could stem from the varied genetic background of patients from different countries. This was an excellent forum for comparing data that could suggest genetic influences on immune function specific for MS.

Northern Europeans with MS are most often DR2$^+$. However, there is a low frequency of DR2 in Turkish MS patients (zero), but high DQ2 and DR14 (6).[11] In contrast DR4 is associated with MS in Sardinia.[12] PHA-activated lymphoid cells from DR4 patients secrete more IFN-γ and TNF-α compared to DR3-positive patients' cells.[12] Serum IFN-γ is lower in active and stable MS than in Turkish controls.[36] In contrast, serum IFN-γ increases before MS exacerbations in Northern European.[37] It is possible that differences in HLA or other genes modify the cytokine profile in MS patients not derived from Northern European stock. These studies show the importance of using appropriately matched control populations, and the difficulties in interpreting immunological data from different groups of MS patients.

Certain cytokines are easier to detect in CSF than in serum, e.g. IFN-γ and IL-10.[38] After IFN-β1a therapy, IL-10 protein increases in CSF more than in serum.[39] In some laboratories, IL-10 is undetectable in the serum or plasma of MS patients treated with IFN-β.[40] Methylprednisolone (i.v.), however, induces IL-10 up to levels of 230 ng/ml.

Serum IL-10 levels are elevated from 48 to 168 hours after an IFN-β injection in MS patients.[39] This differs from an earlier paper on healthy volunteers[41] where serum IL-10 levels rose at 12 and 24 hours after IFN-β injections, but had fallen to baseline by 48 hours. Thus, IFN-β appears to induce more IL-10 in MS than in normal subjects. This contradicts Porrini[42] who showed that IFN-β-induced IL-10 secretion from resting monocytes was not significantly increased in MS compared to controls in vitro.

Migration across endothelial cells

During inflammation, the blood–brain barrier (BBB) becomes leaky, the MRI becomes Gd-+, and cytokines induce adhesion molecules on endothelial cells. There is altered function of endothelial cells and of the pericytes surrounding the post-capillary venules.

Disruption of the BBB

Leakage through the BBB could allow peripheral cytokines and antibodies to affect CNS function. However, BBB dysfunction does not always correspond to inflammation in MS plaques.[43,44] BBB breakdown sometimes precedes morphological changes.[43,44]

T cells from MS patients migrate across a fibronectin barrier twice as fast as normal cells.[45] IFN-β1b therapy initially reduces this migration, but loses efficacy after 3 years (4 of 6 patients were NAb-+). Tissue inhibitor of metalloproteinase (TIMP) also reduced migration and might be targeted as in MS therapy.

Role of adhesion molecules on endothelial and blood cells

CNS microvessels express high levels of adhesion proteins in MS, but also in other inflammatory diseases.[46] Soluble serum intercellular adhesion molecule-1 (ICAM-1), vascular cell adhesion molecule-1 (VCAM-1), L-selectin, and TNF receptor correlates with disease activity[47] and MRI enhancement.[48] IFN-β1b elevates serum VCAM-1, which binds to very late antigen-4 (VLA-4) on lymphocytes and then downregulates VLA-4 expression, possibly blocking inflammation.[49] Serum ICAM (sICAM) levels are already high in MS, but IFN-β1b transiently increases sICAM levels at 3 months;[50] levels are back to baseline by 6 months. Does this sICAM block leucocyte function associated antigen-1 (LFA-1) on immune cells? Clinical trials of antibodies to adhesion molecules are in progress.

Pericytes

Pericytes are small contractile motile cells surrounding blood vessels.[51] White blood cells (WBC) cluster around them in MS, and the pericytes are able to activate the WBC. Activated CD4 cells tend to bind to pericytes, CD8 cells bind to endothelial cells. Inflammatory cytokines activate pericytes and cause them to produce TGF-β. Normal pericytes adhere to precursor, Th0, and Th1 cells, but cytokine-activated pericytes bind to Th2 cells. This suggests that activated pericytes and Th2 cells could inhibit inflammation by secreting TGF-β and binding Th2 cells.

Tissue destruction

Apoptosis

Bcl-2, p53 and Fas proteins are associated with apoptosis of cells. A subpopulation of oligodendroglia in MS plaques stains for Bcl-2.[52] p53 expression is restricted to lesions with prominent loss of oligodendroglia. Patients with progressive MS have more Bcl-2 positive T cells in lesions than RR patients.[52]

Activated T cells release CD95, which inhibits apoptosis.[53] CD95 levels are significantly higher in RRMS (disease activity not stated), and lower in chronic progressive (CP) MS, compared to controls. Thus, the immunology of RRMS and CPMS may differ.

Intravenous methylprednisolone, 10 mg/kg, modestly inhibited EAE and induced apoptosis;[54] 50 mg/kg had more pronounced effects. This would be equivalent to human doses of 700–3500 mg, but rodents are much more sensitive to the effects of glucocorticoids than humans, so the relative dose is even higher. Nevertheless, effects on EAE were not striking. This is surprising because an equivalent dose of dexamethasone profoundly inhibits EAE.[55] Effects of glucocorticoids on activated immune cells in MS lesions bear further investigation.

NEW IMAGING TECHNIQUES

Positron emission tomography (PET) scanning with [^{11}C]PK11195, which binds to benzodiazepine receptors on macrophages, shows increased uptake in inflamed areas during active EAE.[56] In MS, MRI Gd-enhancing regions also light up with this type of PET scanning, but so do some areas of normal-appearing brain. Pathways remote from a lesion bind this ligand, e.g. lateral geniculate and visual cortex in patients with prior optic neuritis.[57] Thus there is widespread inflammation in MS, both in 'normal' brain and in areas possibly affected by retrograde axonal degeneration.

SUPPRESSION OF THE IMMUNE RESPONSE

What shuts off the immune reaction in MS?

Proteolipid protein (PLP)-reactive T-cell clones (?autoreactive) from chronic progressive patients are resistant to dexamethasone-mediated apoptosis.[58] This difficulty in terminating the immune reaction in later stages of MS matches clinical experience—MS patients with longstanding, progressive MS tend to become less responsive to glucocorticoid therapy.

Serum sCD30, shed from Th2 cells and a possible marker of Th2 cell activity, is elevated in RRMS.[59] sCD30 is even higher in primary progressive MS compared to noninflammatory neurological disease. This suggests that activated

Th2 cells are present in MS patients at all times, but their functional role is not clear.

DRUG THERAPY OF MS

IFN-β1a, IFN-β1b, and copaxone all ameliorate MS.

Interferons

The Rebif (IFN-β1a) data were presented at ECTRIMS (also at ANA and ISICR). This is the fourth recent trial showing efficacy of IFNs. It reduced exacerbations by 32% after 2 years, progression by time to 44%, and T2 burden of disease on MRI activity by 14.7%. It is clear that type I IFNs are partially effective therapy in MS.

Two questions arise from the IFN data: (1) which IFN is best, and (2) why does the maximum effect plateau at a 50% reduction of attacks or progression? Depending on how the data are analysed, Betaseron has a more pronounced effect on relapse rate and MRI than Avonex, but Avonex reduced progression more. Rebif was as good or best. Some differences in efficacy may stem from the IFN dose. With Betaseron, 1.6 MU was clinically less effective than 8 MU every other day (q.o.d.), but MRI improvement was approximately equal. With Rebif, 9 MU three times a week (t.i.w.) caused faster improvement on MRI than 3 MU t.i.w. (number and volume of Gd-enhancing lesions).[60] Finally, in the pivotal trial of Rebif, the higher dose (12 MIU t.i.w.) tended to be better at reducing exacerbations, progression, and MRI than the lower dose (6 MIU t.iw.). (The recommended weekly dose for the different preparations is 6 MIU IFN-β1a (Avonex, once per week i.m.), 36 MIU IFN-β1a (Rebif, 12 MIU t.i.w. subcutaneous (s.c.), 28 MIU IFN-β1b (Betaseron, 8 MU q.o.d., s.c.), and 31.5 MU IFN-α2a (Roferon-A, 9 MU q.o.d. i.m.).)

Pharmacokinetic analysis from Serono demonstrates that there is a fall in biological response markers when injections are 1 week apart, but t.i.w. injections yield a continuous elevation of 2'-5' OAS, neopterin, and β2-microglobulin, and a 10-fold decrease in IL-1β, IFN-γ, and TNF-α production.[61] This information from normal volunteers could differ in MS—compare to Rudick and colleagues[39] in MS, vs. Rudick and colleagues[41] in healthy volunteers (above).

IFNs are partially effective in MS. Is this simply because the dose is not high enough, or because immune mechanisms in MS are multifactorial and need to be treated with combinations of drugs? There is evidence of a dose–response, but the beneficial effect of IFNs seems to plateau in both the Betaseron and the Rebif studies. Other factors such as sex, body size and age affect IFN responses. None of them is likely to contribute significantly to efficacy, however; exacerbation-free patients were rare in the 5-year Betaseron study.

Some IFN-β effects on immune function seem to be transient. Reversible changes include matrix metalloprotease inhibition,[45] elevation of sICAM in the serum,[50] and induction of cytokine mRNA.[35] However, the therapeutic effects of IFN-β seem to persist for at least 5 years. After IFN-β1b is discontinued, two-thirds of patients have a return of MRI lesion activity by 3–6 months.[62]

The aetiology of MS is unknown, and the mechanism of action of IFNs in MS is also not clear. New pieces were added to the puzzle in 1997. These included IFN-β-induced reduction of VLA-4[49] and B7-1 on immune cells[30,63] and B7-1 on microglia,[31] elevation of IL-10,[39] and prevention of T-cell penetration of the BBB.[45]

Side-effects of IFNs

Antithyroid antibodies and hypothyroidism appeared in 5 of 19 Italian patients after 2–5 months of IFN-α or IFN-β treatment.[64] Hepatic enzymes increased in all patients after 3-7 months, often associated with positive antinuclear antibody (ANA) or anti-smooth muscle Abs. The most severe problems were with IFN-α, and the report is unclear about whether IFN-β caused any of these side-effects. An increase in liver enzymes is rare with IFN-β1a and, although an increase is sometimes seen with IFN-β1b, it is usually modest.[35] None the less, patients treated with IFNs should be monitored for leucopenia and elevated liver enzymes; tests for thyroid function and ANA may be useful in some patients. Pentoxifylline (Trental©) is a phosphodiesterase inhibitor which elevates cAMP and therefore inhibits Th1 and possibly macrophage responses; 800 mg perorally twice daily prevents most early side-effects of IFN-β1b.[65] Tests of other combinations are in progress.

Neutralizing antibodies (NAb) to IFNs

This is an important issue to patients and financiers. A symposium on IFN-induced NAb was sponsored by Berlex in New York on 24–25 May 1997. Some conclusions were: (1) titres were difficult to compare between different assays and different IFNs; (2) some interferon preparations may be more likely to generate NAb; (3) the effect of NAb was unclear, but if present was often transient.

All of the 11 patients who were NAb positive in the pivotal IFN-β1b trial became NAb negative during a 102-month follow-up in a London, Ontario, clinic.[66]

There may be a pre-existing immune bias in patients who become NAb positive:

In MNC stimulated with pokeweed mitogen (PWM), patients who were high IgG secretors before IFN-β1b treatment were the ones who were likely to develop NAb (9 of 14 patients).[67,68] Low Ig secretors seldom became NAb positive (4 of 15) ($p = 0.04$ by Fisher's exact test). Patients who become NAb positive are more likely to have clinically active MS—before therapy is begun.[69] This may be a partial explanation for the increase in relapses in NAb positive patients in the Betaseron pivotal trial. Similarly, there is a pre-existing trend for excessive MRI activity in patients who are to become NAb positive.[70]

In addition to elevated PWM-induced antibody secretion, MS patients classically have high antimeasles titres. They also frequently have positive ANAs.[71] A predisposition to antibody formation could contribute to the autoantibodies seen during IFN-β therapy.

N Simonian of Biogen reported at ACTRIMS 1997 that serum neopterin, an IFN-induced protein, falls in treated patients who develop NAbs. She also suggested that carbohydrate groups on the IFN-β1a molecule reduced hydrophobicity and prevented formation of aggregates. Fewer aggregates would reduce antigenicity and help prevent NAb formation. In addition, she suggested that oxygenation of the IFN during storage and proximity to the dermis could possibly enhance antigenicity.

A Abdul-Ahad of Serono reported at ACTRIMS that NAb appeared during therapy with IFN-β1a (Rebif). NAb were more common in the low dose group (25%) than in the high dose IFN group (17%). High zone tolerance was invoked as the mechanism.

IVIG

Monthly intravenous immunoglobulin (IVIG) at a low dose, 0.15–0.2 g/kg per month for 2 years, was used in a double-blind trial of 148 patients with RRMS. Eleven of the treated and 17 placebo patients dropped out. IVIG reduced relapses by 59% over 2 years (note that the numbers in table 3 are inconsistent) and progression was 0.35 points less in the treated group compared to placebos, based on a single final EDSS score (i.e. unconfirmed).[72] MRIs were not performed and side-effects were minimal. In a double-blind, crossover trial of 26 patients (1 g/kg per day for 2 days each month for 6 months), IVIG reduced Gd-positive MRI lesions and tended to reduce MRI burden of disease, and exacerbations.[73]

LESSONS FROM RECENT DRUG TRIALS WHICH FAILED

Linomide is a quinolone which enhances antitumor immunity; it also may interfere with TFN-α production. MRI and clinical data suggest that the drug was beneficial in RRMS and SPMS patients. Side-effects were malaise and inflammation of serous linings—joint swelling, pleuritis and pericarditis. Trials were stopped because of nine myocardial infarctions in approximately 1100 study patients (275 of these were placebos without infarctions). The mechanism of the infarctions is unknown, but it may have been inflammatory, and specific to MS patients.

Various questions arise. Are MS patients peculiar in their predisposition to inflammatory pericarditis with this drug? Unfortunately, no immunological studies were performed in parallel with the clinical trial. Linomide has multiple (~30) metabolites—some may be toxic and some beneficial. Were different metabolites responsible for the infarctions and for the improvement in MS? Quinolone antibodies induce mRNA for IFN-γ and TFN-α,[74] and occasionally cause transient worsening of MS symptoms. Does linomide cause serositis with similar induction of cytokines? Why did the drug have robust effects in EAE, but less dramatic benefit in MS?

Soluble TNF receptor (TNFR-Ig fusion protein, Lenercept©) should adsorb serum TFN-α. This drug caused a dose-related worsening of MS in 167 RRMS and SPMS patients. This was surprising because linomide had apparent clinical and MRI benefit in MS (the putative mechanism of action is TNF reduction), and because TNF blockade ameliorates EAE and rheumatoid arthritis. However, there was a warning that TNF blockade would have adverse effects in MS. Antibodies to TNF, effective in rheumatoid arthritis, made MS worse in two patients.[75] This gives rise to the following questions. What is the key immunological difference between MS and rheumatoid arthritis? Was sTNFR acting as a carrier protein and amplifying the toxic effect of TNF? Conversely, is TFN-α beneficial in the overall immune reaction in MS—could it be involved in apoptosis of activated T cells?

Oral myelin was ineffective in 515 patients with RRMS, EDSS of 0–4.5, treated for 24–30 months. Experiments in rodents and a post hoc analysis of pilot data in humans[76] had suggested that bovine myelin might work in DR2 males. However, trends for efficacy were strongest in DR2$^+$ males in the phase III trials, with a slight decrease in burden of disease on MRI.[77] (note that IFN-β is much more effective on MRI measures). Combination trials (IFN-β plus oral myelin) are under consideration.

Questions include: is myelin the antigenic trigger in MS? Was this the optimal dose of oral myelin in MS?

Sulfasalazine significantly ameliorated MS at 18 months, but at 36 months, the trend was reversed.[78] An important lesson was that 2 or 3 year trials are essential for evaluating MS therapies.

The rationale for a trial using IVIG for recently acquired weakness was that Ig treatment induced remyelination in the Theiler's model of MS. There was no difference in a group of 63 patients on IVIG or placebo.[79]

Bimonthly pulses of intravenous methylprednisolone had no effect on progression in 109 SPMS patients.[80] This confirms many prior studies of glucocorticoid therapy in MS.

Possibly effective therapies

Cladribine has been effective in two out of three trials in patients with progressive MS; for positive trials see Sipe and colleagues;[81,82] for negative trials see Rice.[83] The two positive trials showed improvement in EDSS and MRI. The negative trial included 30% primary progressive patients, and had no clinical benefit, but T1 lesions on MRI decreased. The drug causes a drop in T-cell counts which lasts up to 2 years.

The dose has recently been reduced to 0.07 mg/kg per day (s.c.) for 5 days for 6 months. Early trials with indwelling access lines and higher drug doses. Subcutaneous cladribine, at low doses of 0.07 mg/kg per day for 5 days for 4 months was well tolerated, but did not affect EDSS in this small sample.[84] Oral cladribine, 0.14 mg for 5 days for 4–6 months, reduced absolute lymphocyte counts in three patients.[85]

T-cell vaccination uses lymphacytapheresis to remove MNC, followed by 4 days of MNC stimulation with bovine brain antigens, 1 hour mitomycin C, then reinfusion of treated MNC). In 15 patients T-cell vaccination stabilized disease in all, and improved disease in 10 of 15 patients on EDSS and MRI measures. Serum IFN-γ levels fell and IL-4 levels rose.[86]

WHICH FUTURE THERAPIES ARE REASONABLE FOR TREATMENT OF MS?

Studies of T-cell receptor peptide vaccination, T-cell vaccination, and infusion of antibodies to adhesion molecules (LFA-1, VLA-4) are in progress.

The B7-1 (or B7-2) costimulatory molecule, in addition to the TCR, is necessary for T-cell activation. B7-1 is elevated on B cells in MS during active disease, and levels fall during IFN-β therapy.[63] Also, the CD40-ligand (CD40L) on T cells interacts with APCs to induce IL-12, and in turn IFN-γ. Anti-B7 antibodies (or CTLA4-Ig), possibly in combination with anti-CD40, is a potential treatment for MS, but studies in MS have not been started.

In contrast to limited studies in MS, B7 and CD40L have been extensively investigated in EAE. Blockade of B7 and CD40L inhibits EAE. Anti-CD40L Ab on the day of immunization, followed by CTLA4-Ig fusion protein on Day 2, significantly inhibits EAE.[87]

IFN-tau is as effective as IFN-β (using equivalent antiviral units) in inhibiting ConA-induced lymphocyte proliferation, IFN-γ-induced MHC class II protein expression on endothelial cells, and microglial APC function.[88] These data confirm work from the H. Johnson laboratory.[89] IFN-tau is much less toxic than IFN-β and crosses species barriers, making it potentially useful in human therapy. Also, combinations of IFN-β with cAMP agonists and with vitamin A are being studied. There is potential synergy between many of these therapies—knowledge of their mechanisms of action would be helpful.

ANIMAL MODELS

At ECTRIMS, presentations by Olson and Hohlfeld suggested that EAE was not always a good model for studying therapies in MS, but that it might be more relevant as a model for apoptosis and for regeneration. TNF-α and TNF-β worsen EAE and cause apoptosis of cultured oligodendroglia.[90] IFN-β prevents TNF-induced apoptosis of oligodendroglia in vitro, and could help preserve oligodendroglia in MS. IFN-γ also induces apoptotic death of oligodendroglia.[91] The apoptosis is reversed by anti-IFN-γ and by leukaemia inhibitory factor (LIF). IFN-β was not studied, but induces LIF[35] and might also prevent IFN-γ-induced apoptosis of oligodendroglia.

Gene therapy of EAE is possible with nonreplicative herpes virus vectors containing IL-4 and β-Gal genes. The vector is injected into the cisterna magna of Balb/c mice. Transfection of the IL-4 gene is localized to ependymal cells. Secretion of IL-4 by these cells decreases EAE, probably by bathing the brain with IL-4. This technique could also be used in the CNS to produce growth factors for oligodendroglia.

AAN—Boston, 15–17 April 1997
ENS—Rhodes, 14–18 June 1997
ACTRIMS—San Diego, 28 September 1997
ANA—San Diego, 28 September–1 October 1997
ECTRIMS—Istanbul, 2–5 November 1997

REFERENCES

1. Lauer K, Wahl A. Specific dietary items in relation to the risk of multiple sclerosis: a case-control study. *Multiple Sclerosis* 1997; **3**: 282.
2. Segal BM, Shevach EM. Infectious agents promote the development of autoimmune disease of the central nervous system by inducing IL-12 production. *Neurology* 1997; **48**: A383.
3. Constantinescu CS, Hilliard BA, Wysocka M et al. Interleukin-12 is involved in spontaneous and superantigen-induced relapses in experimental allergic encephalomyelitis. *Neurology* 1997; **48**: A114.
4. Rapp NS, Gilroy J, Lerner AM. Role of bacterial infection in exacerbation of multiple sclerosis. *Am J Phys Med Rehab* 1995; **4**: 415–418.
5. Ventre J-J, Loupi E, Debois H et al. Central nervous system demyelination and hepatitis B virus vaccination. The French experience about Genhevac B®. *Multiple Sclerosis* 1997; **3**: 309.
6. Carrigan DR, Harrington D, Knox KK. Subacute leukoencephalitis caused by CNS infection with human herpesvirus-6 manifesting as acute multiple sclerosis. *Neurology* 1996; **47**: 145–148.
7. Nakawatase TV, Novoa LJ, Nagra RM et al. Rapidly progressive demyelinating lesions in three young adults—can this be due to an

overreactivation of HHV-6? *Multiple Sclerosis* 1997; **3**: 403.

8. Challoner PB, Smith KT, Parker JD et al. Plaque-associated expression of human herpesvirus 6 in multiple sclerosis. *Proc Natl Acad Sci USA* 1995; **92**: 7440–7444.
9. Tourtellotte WW, Nagra RM, Darvish R. HHV-6 expression in multiple sclerosis plaques and surrounding normal white and gray matter: preliminary negative study. *Multiple Sclerosis* 1997; **3**: 403.
10. Lycke J, Svennerholm B, Hjelmquist E et al. Acyclovir treatment of relapsing–remitting multiple sclerosis. A randomized, placebo-controlled, double-blind study. *J Neurol* 1996; **243**: 214–224.
11. Altintaş A, Yılmaz E, Kantarcı O et al. HLA typing in Turkish MS patients. *Multiple Sclerosis* 1997; **3**: 321.
12. Sotgiu S, Serra C, Marrosu MG et al. HLA-DR4 haplotype influences the cytokine production in Sardinian MS patients. *Multiple Sclerosis* 1997; **3**: 322.
13. Kira J, Kanai T, Nishimura Y et al. Western versus Asian types of multiple sclerosis: immunogenetically and clinically distinct disorders. *Ann Neurol* 1996; **40**: 569–574.
14. Schwid SR, Goodman AD, Mattson DH. The cause of osteoporosis in multiple sclerosis. *Ann Neurol* 1997; **42**: 422.
15. Karussis D, Ashkenazi A, Leker R et al. Primary antiphospholipid syndrome mimicking—clinically and radiologically—multiple sclerosis. *Neurology* 1997; **48**: A425.
16. Cordoliani MA, Michon-Pasturel U, Rerat K et al. Lack of association between multiple sclerosis and antiphospholipid antibodies. *J Neurol* 1997; **244**: S76.
17. Zorgdrager A, De Keyser J. Menstrually related worsening of symptoms in multiple sclerosis. *J Neurol Sci* 1997; **149**: 95–97.
18. Rovaris M, Filippi M, Falautano M et al. Correlations between brain MRI measures of demyelination/axonal loss and patterns of cognitive disturbances in multiple sclerosis. *Multiple Sclerosis* 1997; **3**: 265.
19. Mendozzi L, Pippolo L, Caimi AR et al. Verbal and visuospatial working memory in R–R and C–P MS patients. *Multiple Sclerosis* 1997; **3**: 303.
20. Idiman E, Yener GG, Özakbaş S et al Cognitive tests and beta interferon 1a in multiple sclerosis. *Multiple Sclerosis* 1997; **3**: 276.
21. Pliskin NH, Hamer DP, Goldstein DS et al. The effects of interferon-beta on cognitive function in multiple sclerosis patients receiving interferon β-1B. *Neurology* 1996; **47**: 1463–1468.
22. Martino G, Grohovaz F, Brambilla E et al. Proinflammatory cytokines regulate antigen-independent T cell activation by two separate calcium signaling pathways in multiple sclerosis patients. *Multiple Sclerosis* 1997; **3**: 312.
23. Grimaldi LME, Martino G, Filippi M et al. Interferon (IFN)-γ-induced intracellular calcium increase in T lymphocytes from patients with multiple sclerosis precedes clinical exacerbation and detection of active lesions on MRI. *Multiple Sclerosis* 1997; **3**: 316.
24. Çelet B, Saruhan-Direskeneli G, Tasçı B et al. Humoral immune response to α B-crystallin in multiple sclerosis. *Multiple Sclerosis* 1997; **3**: 315.
25. van Sechel-Plomp AC, Bajramovic JJ, Tielemans MJC et al. Activation of autoreactive helper T cells by virus-induced presentation of a self antigen. *Multiple Sclerosis* 1997; **3**: 272.
26. van Noort JM, van Sechel AC, Bajramovic JJ et al. The small heat-shock protein alpha B-crystallin as candidate autoantigen in multiple sclerosis. *Nature* 1995; **375**: 798–801.
27. Kastrukoff LF, Morgan N, Zecchini D et al. A role for natural killer (NK) cells in the immunopathogenesis of multiple sclerosis. *Neurology* 1997; **48**: A61.
28. Diaz-Villoslada P, Koehler NKU, Shih AC et al. T-cell responses to myelin oligodendrocyte protein and other myelin antigens in multiple sclerosis. *Ann Neurol* 1997; **42**: 459–460.
29. Heidendreich F, Windhagen A, Maniak S. Costimulatory molecules B7-1 and B7-2 on CSF cells in multiple sclerosis and optic neuritis. *Multiple Sclerosis* 1997; **3**: 311.
30. Svenningsson A, Dotevall L, Stemme S et al. Increased expression of B7-1 costimulatory molecule on cerebrospinal fluid cells of patients with multiple sclerosis and infectious central nervous system disease. *J Neuroimmunol* 1997; **75**: 59–68.
31 Genç K, Altungöz O, Pekçetin Ç. The effect of IFNβ on IFNγ-induced B7 costimulation molecules expression on microglial cells in vitro. *Multiple Sclerosis* 1997; **3**: 312.
32. Jurewicz AM, Walczak A, Selmaj KW. HSP recognition by γδ T cells in MS. *Multiple Sclerosis* 1997; **3**: 272.

33. Kivisäkk P, Matusevicius D, Fredrikson S et al. IL-15 mRNA expression is upregulated in mononuclear cells in multiple sclerosis. *Multiple Sclerosis* 1997; **3**: 271.
34. Rieckmann P, Albrecht M, Kitze B et al. Cytokine mRNA levels in mononuclear blood cells from patients with multiple sclerosis. *Neurology* 1994; **44**: 1523–1526.
35. Byskosh PV, Reder AT. Interferon-β effects on cytokine mRNA in peripheral mononuclear cells in multiple sclerosis. *Multiple Sclerosis* 1996; **1**: 262–269.
36. Altintaş A, Kantarcı O, Hekim N et al. Serum and CSF cytokine levels in different forms of multiple sclerosis. *Multiple Sclerosis* 1997; **3**: 313.
37. Beck J, Rondot P, Catinot L et al. Increased production of interferon gamma and tumor necrosis factor precedes clinical manifestation in multiple sclerosis: do cytokines trigger off exacerbations? *Acta Neurol Scand* 1988; **78**: 318–323.
38. Sindic CJM, Van Laere V, Monteyne P. Cytokine mRNA expression in CSF and peripheral blood mononuclear cells in multiple sclerosis. *Multiple Sclerosis* 1997; **3**: 272.
39. Rudick RA, Lee J-C, Peppler R et al. Cytokine changes with IFNβ-1A (Avonex©) treatment: results from controlled clinical trials. *Multiple Sclerosis* 1997; **3**: 276.
40. Coquerel A, Chevallier F, Mihout B et al. Blood interleukin-10 is not increased with interferon therapy in multiple sclerosis. *J Neurol* 1997; **244**: S97.
41. Rudick RA, Ransohoff RM, Peppler R et al. Interferon beta induces interleukin-10 expression: relevance to multiple sclerosis. *Ann Neurol* 1996; **40**: 618–627.
42. Porrini AM, Gambi D, Reder AT. Interferon effects on interleukin-10 secretion. Mononuclear cell response to interleukin-10 is normal in multiple sclerosis patients. *J Neuroimmunol* 1995; **61**: 27–34.
43. Filippi M, Rocca MA, Martino G et al. Magnetization transfer changes in the normal appearing white matter precede the appearance of enhancing-lesions in patients with multiple sclerosis. *Ann Neurol* 1998; **43**: 809–814.
44. Li D, Zhao G, Koopmans RA et al. Can morphological changes in MRI active lesions occur prior to their blood–brain barrier breakdown in MS? *Neurology* 1997; **48**: A311.
45. Uhm JH, Dooley NP, Stuve O et al. Migratory behaviour of T lymphocytes isolated from MS patients undergoing treatment with β-interferon (IFN-β1b). *Neurology* 1997; **48**: A80.
46. Cannella Braine CS. The adhesion molecule and cytokine profile of multiple sclerosis lesions. *Ann Neurol* 1995; **37**: 424–435.
47. Dore-Duffy P, Newman W, Balabanov R et al. Circulating, soluble adhesion proteins in cerebrospinal fluid and serum of patients with multiple sclerosis: correlation with clinical activity. *Ann Neurol* 1995; **37**: 55–62.
48. Hartung H-P, Reiners K, Archelos JJ et al. Circulating adhesion molecules and tumor necrosis factor receptor in multiple sclerosis: correlation with magnetic resonance imaging. *Ann Neurol* 1995; **38**: 186–193.
49. Calabresi PA, Pelfrey CM, Tranquill LR et al. VLA-4 expression on peripheral blood lymphocytes is downregulated after treatment of multiple sclerosis with interferon beta. *Neurology* 1997; **49**: 1111–1116.
50. Karabudak R, Kilinç M, Saatçi I. Serial analysis of sICAM and TNFα in patients with relapsing remitting multiple sclerosis during IFNβ-1b treatment. *Multiple Sclerosis* 1997; **3**: 276.
51. Dore-Duffy P, Balabanov R. The immune potential of the CNS microvascular pericyte. Role of the blood–brain barrier in inflammatory disease. *Neurology* 1997; **48**: A383–A384.
52. Brück W, Kuhlman T, Zettl UK et al. Bcl-2 expression by oligodendrocytes in multiple sclerosis lesions. *Multiple Sclerosis* 1997; **3**: 309.
53. Zipp F, Weller M, Dichgans J et al. Elevated CD95 (APO-1/Fas) serum levels in relapsing–remitting multiple sclerosis (MS). *Neurology* 1997; **48**: A426.
54. Schmidt J, Gold R, Hartung HP et al. Corticosteroid pulse therapy in experimental autoimmune encephalomyelitis (EAE): standard methylprednisolone therapy is not sufficient to augment T cell apoptosis in situ. *Neurology* 1997; **48**: A422.
55. Reder AT, Thapar M, Jensen M. A fall in serum glucocorticoids provokes experimental allergic encephalomyelitis—implications for treatment of inflammatory brain disease. *Neurology* 1994; **44**: 2289–2294.
56. Reutens DC, Vowinckel E, Owens T et al. In vivo and in vitro binding of the peripheral benzodiazapine receptor ligand PK11195 in active lesions of multiple sclerosis and experimental allergic encephalomyelitis. *Neurology* 1997; **48**: A114.

57. Banati RB, Myers R, Goerres G et al. [^{11}C] PK11195 PET-imaging of microglial activation in multiple sclerosis. *Neurology* 1997; **48**: A313.
58. Correale J, Gilmore W, Welsh J et al. Autoreactive proteolipid protein specific T cell clones from chronic progressive multiple sclerosis patients are resistant to dexamethasone-mediated apoptosis. *Neurology* 1997; **48**: A382.
59. McMillan SA, McDonnell GV, Douglas JP et al. Elevated levels of soluble CD30 in multiple sclerosis. *Multiple Sclerosis* 1997; **3**: 317.
60. Pozzilli C, Bastianello S, Koudriavtseva T et al. Magnetic resonance imaging changes with recombinant human interferon-beta-1a: a short term study in relapsing–remitting multiple sclerosis. *J Neurol Neurosurg Psychiatry* 1996; **61**: 251–258.
61. Munafo A, Spertini F, Rothuisen L et al. Pharmacodynamic response to r-hIFN-β 1a administered subcutaneously once-a-week (qw) or three-times a week (tiw), over one month. *Multiple Sclerosis* 1997; **3**: 343.
62. Calabresi PA, Frank JA, Maloni HW et al. Association between neutralizing antibodies to interferon beta and contrast enhancing lesions in multiple sclerosis patients. *Neurology* 1997; **48**: A80.
63. Genç K, Dona DL, Reder AT. Increased CD80$^+$ B cells in active multiple sclerosis, and reversal by IFNβ-1b therapy. *J Clin Invest* 1997; **99**: 2664–2671.
64. Oggero A, Bongioanni MR, Marzano A et al. Thyroid and liver autoimmunity during interferon (IFN) treatment for multiple sclerosis (MS) may be at times lethal. *Neurology* 1997; **48**: A244–A245.
65. Rieckmann P, Weber F, Günther A et al. The phosphodiesterase inhibitor pentoxifylline reduces early side effects of interferon-β 1b treatment in patients with multiple sclerosis. *Neurology* 1996; **47**: 604.
66. Rice GPA. The evolution of neutralizing antibodies in patients taking beta interferon 1b. *Multiple Sclerosis* 1997; **3**: 344.
67. Oger JJF, Vorobeychick G, Al-Fahim A et al. Neutralizing antibodies in Betaseron-treated MS patients and in vitro immune function before treatment. *Neurology* 1997; **48**: A80.
68. Oger J, Vorobeychick G, Paty DW. IgG secretion in vitro in relation with antibody status in MS patients treated with interferon beta 1b. *Multiple Sclerosis* 1997; **3**: 406.
69. Petkau J, White R. Neutralizing antibodies and the efficacy of interferon beta 1B in relapsing–remitting multiple sclerosis. *Multiple Sclerosis* 1997; **3**: 402.
70. Calabresi PA, Frank JA, Maloni HW et al. Association between neutralizing antibodies to interferon beta and contrast enhancing lesions in multiple sclerosis patients. *Neurology* 1997; **48**: A80.
71. Collard RC, Koehler RPM, Mattson DH. Frequency and significance of antinuclear antibodies in multiple sclerosis. *Neurology* 1997; **49**: 857–861.
72. Fazekas F, Deisenhammer F, Strasser-Fuchs S et al. Randomised placebo-controlled trial of monthly intravenous immunoglobulin therapy in relapsing–remitting multiple sclerosis. *Lancet* 1997; **349**: 589–593.
73. Sørensen PS, Wanscher B, Schreiber K et al. Effect of intravenous immunoglobulin (IVIG) on gadolinium enhancing lesions on MRI in multiple sclerosis (MS): final results of a double-blind cross-over trial. *Multiple Sclerosis* 1997; **3**: 268.
74. Riesbeck K, Sigvardsson M, Leanderson T et al. Superinduction of cytokine gene transcription by ciprofloxacin. *J Immunol* 1994; **153**: 343–352.
75. van Oosten BW, Barkhof F, Truyen L et al. Increased MRI activity and immune activation in two multiple sclerosis patients treated with the monoclonal anti-tumor necrosis factor antibody cA2. *Neurology* 1996; **47**: 1531–1534.
76. Weiner HL, Mackin GA, Matsui M et al. Double-blind pilot trial of oral tolerization with myelin antigens in multiple sclerosis. *Science* 1993; **259**: 1321–1324.
77. Francis G, Evans A, Panitch H. MRI results of a phase III trial or oral myelin in relapsing–remitting multiple sclerosis. *Ann Neurol* 1997; **42**: 467.
78. Noseworthy JH, O'Brien PC, The Mayo Clinic–Canadian Cooperative MS study group et al. The Mayo Clinic–Canadian cooperative study of sulfasalazine (Salazopyrin EN) in active multiple sclerosis: preliminary report. *Neurology* 1997; **48**: A340.
79. Noseworthy JH, Weinshenker BG, O'Brien PC et al. Intravenous immunoglobulin does not reverse recently acquired, apparently permanent weakness in multiple sclerosis. *Ann Neurol* 1997; **42**: 421.
80. Goodkin DE, Kinkel RP, Weinstock-Guttman B et al. A randomized, double-masked, dose-comparison, phase II study of bimonthly intravenous methylprednisolone (IVMP) to modify progression of disability in patients with secondary progressive multiple sclerosis (SPMS). *Neurology* 1997; **48**: A339.

81. Sipe JC, Romine JS, Koziol JA et al. Cladribine in treatment of chronic progressive multiple sclerosis. *Lancet* 1994; **344**: 9–13.
82. Sipe JC, Romine JS, Koziol J et al. Cladribine improves relapsing–remitting MS: a double blind, placebo controlled study. *Neurology* 1997; **48**: A340.
83. Rice GR, Cladribine Group. Cladribine and chronic progressive multiple sclerosis: the results of a multi-centre trial. *Neurology* 1997; **48:** 1730.
84. O'Connor PW, Selby R, Brandwein J. Safety and tolerability of subcutaneous cladribine therapy in chronic progressive multiple sclerosis. *Neurology* 1997; **48**: A175.
85. Ellison GW, Myers LW. Oral cladribine for multiple sclerosis. *Neurology* 1997; **48**: A174.
86. Moviglla GA, Varela O, Memolli M et al. Lymphocyte autovaccine for multiple sclerosis and other demyelinating autoimmune diseases: results in a phase I-II clinical trial. *Ann Neurol* 1997; **42**: 461.
87. Schaub M, Chandraker A, Sayegh MH et al. Synergistic effect of CD40L/CD40 and CD28/B7 blockade in murine EAE. *Neurology* 1997; **48**: A420.
88. Khan OA, Jiang H, Subramaniam PS et al. Effect of recombinant ovine interferon-tau on human T-cell responses and HLA-expression: potential for therapy in multiple sclerosis. *Neurology* 1997; **48**: A245.
89. Genç K, Altungöz O, Pekçetin Ç. The effect of IFNβ on TNFα- and TNFβ-induced apoptotic death of oligodendrocytes. *Multiple Sclerosis* 1997; **3**: 275.
90. Vartanian T, Li Y, Zhao M et al. Interferon-γ-induced oligodendrocyte cell death: implications for the pathogenesis of multiple sclerosis. *Mol Med* 1995; **1**: 732–743.
91. Furlan R, Galbiati F, Poliani PL et al. A gene therapy approach using herpetic vectors for the treatment of experimental demyelination. *Multiple Sclerosis* 1997; **3**: 278.

Index

Page numbers in *italic* refer to illustrations.